NAPLEX®

THE COMPLETE GUIDE TO LICENSING EXAM CERTIFICATION FOR PHARMACISTS

NAPLEX®

THE COMPLETE GUIDE TO LICENSING EXAM CERTIFICATION FOR PHARMACISTS

Steven T. Boyd, PharmD, BCPS, CDE
Amie McCord Brooks, PharmD, BCPS, CDE
Karen Nagel-Edwards, BS Pharm, PhD
Cynthia Sanoski, BS, PharmD, FCCP, BCPS

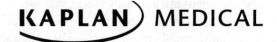

This publication is designed to provide accurate and authoritative information in regard to the subject matter covered. It is sold with the understanding that the publisher is not engaged in rendering legal, accounting, or other professional service. If legal advice or other expert assistance is required, the services of a competent professional should be sought.

© 2008 Steven T. Boyd, Amy McCord Brooks, Karen Nagel-Edwards, Cynthia Sanoski

Published by Kaplan Publishing, a division of Kaplan, Inc.
1 Liberty Plaza, 24th Floor
New York, NY 10006

Printed in the United States of America

10 9 8 7 6 5 4 3 2

ISBN-13: 978-1-4277-9576-2

Kaplan Publishing books are available at special quantity discounts to use for sales promotions, employee premiums, or educational purposes. Please email our Special Sales Department to order or for more information at kaplanpublishing@kaplan.com, or write to Kaplan Publishing, 1 Liberty Plaza, 24th Floor, New York, NY 10006.

About the Authors

Steven T. Boyd, PharmD, BCPS, CDE, is an associate professor of clinical pharmacy at Xavier University. He received his Doctor of Pharmacy degree from the University of Nebraska and completed a primary care residency at the University of Mississippi. Dr. Boyd's primary and current research endeavors have focused on diabetes, weight loss, student education, medication therapy management, and pharmacoeconomic outcomes at employer worksites. He is a board-certified pharmacotherapy specialist, clinical pharmacist at Causey's Pharmacy and serves as an instructor with Kaplan Medical, performing multiple NAPLEX reviews across the country.

Amie McCord Brooks, PharmD, BCPS, CDE, is an associate professor of pharmacy practice at the St. Louis College of Pharmacy and a clinical pharmacy specialist in ambulatory care at St. Louis County Department of Health. She previously worked as an assistant professor of pharmacy practice at Midwestern University Chicago College of Pharmacy and clinical pharmacy specialist in endocrinology at Dreyer Medical Clinic. Dr. Brooks is a board-certified pharmacotherapy specialist and a certified diabetes educator.

Karen Nagel-Edwards, BS Pharm, PhD, is an associate professor of pharmaceutical sciences at Midwestern University Chicago College of Pharmacy, where she teaches courses in pharmaceutics, compounding, and biotechnology. She has held national and local offices in pharmacy organizations, including chair of the AACP Laboratory Special Interest Group, pharmaceutics section secretary in AACP, treasurer and chair of the AAPS Chicago discussion group. Her research interests include herbal product analysis and pharmacy education.

Cynthia Sanoski, BS, Pharm.D., FCCP, BCPS, is the chair of the department of pharmacy practice at the Jefferson School of Pharmacy at Thomas Jefferson University. Dr. Sanoski received her Doctor of Pharmacy degree from the Ohio State University, and subsequently completed a two-year fellowship in cardiovascular pharmacotherapy at the University of Illinois at Chicago. She is also a board-certified pharmacotherapy specialist and a fellow of the American College of Clinical Pharmacy. Dr. Sanoski serves as an instructor with Kaplan Medical, teaching NAPLEX review courses for graduating pharmacy students across the country.

The authors wish to thank the following test item writers: LeAnn C. Boyd, Pharm.D., BCPS, CDE; Elizabeth Langan, M.D.; Amy Miller, Pharm.D., BCPS; and Stacey Thacker, Pharm.D.

AVAILABLE ONLINE

Free Additional Practice

kaptest.com/booksonline

As owner of this guide, you are entitled to get more practice and help online. Log on to kaptest.com/booksonline to access additional NAPLEX® practice questions. Access to this selection of online NAPLEX® practice material is free of charge to purchasers of this book. You'll be asked for a specific password derived from the text in this book, so have your book handy when you log on.

For Any Test Changes or Late-Breaking Developments

kaptest.com/publishing

The material in this book is up-to-date at the time of publication. However, the NABP® may have instituted changes in the test after this book was published. Be sure to carefully read the materials you receive when you register for the test. If there are any important late-breaking developments—or any changes or corrections to the Kaplan test preparation materials in this book—we will post that information online at kaptest.com/publishing.

Feedback and Comments

kaplansurveys.com/books

We'd love to hear your comments and suggestions about this book. We invite you to fill out our online survey form at kaplansurveys.com/books. Your feedback is extremely helpful as we continue to develop high-quality resources to meet your needs.

Table of Contents

PART ONE: Overview

How to Use This Book   xi

Introduction and Test-Taking Strategies   xiii

PART TWO: Review of Therapeutics

CHAPTER 1:   Cardiovascular Disorders . . . . 2.5 hr   3

CHAPTER 2:   Infectious Diseases. . . . . 3 hr   45

CHAPTER 3:   Pulmonary Disorders . . . . 30 min   89

CHAPTER 4:   Endocrine Disorders . . . . 45 min   105

CHAPTER 5:   Neurological Disorders . . . . 45 min   127

CHAPTER 6:   Gastrointestinal Disorders . . . . 45 min   155

CHAPTER 7:   Oncology. . . . . 1 hr   175

CHAPTER 8:   Psychiatric Disorders. . . . . 45 min   201

CHAPTER 9:   Bone and Joint Disorders . . . . 40 min   229

CHAPTER 10:   Pain Management . . . . 30 min   253

CHAPTER 11:   Ophthalmologic Disorders. . . . . 10 mm   267

CHAPTER 12:   Hematologic Disorders . . . . 45 min   277

CHAPTER 13:   Dermatologic Disorders . . . . 30 min   291

CHAPTER 14:   Antidotes. . . . . 15 min   303

CHAPTER 15:   Gynecologic, Obstetric and Urologic Disorders . . . . 45 min   315

CHAPTER 16:   Clinical Lab Test. . . . . 20 min   341

CHAPTER 17:   Over-the-Counter Medications . . . . 75 min   349

PART THREE: Pharmaceutical Sciences, Mathematics, and Biostatistics

CHAPTER 18: Pharmaceutics .... *1.5 hr* . 377

CHAPTER 19: Biopharmaceutics. .... *2-3 hr* . 401

CHAPTER 20: Pharmacokinetics and Graph Interpretation .... *2 hr* ... 419

CHAPTER 21: Calculations .... *1 hr* 435

CHAPTER 22: Biostatistics. .... *15 min* . 455

PART FOUR: Resources and Policy

CHAPTER 23: Drug Information .... *30 mn* . 465

CHAPTER 24: Health Policy. .... *30 mn* . 475

PART FIVE: Full-Length Practice Test

Answer Grid. 491

Full-Length Practice Test 495

Answer Explanations 533

PART SIX: Appendix

Top 200 Generic Drugs 560

Top 200 Name Brand Drugs 562

Index 565

PART ONE

Overview

How to Use This Book

Congratulations! You've taken the first step to prepare yourself for the NAPLEX®. This book contains the information you want and need to do your best.

The NAPLEX® is a computer-adaptive examination consisting of 185 questions. To assist you in preparing for the test-taking experience, this book offers two complete practice examinations of 185 questions each. One practice exam, along with answer explanations, is included in the text of this book. A second test is available as an online companion.

This content of this book is designed to provide a concentrated and concise review of the competency areas tested on the exam. This book is not intended to replace standard textbooks in pharmacy. Rather, it should serve as a primary tool in the weeks and months prior to taking the exam. Since it is not practical to re-read textbooks, you will need a resource that will provide concise, focused review. This book fills that need.

This book covers all of the areas tested on the NAPLEX® and features an efficient time-management tool to ensure adequate preparation. Each chapter includes an *estimated time for review*, prepared by the authors. These are only suggested rates; certainly, the study rate will vary based on your own level of comfort with the subject matter. By gauging yourself, however, you will be able to practice for test day, when your time on the computer will be limited.

The review is arranged by disease states, focusing on the following:

- Definitions of the disease
- Diagnosis
- Signs and Symptoms
- Guidelines
- Guidelines Summary
- Medication Charts
- Storage & Administration Pearls
- Patient Education Pearls

Each chapter also contains a few practice questions, allowing you to apply the information you have just reviewed. The appendix at the end of the book provides tables of the top 200 prescription drugs, listed by both trade and generic names, which will help you with your memorization skills.

Practice Test 1 should be taken prior to the beginning of your study period. Then, use the results to identify areas of strength and weakness and to tailor an individualized study plan. For example, if you score below average on questions related to oncology therapeutics, plan to spend some additional days studying this subject. Likewise, if cardiovascular therapeutics was the area in which you scored the highest, you may want to leave this section for last.

Kaplan suggests that areas in which you feel weakest should be studied first; in this way, you can spend additional review time on difficult concepts. Both of the practice tests should be taken in quiet areas—dedicate four hours for each test.

It is advisable to take the practice exam at a library and to limit distractions. The goal is to simulate examlike conditions and to obtain data that will help structure an effective study plan.

As you work through the items, pay particular attention to the explanations. Often, studying the explanations is one of the most valuable study resources. Note that for difficult questions, explanations have been provided that explain the reasoning for not choosing the incorrect answer choices. Use this information to understand the rationale behind eliminating each distracter. The online companion to this book includes animated flashcards to help you with self-assessment on the material prior to the final practice test.

Finally, take Practice Test 2 a week or two prior to your exam date. Test 2 should be taken once the majority of your study has been completed. Test 2 is provided as an online companion to this book and also contains 185 unique questions. Our intention–and our hope—is that this book will be an integral part of your preparation for the NAPLEX®.

Best of luck to you on your journey toward a successful career as a pharmacist!

Introduction and Test-Taking Strategies

WHAT IS THE NAPLEX®?

NAPLEX stands for North American Pharmacist Licensure Examination. The NAPLEX is issued by the National Association of Boards of Pharmacy (NABP®) and is utilized by the boards of pharmacy as part of their assessment of competence to practice pharmacy. NABP represents each of the 50 states in the United States, the District of Columbia, and the five U.S. territories. South Africa, New Zealand, Australia, and Canada also utilize the NAPLEX for licensure.

These boards of pharmacy have a mandate to protect the public from unsafe and ineffective pharmacy care, and each board has been given responsibility to regulate the practice of pharmacy in its respective state. In fact, the NAPLEX is often referred to as "The Boards" or "State Boards."

Each state requires applicants to take and pass the NAPLEX in order to obtain a license to practice as a registered pharmacist. The NAPLEX has only one purpose: to determine if it is safe for you to begin practicing as an entry-level pharmacist.

To take the NAPLEX, you must meet the eligibility requirements of the board of pharmacy from which you seek licensure. The board will determine your eligibility in accordance with the jurisdiction's requirements. If you are determined to be eligible, the board will notify NABP of your eligibility. Once that happens, a letter will be issued to you by Pearson VUE, the test administrator, with information about how to schedule your testing appointment.

CONTENT AND STRUCTURE

The NAPLEX is a computer-adaptive test that consists of 185 multiple-choice questions. Of these, 150 questions will be used to calculate your test score. The remaining 35 items serve as experimental questions and do not affect your score.

The NAPLEX is not a test of achievement or intelligence, nor is it designed for pharmacists with years of experience. The questions do not involve high-tech clinical pharmacy or equipment. Note, too, that you will not be tested on all the content you were taught in pharmacy school.

Many of the questions on the NAPLEX are asked in a scenario-based format (i.e., patient profiles with accompanying test questions). To properly analyze and answer the questions, you must refer to the information provided in the patient profile. Other questions are answered solely from the information provided in the question.

There is also a combined-response type question, otherwise called the K question. This type of question includes three Roman-numeral choices. For example:

> Ideally, Lovastatin affects blood lipids by which of the following?
>
> I. Increasing HDLs
> II. Decreasing LDLs
> III. Decreasing triglycerides

The standard response format has been:

- (A) I only
- (B) III only
- (C) I and II only
- (D) II and III only
- (E) I, II, and III

K questions can seem confusing if you haven't tackled them before. These are actually a series of true/false questions packaged together. For each question, focus on whether each of the three given statements (I, II, and III) is true or false.

HOW IS THE NAPLEX SCORED, AND WHAT SCORE DO YOU NEED TO PASS?

Your NAPLEX score is a scaled score, not a number-correct score or a percentile score. The scoring scale ranges from 0 to 150. **The minimum passing score is 75**. The algorithms for determining your scaled score are highly confidential and are not released to the public.

Candidates who fail to answer at least 162 of the 185 questions will not receive any score. Since the computer format requires that you answer every question on the screen, the only way you could answer only 162 would be to stop short before the end of the exam. If you complete at least 162 questions but fewer than 185, you will receive a penalty, and your score will be adjusted to reflect the number of questions that remained unanswered. It is certainly in your best interest to answer all questions presented.

NABP will forward your NAPLEX score to the board of pharmacy from which you are seeking licensure. NABP **does not** provide scores to candidates, and score results **are not** released at the test center.

WHAT IF YOU FAIL THE NAPLEX?

First of all, it's unlikely you will fail. Be positive! Currently, the passage rate is approximately 93%. Candidates who receive a failing score on the NAPLEX will automatically be provided with a diagnostic report that indicates their relative performance in each major competency area. The board of pharmacy will notify the candidates of the NAPLEX results and diagnostic report.

THE CAT FORMAT

What Is a CAT?

A computer-adaptive test (CAT) is quite different from a paper-and-pencil test. Each CAT is assembled interactively based on the accuracy of the candidate's response to the questions. This ensures that the questions you are answering are not "too hard" or "too easy" for your skill level. Your first question will be relatively easy; that is, below the level of minimum competency. If you answer that question correctly, the computer selects a slightly more difficult question. If you answer the first question incorrectly, the computer selects a slightly easier question. By continuing to do this as you answer questions, the computer is able to calculate your level of competence.

Because the CAT presents questions on the basis of your responses to previous questions, **you may not change an answer once you have confirmed an answer choice. Likewise, you may not go back to review a question once you have moved on to the next questions.** You must answer **all** questions in the order in which they are presented, and you may not skip a question.

Exam questions are chosen for you on the basis of your answers to previous questions, so you cannot skip a question or return to an earlier one for review. Once you have confirmed an answer choice and have moved on to the next question, you cannot return to the previous question to change your answer.

In a CAT, the questions are adapted to your ability level. The computer selects questions that represent all areas of pharmacy, as defined by the NAPLEX test plan and by the level of item difficulty. Each question is self-contained, so all of the information you need to answer a question is presented on the computer screen. This difficulty-level determination will then be used to calculate your score.

Strategies for Success with a CAT

1. There is a timer at the top of the computer screen to help you pace yourself. You can hide it if it distracts you—but since the test is timed, you might find it helpful for pacing. You have **4 hours and 15 minutes** to complete all 185 questions.

2. There will be only a few other test-takers in the room with you. It will not be like taking an exam in a massive lecture hall with distractions everywhere.

3. There is a 10-minute break at the two-hour time point. Make sure to take that break! You need to rest your brain. And while the average candidate takes 2.5 to 3 hours to complete the exam, there are no bonus points for finishing early.

4. You will find the CAT much more convenient for your schedule than the pencil-and-paper exam. The CAT is offered at hundreds of centers almost every day of the year.

5. It is possible that questions involving mathematical calculations will be weighted more heavily than other questions. Spend extra time solving them, but limit yourself to a maximum of 5 or 6 minutes each.

6. If a question calls for a calculation or a certain mechanism, scratch a rough image. Having a crude diagram to look at, rather than having to imagine it from the computer screen, will help you to see what you're dealing with. Such notes also often stimulate more recall.

7. Look for key words in questions. Words such as "most likely" may help you eliminate some choices even when you don't have comprehensive recall—the most likely choice is probably the one that is most familiar as you review the choices.

8. You cannot cross off an answer choice and banish it from your sight (it's on a computer screen, after all), so you have to be disciplined about not reconsidering choices you've already eliminated.

NAPLEX REGISTRATION

The NAPLEX is administered year-round on business days. There are several steps in registering for the exam. As of this printing, the fee for the exam is $465. (Also, be sure to check with your local board of pharmacy for its fees.)

- **First Step:**
  - Contact the board of pharmacy in the state in which you want to be licensed. The state board will issue paperwork and instructions that determine your eligibility, and will notify the NABP. You will then be issued an Authorization to Test, as well as other documents, including:
    » Test authorization number
    » Expiration date
    » Range of dates during which you can take the NAPLEX
- **Second Step:**
  - Once you receive your authorization packet from the NABP, you can call or register online at Pearsonvue to choose your testing center to schedule your test date. You will need your Authorization to Test information to schedule a testing date.
  - For more information about registration, go to:
    » NABP   http://www.nabp.net
    » Pearson Vue   http://www.pearsonvue.com/

TAKING THE EXAM

There is no time limit for each individual question; however, you have a total of four hours and 15 minutes to complete the exam. This does not include the beginning tutorial or the 10-minute break given after the first two hours of testing.

Remember, every question counts. There is no warm-up time, so it is important for you to be ready to answer questions correctly from the very beginning. Concentration is also key. You need to give your best thinking to each question.

ON THE DAY OF THE EXAM

1. Arrive at the test center at least 30 minutes before your scheduled testing time to allow for check-in. If you arrive late, you may be required to forfeit your appointment. **If you forfeit your appointment, your testing fee will not be refunded.**

2. Bring two forms of identification: a picture ID that includes your signature and a second form of ID. You will be required to show these IDs for entry. Your thumbprint will also be required when you enter the testing room.

3. You will be provided with laminated note boards, which may be replaced as needed during testing. You will not be allowed to take your own scratch paper or pencil into the testing room.

4. An on-screen, five-function calculator can be activated during the test administration for your use. You may also request a hand-held, five-function calculator from the test administrator.

5. The seating time for the exam is four hours and 15 minutes with a 10-minute mandatory break after approximately two hours of testing time. Any voluntary breaks will be subtracted from your testing time.

NAPLEX BLUEPRINT

The questions on the NAPLEX involve integrated pharmacy content. The NAPLEX Competency Statements provide a blueprint of the topics covered on the exam. Reviewing these statements will assist you in preparation for the exam.

- **Competence Area 1:** Assure Safe and Effective Pharmacotherapy and Optimize Therapeutic Outcomes (over 54% of exam).

- **Competence Area 2:** Assure Safe and Accurate Preparation and Dispensing of Medications (35% of exam).

- **Competence Area 3:** Provide Health Care Information and Promote Public Health (about 11% of exam).

For specific subcategories under each competence areas, go to **www.nabp.net**.

KAPLAN) MEDICAL

TEST-TAKING STRATEGIES

As you review each section ahead, it is important to focus on your own areas of weakness. To help you do so, keep the following in mind:

Key Steps toward Preparedness

- Assess your strengths and weaknesses. Review your weakest subjects first.
- Focus heavily on the Top 200 drugs. Use the online flashcard component that accompanies this book and spend extra time reviewing the Top 200. These are important.
- Practice calculations to increase your confidence.
- Schedule extra time before your testing date to revisit your weaker areas.
- Complete the practice test under real exam conditions.
- Order and complete the Pre-NAPLEX exam, available from NABP.
- When you review the practice exam, make sure you understand why your incorrect answer choices were incorrect.
- Be sure you understand why you missed a question. Did you simply forget a fact? Choose your answer too quickly? Misunderstand the question? Miss an important clue within the question? Finally, do you keep making the same mistakes over and over? If so, it is important to spend more time on those areas.

Guessing

During the exam, there are sure to be some questions that stump you. For those, just narrow down the choices and take your best guess. You don't want to spend too much time analyzing a question you do not know and then run out of time toward the end of the exam. Remember, you cannot simply leave a question blank, so in some shape or form you'll have to take your best guess.

Keep in mind that 35 experimental questions are not calculated into your score, so if you answer a few questions incorrectly, it's possible that they won't be scored at all.

When you just don't know the answer: narrow the answer choices to two likely choices, then use the "upper, then lower" decision rule to select one of them. This rule means you alternate your guess, using the upper choice the first time you are stuck, then the lower choice the next time you are stuck. This technique helps keep you moving forward.

Positive Attitude

The most important decision you can make in your studying process is to have a positive attitude, especially on exam day. Remember this:

- The odds are on your side; around 93% of pharmacy graduates pass the NAPLEX.
- This is a minimal competency exam.
- You spent a minimum of six years in school to become a pharmacist. If you could do that, you can conquer this exam!

You **are** prepared, and this book is a tool to increase your confidence.

Part Two

Review of Therapeutics

Cardiovascular Disorders

1

This chapter covers the following diseases:

- **Hypertension**
- **Dyslipidemia**
- **Heart failure**
- **Ischemic heart disease**

The text also provides an overview of the anti-arrhythmic drugs commonly used in clinical practice.

 Suggested Study Time: **2.5 hours**

HYPERTENSION

Definitions

Hypertension (HTN) is defined as a systolic blood pressure (SBP) >140 mmHg, a diastolic blood pressure (DBP) >90 mmHg, or any patient requiring antihypertensive therapy. Most patients with HTN have primary (essential) HTN (due to unknown cause, likely genetic), while less than 10% have secondary HTN (due to chronic kidney disease [CKD], pheochromocytoma, Cushing's syndrome, or medications [nonsteroidal anti-inflammatory drugs (NSAIDs), corticosteroids, cyclosporine, tacrolimus, sibutramine, estrogens, erythropoietin, venlafaxine, sympathomimetics, cocaine]).

Diagnosis

- Normal blood pressure (BP): SBP <120 mmHg and DBP <80 mmHg
- Prehypertension: SBP 120–139 mmHg or DBP 80–89 mmHg

- Hypertension is categorized into two stages:
  - Stage 1 HTN: SBP 140–159 mmHg or DBP 90–99 mmHg
  - Stage 2 HTN: SBP ≥160 mmHg or DBP ≥100 mmHg

Signs and Symptoms

- Can develop target organ damage with chronic, uncontrolled HTN:
  - Cardiac
    - » Angina, myocardial infarction (MI), history of coronary revascularization (e.g., percutaneous coronary intervention [PCI], coronary artery bypass graft [CABG] surgery), left ventricular hypertrophy (LVH), left ventricular (LV) dysfunction (i.e., heart failure [HF])
  - Cerebrovascular
    - » Stroke, transient ischemic attack (TIA)
  - Renal
    - » CKD
  - Ophthalmologic
    - » Retinopathy, blindness
  - Vascular
    - » Peripheral arterial disease (PAD)

Guidelines

Seventh Joint National Committee on the Detection, Evaluation, and Treatment of High Blood Pressure (JNC 7), *JAMA*, no. 289 (2003): 2560–71. www.nhlbi.nih.gov/guidelines/hypertension.

Guidelines Summary

- BP goals:
  - Uncomplicated HTN: <140/90 mmHg
  - Diabetes or CKD: <130/80 mmHg
- Lifestyle modifications: weight loss (goal body mass index [BMI] 18.5–24.9 kg/m^2), diet rich in fruits, vegetables, and low-fat dairy products with ↓ saturated and total fat, ↓ sodium (Na$^+$) intake (≤2.4 g/day), ↑ physical activity (30 minutes most days of the week), moderation of alcohol use (≤1 ounce of ethanol/day), smoking cessation
- Pharmacologic therapy:
  - Initial antihypertensive drug selection: Based upon degree of BP elevation and whether compelling indications are present

- Compelling indications for specific antihypertensive drug therapy:
  - » HF: Diuretic, angiotensin-converting enzyme inhibitor (ACE-I), β-blocker (carvedilol, metoprolol, or bisoprolol), angiotensin II receptor blocker (ARB), aldosterone antagonist
  - » Post-MI: β-blocker, ACE-I, aldosterone antagonist
  - » High coronary disease risk: β-blocker, ACE-I, diuretic, calcium channel blocker (CCB)
  - » Diabetes mellitus (DM): ACE-I, ARB, diuretic, β-blocker, CCB
  - » CKD: ACE-I, ARB
  - » Recurrent stroke prevention: ACE-I, diuretic
- Management of pre-HTN:
  - » No compelling indication present → Lifestyle modifications only
  - » If patient has CKD or DM → Treat with drugs listed for these compelling indications (see above)
- Management of HTN:
  - » No compelling indication present:
    - Stage 1 HTN → Initiate thiazide diuretic (may also consider ACE-I, ARB, β-blocker, CCB, or combination of these drugs)
    - Stage 2 HTN → Initiate two antihypertensive drugs (one of the drugs should be a thiazide diuretic)
  - » Compelling indication present:
    - Use drugs indicated for these specific conditions (see above)

Diuretics

Thiazide Diuretics – inhibit Na+ reabsorption in the distal convoluted tubule

Generic	Brand	Dose	Contra-indications	Primary Side Effects	Key Monitoring	Pertinent Drug Interactions	Med Pearl	Top 200
Chlorothiazide	Diuril	500–2,000 mg/day	Sulfa allergy	• Hypokalemia • Hypomagnesemia • Hyponatremia • Hypercalcemia • Hyperglycemia • Hyperuricemia	• BP • Electrolytes • Blood urea nitrogen (BUN)/serum creatinine (SCr) • Blood glucose • Uric acid	• May ↑ risk of lithium toxicity • May ↓ effect of antidiabetic agents • NSAIDs ↓ antihypertensive effects	• Synergistic effect with other antihypertensives • Not effective (except metolazone) when creatinine clearance (CrCl) <30 mL/min; use loop diuretics • Have ceiling dose (unlike loop diuretics)	No
Chlorthalidone	Thalitone	12.5–100 mg/day						No
Hydrochlorothiazide	Microzide	12.5–50 mg/day						Yes
Indapamide	Lozol	1.25–5 mg/day						Yes
Metolazone	Zaroxolyn	2.5–5 mg/day						Yes

Loop Diuretics – inhibit Na+ reabsorption in the ascending limb of loop of Henle (should only be used for HTN in patients with renal insufficiency [maintains efficacy when CrCl <30 mL/min], severe edema or HF) (see HF section for further details)

Potassium-Sparing Diuretics – inhibit Na+ reabsorption in the collecting ducts

Generic	Brand	Dose	Contra-indications	Primary Side Effects	Key Monitoring	Pertinent Drug Interactions	Med Pearl	Top 200
Amiloride	Only available generically	5–10 mg/day	• Hyperkalemia • CKD	Hyperkalemia	BP Potassium (K+) BUN/SCr	Use with K+ supplements, ACE-Is, ARBs, or NSAIDs may ↑ risk of hyperkalemia	• Not used often as monotherapy (weak antihypertensives) • Often used with hydrochlorothiazide to ↓ K+ loss	No
Triamterene	Dyrenium	50–100 mg/day						No

Combination products:
Triamterene/hydrochlorothiazide (Dyazide, Maxzide)
Amiloride/hydrochlorothiazide (Moduretic)

Aldosterone Receptor Antagonists – have similar mechanism of action to K+-sparing diuretics (also block the effects of aldosterone) (not used often for HTN) (see HF section for further details)

Combination products:
Spironolactone/hydrochlorothiazide (Aldactazide)

β-Blockers

Mechanism of action – ↓ cardiac output (CO) by negative inotropic (↓ contractility) and negative chronotropic (↓ heart rate [HR]) effects

- Cardioselective – bind more to β₁ than β₂ receptors (at low doses); less likely to cause bronchoconstriction or vasoconstriction at low doses (safer to use in patients with asthma, chronic obstructive pulmonary disease [COPD], PAD, or DM); cardioselectivity may be lost at higher doses)
  - Bisoprolol, atenolol, metoprolol, betaxolol, acebutolol (BAMBA)
- Intrinsic sympathomimetic activity (ISA) – have partial β-receptor agonist activity
  - Carteolol, acebutolol, pindolol, penbutolol (CAPP)
- Lipophilic vs. hydrophilic – lipophilic (propranolol, metoprolol, carvedilol, labetalol, pindolol) more likely to cause central nervous system (CNS) side effects (e.g., depression, fatigue)

Cardioselective:

Generic	Brand	Dose	Contraindications	Primary Side Effects	Key Monitoring	Pertinent Drug Interactions	Med Pearl	Top 200
Acebutolol	Sectral	200–1,200 mg/day	• ≥2nd degree heart block (in absence of pacemaker) • HF (except metoprolol or bisoprolol)	• Bradycardia/heart block • HF exacerbation • Bronchospasm • Cold extremities • Fatigue • ↓ exercise tolerance • Depression • Glucose intolerance • Mask hypoglycemia (in patients with DM)	• BP • HR • S/S HF • Blood glucose (in patients with DM)	Use with other negative chronotropes (e.g., digoxin, verapamil, diltiazem, or clonidine) may ↑ risk of bradycardia)	Abrupt discontinuation may cause angina, MI or hypertensive emergency; need to taper over 2 wks	No
Atenolol	Tenormin	25–100 mg/day						Yes
Betaxolol	Kerlone	5–20 mg/day						No
Bisoprolol	Zebeta	2.5–20 mg/day						No
Metoprolol	• Tartrate: Lopressor (2x daily) • Succinate: Toprol XL (1x daily)	25–400 mg/day						Yes

Nonselective:

Generic	Brand	Dose	Contraindications	Primary Side Effects	Key Monitoring	Pertinent Drug Interactions	Med Pearl	Top 200
Carvedilol	Coreg, Coreg CR	Immediate-release (IR): 12.5–50 mg/day (in two divided doses) Controlled-release (CR): 20–80 mg/day (1x daily)	• ≥2nd degree heart block (in absence of pacemaker) • HF (except carvedilol)	Same as with selective β-blockers	Same as with selective β-blockers	Same as with selective β-blockers	• Same as with selective β-blockers • Labetalol and carvedilol also have α₁-blocking properties	Yes
Labetalol	Trandate	200–2,400 mg/day						Yes
Nadolol	Corgard	20–320 mg/day						Yes
Pindolol	Visken	5–60 mg/day						No
Propranolol	Inderal, Inderal LA, InnoPran XL	80–640 mg/day (IR given 2–3x daily; extended-release [ER] given 1x daily)						Yes
Timolol	Blocadren	20–60 mg/day						No

Combination products:

Atenolol/chlorthalidone (Tenoretic)	Nadolol/bendroflumethiazide (Corzide)
Bisoprolol/hydrochlorothiazide (Ziac)	Propranolol/hydrochlorothiazide (Inderide)
	Metoprolol/hydrochlorothiazide (Lopressor HCT)

Angiotensin-Converting Enzyme Inhibitors

Mechanism of action – inhibit ACE and prevent the conversion of angiotensin I to angiotensin II → vasodilation, ↓ aldosterone production; also inhibit degradation of bradykinin

Generic	Brand	Dose	Contraindications	Primary Side Effects	Key Monitoring	Pertinent Drug Interactions	Med Pearl	Top 200
Benazepril	Lotensin	5–40 mg/day	• Pregnancy • History of angioedema or renal failure with prior use • Hyperkalemia • Bilateral renal artery stenosis	• Hyperkalemia • Renal insufficiency • Cough (dry) • Angioedema	• BP • BUN/SCr • K+	• Use with ARBs, K+ supplements, K+-sparing diuretics, aldosterone receptor antagonists, or NSAIDs may ↑ risk of hyperkalemia • May ↑ risk of lithium toxicity	• Captopril has shortest duration of action • If patient has intolerable dry cough, may switch to ARB • Hyperkalemia and renal insufficiency also likely to occur with ARBs (risk of angioedema cross sensitivity with ARBs controversial)	Yes
Captopril	Capoten	12.5–450 mg/day						Yes
Enalapril	Vasotec	2.5–40 mg/day						Yes
Fosinopril	Monopril	5–80 mg/day						Yes
Lisinopril	Prinivil, Zestril	2.5–0 mg/day						Yes
Quinapril	Accupril	10–80 mg/day						Yes
Moexipril	Univasc	3.75–0 mg/day						No
Perindopril	Aceon	4–16 mg/day						No
Ramipril	Altace	1.25–20 mg/day						Yes
Trandolapril	Mavik	0.5–4 mg/day						No

Combination products:

Benazepril/amlodipine (Lotrel)
Benazepril/hydrochlorothiazide (Lotensin HCT)
Captopril/hydrochlorothiazide (Capozide)

Enalapril/hydrochlorothiazide (Vaseretic)
Fosinopril/hydrochlorothiazide (Monopril HCT)
Lisinopril/hydrochlorothiazide (Prinzide, Zestoretic)

Moexipril/hydrochlorothiazide (Uniretic)
Quinapril/hydrochlorothiazide (Accuretic, Quinaretic)
Trandolapril/verapamil (Tarka)

Cardiovascular Disorders

Angiotensin II Receptor Blockers

Mechanism of action – inhibit the binding of angiotensin II to the angiotensin type 1 (AT_1) receptor → vasodilation, ↓ aldosterone production; no effect on bradykinin

Generic	Brand	Dose	Contraindications	Primary Side Effects	Key Monitoring	Pertinent Drug Interactions	Med Pearl	Top 200
Candesartan	Atacand	4–32 mg/day	Same as for ACE-Is	Same as for ACE-Is (except no cough)	Same as for ACE-Is	• Use with ACE-Is, K+ supplements, K+-sparing diuretics, aldosterone receptor antagonists, or NSAIDs may ↑ risk of hyperkalemia • May ↑ risk of lithium toxicity	Hyperkalemia and renal insufficiency also likely to occur with ACE-Is (risk of angioedema cross-sensitivity with ACE-Is is controversial)	Yes
Eprosartan	Teveten	400–800 mg/day						No
Irbesartan	Avapro	75–300 mg/day						Yes
Losartan	Cozaar	25–100 mg/day						Yes
Olmesartan	Benicar	20–40 mg/day						Yes
Telmisartan	Micardis	20–80 mg/day						Yes
Valsartan	Diovan	80–320 mg/day						Yes

Combination products:

Candesartan/hydrochlorothiazide (Atacand HCT)
Eprosartan/hydrochlorothiazide (Teveten HCT)
Irbesartan/hydrochlorothiazide (Avalide)
Losartan/hydrochlorothiazide (Hyzaar)
Olmesartan/amlodipine (Azor)
Olmesartan/hydrochlorothiazide (Benicar HCT)
Telmisartan/hydrochlorothiazide (Micardis HCT)
Valsartan/amlodipine (Exforge)
Valsartan/hydrochlorothiazide (Diovan HCT)

Renin Inhibitor

Mechanism of action – inhibits renin and prevents the conversion of angiotensinogen to angiotensin I, which then ↓ production of angiotensin II

Generic	Brand	Dose	Contraindications	Primary Side Effects	Key Monitoring	Pertinent Drug Interactions	Med Pearl	Top 200
Aliskiren	Tekturna	150–300 mg/day	• Pregnancy • History of ACE-I or ARB-induced angioedema • Hyperkalemia • Bilateral renal artery stenosis	• Headache • Dizziness • Diarrhea • May also cause hyperkalemia and renal insufficiency	• BP • BUN/SCr • K+	• Use with ACE-Is, ARBs, K+ supplements, K+-sparing diuretics, aldosterone receptor antagonists, or NSAIDs may ↑ risk of hyperkalemia • Atorvastatin, ketoconazole, or cyclosporine may ↑ effects	• Use with caution in patients with CrCl <30 mL/min • Avoid taking with high-fat meals • Should not use with cyclosporine	No

Calcium Channel Blockers

Mechanism of action – bind to L-type channels in heart and coronary/peripheral arteries to block inward movement of calcium (Ca^{2+}) → vascular smooth-muscle relaxation (vasodilation); all (except for amlodipine and felodipine) have negative inotropic effects (↓ contractility)
- Dihydropyridines (DHPs) – more selective to vasculature; more potent vasodilators; have no effect on cardiac conduction
- Non-DHPs – cause less peripheral vasodilation than DHPs; negative chronotropic properties (↓ HR)

Generic	Brand	Dose	Contra-indications	Primary Side Effects	Key Monitoring	Pertinent Drug Interactions	Med Pearl	Top 200
DHPs:								
Amlodipine	Norvasc	2.5–10 mg/day	None	• Reflex tachycardia • Headache • Flushing • Peripheral edema • Gingival hyperplasia • HF exacerbation (except amlodipine and felodipine)	• BP • HR • S/S HF	• CYP3A4 inhibitors may ↑ effects • CYP3A4 inducers may ↓ effects	• Sublingual nifedipine should not be used → may ↑ risk of MI, death • Do not use grapefruit juice	Yes
Felodipine	Plendil	2.5–20 mg/day						Yes
Isradipine	DynaCirc CR	5–10 mg/day						No
Nicardipine	Cardene, Cardene SR	60–120 mg/day (IR given 3x daily; sustained-release [SR] given 2x daily)						No
Nifedipine	Adalat CC, Afeditab CR, Nifediac CC, Nifedical XL, Procardia XL	30–180 mg/day						Yes
Nisoldipine	Sular	10–40 mg/day						Yes
Non-DHPs:								
Diltiazem	Cardizem CD, Cardizem LA, Cartia XT, Dilacor XR, Taztia XT, Tiazac	120–540 mg/day	• ≥2nd degree heart block (in absence of pacemaker) • Systolic HF	• Bradycardia/heart block • Constipation • Peripheral edema • Gingival hyperplasia • HF exacerbation	• BP • HR • S/S HF	• Same as for DHPs • Use with other negative chronotropes (e.g., digoxin, β-blockers, or clonidine) may ↑ risk of bradycardia • May ↑ effect/toxicity of CYP3A4 substrates • May ↑ risk of digoxin toxicity	• Do not use grapefruit juice	Yes
Verapamil	Calan, Calan SR, Covera-HS, Isoptin SR, Verelan, Verelan PM	120–360 mg/day (IR given 2–3x daily; SR given 1–2x daily)						Yes

α₁-Receptor Antagonists

Mechanism of action – block the α_1 receptor on peripheral blood vessels → arterial and venous vasodilation

Generic	Brand	Dose	Contraindications	Primary Side Effects	Key Monitoring	Pertinent Drug Interactions	Med Pearl	Top 200
Doxazosin	Cardura	1–16 mg/day	Should not be used with phosphodiesterase (PDE)-5 inhibitors (e.g., sildenafil, tadalafil, vardenafil) → ↑ risk of hypotension	• Orthostatic hypotension • Reflex tachycardia • Peripheral edema • Headache • Drowsiness	• BP • HR	• ↑ risk of hypotension with PDE-5 inhibitors (avoid concurrent use)	• ALLHAT trial → 25% ↑ in cardiovascular events with doxazosin • Should not be used as 1st-line therapy (even in patients with benign prostatic hyperplasia)	Yes
Prazosin	Minipress	1–20 mg/day						No
Terazosin	Hytrin	1–20 mg/day						Yes

Central α₂-Receptor Agonists

Mechanism of action – stimulate α_2 receptors in brain → ↓ sympathetic outflow (release of norepinephrine) → ↓ BP and HR

Generic	Brand	Dose	Contraindications	Primary Side Effects	Key Monitoring	Pertinent Drug Interactions	Med Pearl	Top 200
Clonidine	Catapres, Catapres-TTS	Oral: 0.2–2.4 mg/day Transdermal: 0.1–0.3 mg weekly		• Sedation • Orthostatic hypotension • Depression • Peripheral edema • Dry mouth • Bradycardia	• BP • HR • Liver function tests (LFTs) (methyldopa)	Use with other negative chronotropes (e.g., digoxin, verapamil, diltiazem, or β-blockers) may ↑ risk of bradycardia	• Patch should be applied once weekly • Abrupt discontinuation (especially in presence of β-blockers) may cause angina, MI or hypertensive emergency; need to taper over 2 wks • When starting patch, overlap with oral for 2–3 days, then discontinue oral	Yes
Methyldopa	Aldomet	250–1,000 mg/day	Methyldopa: Liver disease	• Hepatitis (methyldopa)				No

Direct Vasodilators

Mechanism of action – ↑ cyclic GMP → arterial vasodilation

Generic	Brand	Dose	Contraindications	Primary Side Effects	Key Monitoring	Pertinent Drug Interactions	Med Pearl	Top 200
Hydralazine	Apresoline	25–300 mg/day	• Acute MI • Aortic dissection	• Reflex tachycardia • Orthostatic hypotension • Peripheral edema • Lupus-like syndrome (hydralazine) • Hirsutism (minoxidil)	• BP • HR • S/S lupus (e.g., stabbing chest pain, joint pain, fever, rash)	None	Used for refractory HTN (should not be used as 1st-line therapy)	Yes
Minoxidil	Loniten	2.5–100 mg/day						No

Storage and Administration Pearls

- When initiating antihypertensive drug therapy in the elderly, initiate at a low dose and slowly titrate to achieve goal BP ("start low and go slow").

Patient Education Pearls

- Diuretics should be taken in the morning to avoid nocturia.
- Patients receiving diuretics should wear sunscreen and protective clothing. Also, they should report any episodes of muscle cramps, as this may be a symptom of hypokalemia or hypomagnesemia.
- Patients receiving K^+-sparing diuretics, aldosterone antagonists, ACE-Is, or ARBs should avoid excessive intake of foods high in K^+ (e.g., green leafy vegetables, potatoes, apricots, bananas, dates, oranges, avocados) and K^+-containing salt substitutes.
- α_1-receptor antagonists should be taken at bedtime to minimize the risk of developing orthostatic hypotension.
- A patient receiving α_1-receptor antagonists, α_2-receptor agonists, or direct vasodilators should rise slowly from a sitting position.
- A patient receiving ACE-Is or ARBs should call 911 immediately if she experiences lip, tongue, or facial swelling or has difficulty breathing.
- ACE-Is, ARBs, and renin inhibitors should be avoided in pregnant patients. Antihypertensive drugs that can be safely used in pregnancy include methyldopa, labetalol, or CCBs.

Definitions

Dyslipidemia can refer to any lipid disorder. Hyperlipidemia refers to an $\uparrow$ blood concentration of a lipid such as cholesterol or triglycerides (TGs). Dyslipidemia ($\uparrow$ total cholesterol [TC], low-density lipoprotein cholesterol [LDL-C] and TGs and $\downarrow$ high-density lipoprotein cholesterol [HDL-C]) can predispose patients to the development of cardiovascular, cerebrovascular, or PAD. While most forms of dyslipidemia are due to genetic factors, certain drugs may also cause elevated lipid concentrations, including β-blockers, diuretics, corticosteroids, isotretinoin, protease inhibitors, cyclosporine, and estrogens.

Diagnosis

Classification of TC, LDL-C, HDL-C, and TGs

TC	*HDL-C*
• <200 mg/dL → Desirable • 200–239 mg/dL → Borderline high • ≥240 mg/dL → High	• <40 mg/dL → Low • ≥60 mg/dL → High
LDL-C	*TGs*
• <100 mg/dL → Optimal • 100–129 mg/dL → Near/above optimal • 130–159 mg/dL → Borderline high • 160–189 mg/dL → High • ≥190 mg/dL → Very high	• <150 mg/dL → Normal • 150–199 mg/dL → Borderline high • 200–499 mg/dL → High • ≥500 mg/dL → Very high (↑ risk for pancreatitis)

- Fasting lipid profile should be obtained in adults ≥20 years every 5 years.

- The Friedwald LDL equation (applies if TG <400 mg/dL) is LDL = TC – (HDL-C + TG/5).

- To determine LDL-C goal and appropriate lipid-lowering therapy, a risk factor assessment should be performed.

  - Major risk factors for coronary heart disease (CHD) (count-up risk factors) are:

    » Age ≥45 years (males), ≥55 years (females)

    » Cigarette smoking

    » HTN (BP >140/90 mmHg or on antihypertensive therapy)

    » HDL-C <40 mg/dL

    » Family history of premature CHD (male first-degree relative <55 years, female first-degree relative <65 years)

  - A negative risk factor (if present, subtract one risk factor from total count above) is:

    » HDL-C ≥60 mg/dL

  - Patient's risk factors should be counted up. If ≥2 risk factors, Framingham risk score (FRS) should be calculated. You do not need to calculate FRS in patients with 0–1 risk factors, or those with established CHD (angina, MI, history of PCI/CABG surgery). You will not need to calculate FRS for exam!

  - CHD-risk equivalents (confer the same degree of risk for developing a CHD event as an individual who has established CHD) are:

    » PAD

    » Abdominal aortic aneurysm

    » Symptomatic carotid artery disease (i.e., stroke, TIA)

    » DM

    » Stage 5 CKD

    » Multiple (≥2) risk factors that confer ≥20% risk of CHD at 10 years (as determined by FRS)

Signs and Symptoms

Most patients with hyperlipidemia have no signs/symptoms.

Guidelines

National Cholesterol Education Program (NCEP) Adult Treatment Panel III. *Circulation*, no. 110 (2004), 227–239. http.nhlbi.nih.gov/guidelines/cholesterol/index.htm.

Guidelines Summary

Risk Category	LDL-C Goal
CHD or CHD risk equivalent	<100 mg/dL (<70 mg/dL reasonable for patients with CHD, PAD, atherosclerotic aortic disease, stroke/TIA, or DM)
Multiple (≥2) risk factors	<130 mg/dL (<100 mg/dL optional goal for patients with FRS of 10–20%)
0–1 risk factors	<160 mg/dL

- Lifestyle modifications (to be initiated in all patients): Therapeutic lifestyle changes, weight loss, ↑ physical activity, use of plant stanols/sterols (may help ↓ LDL-C)
- Pharmacologic therapy
  - Selection of drug therapy should be based on lipid abnormality.
  - Achieving LDL-C goal should be the primary goal for all patients, except for when TG >500 mg/dL (↓ TG to <500 mg/dL then becomes the primary goal).
  - For HMG-CoA reductase inhibitors (statins), select dose that will achieve %. LDL-C reduction that will get patient to their LDL-C goal.
    - » % LDL-C reduction: [(Baseline LDL-C – Goal LDL-C)/Baseline LDL-C] × 100

Lipid-Lowering Effects of Various Drug Classes

Drug Class	Effect on LDL-C	Effect on HDL-C	Effect on TGs
Bile acid resins	↓ 15–30%	↑ 3–5%	↑ 1–10%
Niacin	↓ 5–25%	↑ 15–35%	↓ 20–50%
Fibric acid derivatives	↓/↑ 5–20%	↑ 10–20%	↓ 20–50%
Statins	↓ 18–55%	↑ 5–15%	↓ 7–30%
Cholesterol absorption inhibitors	↓ 15–20%	↑ 1%	↓ 8%

Bile Acid Resins

Mechanism of action – bind bile acids in intestines, forming insoluble complex that is excreted in feces → ↓ in bile acids causes liver to convert cholesterol into bile acids, which then → ↓ cholesterol stores → ↑ demand for cholesterol in liver → upregulation of LDL receptors → ↑ LDL-C clearance from bloodstream

Generic	Brand	Dose	Contra-indications	Primary Side Effects	Key Monitoring	Pertinent Drug Interactions	Med Pearl	Top 200
Cholestyramine	Prevalite, Questran	4–24 g/day	Complete biliary obstruction	• Constipation • Bloating • Abdominal pain • Nausea/vomiting (N/V) • Flatulence • ↑ TGs	Lipid panel	Bind to and ↓ absorption of many drugs (e.g., warfarin, digoxin, thiazides, levothyroxine)	• Used to ↓ LDL-C • Can be used in patients with liver disease • Use with caution in patients with ↑ TGs • Colesevelam has fewer gastro-intestinal (GI) side effects and drug interactions	No
Colesevelam	WelChol	3.75 g/day						No
Colestipol	Colestid	• Granules: 5–30 g/day • Tablets: 2–16 g/day						No

Niacin

Mechanism of action – reduces production of VLDL in liver → ↓ synthesis of LDL-C

Generic	Brand	Dose	Contra-indications	Primary Side Effects	Key Monitoring	Pertinent Drug Interactions	Med Pearl	Top 200
Niacin	Niaspan; also available as over-the-counter (OTC) product	500–3,000 mg/day	• Hepatic dysfunction • Active gout • Active peptic ulcer disease	• Flushing/itching • Nausea • Orthostatic hypotension • ↑ LFTs • Myopathy • Hyperuricemia • Hyperglycemia	• Lipid panel • LFTs • Creatine kinase (CK) (if muscle aches) • Uric acid • Blood glucose (if patient has DM)	None significant	• Used to ↓ LDL-C, ↓ TGs, and ↑ HDL-C • Most effective drug for ↑ HDL-C • Do not ↑ dose by >500 mg in 4-week period • Avoid use of OTC SR products (↑ risk of hepatotoxicity)	Yes

Combination product: Niacin/lovastatin (Advicor)   Niacin/simvastatin (Simcor)

Fibric Acid Derivatives

Mechanism of action – ↑ activity of lipoprotein lipase → ↑ catabolism of VLDL → ↓ TGs

Generic	Brand	Dose	Contra-indications	Primary Side Effects	Key Monitoring	Pertinent Drug Interactions	Med Pearl	Top 200
Fenofibrate	Antara, Lipofen, Lofibra, TriCor, Triglide	43–200 mg/day (depending on brand)	• Hepatic dysfunction • Severe renal dysfunction • Gallbladder disease	• N/V • Abdominal pain • Diarrhea • ↑ LFTs • Myopathy	• Lipid panel • LFTs • CK (if patient has muscle aches)	• Avoid using gemfibrozil with statins (↑ risk of myopathy) • ↑ effects of warfarin and sulfonylureas • ↓ cyclosporine levels	• Used to ↓ TGs and/or ↑ HDL-C • When adding to statin, fenofibrate preferred • Adjust dose in renal insufficiency	Yes
Gemfibrozil	Lopid	1,200 mg/day						Yes

Omega-3 Polyunsaturated Fatty Acids (Fish Oil)

Mechanism of action — ↓ production of TGs in the liver

Generic	Brand	Dose	Contraindications	Primary Side Effects	Key Monitoring	Pertinent Drug Interactions	Med Pearl	Top 200
Omega-3-Acid Ethyl Esters	Lovaza; also available as OTC product	2–4 g/day	Fish allergy	Belching ("fishy taste") Dyspepsia	Lipid panel	May ↑ risk of bleeding with antiplatelets or warfarin	• Used to ↓ TGs • May ↑ LDL-C	Yes

HMG-CoA Reductase Inhibitors (Statins)

Mechanism of action — inhibit HMG-CoA reductase → prevent the conversion of HMG-CoA to mevalonate (rate-limiting step in cholesterol synthesis)

Generic	Brand	Dose	Contraindications	Primary Side Effects	Key Monitoring	Pertinent Drug Interactions	Med Pearl	Top 200
Atorvastatin	Lipitor	10–80 mg/day	• Hepatic dysfunction • Pregnancy	• ↑ LFTs • Myopathy • N/V • Constipation	• Lipid panel • LFTs • CK (if patient has muscle aches)	• Atorvastatin, lovastatin, rosuvastatin, and simvastatin are CYP3A4 substrates; CYP3A4 inhibitors may ↑ risk of side effects; may ↑ effects of warfarin • Fluvastatin metabolized by CYP2C9; may ↑ effects of warfarin • Pravastatin not metabolized by CYP enzymes	• Most effective drugs for ↓ LDL-C • Lower maximum dosage of simvastatin and lovastatin when used with amiodarone, verapamil, fibrates, cyclosporine, or niacin • Adjust rosuvastatin dose in patients with CrCl <30 mL/min	Yes
Fluvastatin	Lescol, Lescol XL	20–80 mg/day						Yes
Lovastatin	Altoprev, Mevacor	20–80 mg/day						Yes
Pravastatin	Pravachol	10–80 mg/day						Yes
Simvastatin	Zocor	10–80 mg/day						Yes
Rosuvastatin	Crestor	5–40 mg/day						Yes

Combination products: Atorvastatin/amlodipine (Caduet)   Simvastatin/ezetimibe (Vytorin)

Cholesterol Absorption Inhibitor

Mechanism of action — prevents absorption of cholesterol from small intestine

Generic	Brand	Dose	Contraindications	Primary Side Effects	Key Monitoring	Pertinent Drug Interactions	Med Pearl	Top 200
Ezetimibe	Zetia	10 mg/day	None	• Headache • Diarrhea	Lipid panel	• Cyclosporine and fibrates may ↑ effects • ↑ cyclosporine levels • ↑ effects of warfarin	• Used to ↓ LDL-C • Can add to statin to further ↓ LDL-C or if dose-limiting side effects occur with statin	Yes

Storage and Administration Pearls

- Bile acid resins
  - Cholestyramine available as powder; colestipol available as granules and tablets; colesevelam available as tablets
  - Should be administered with meals
  - Powder can be mixed in applesauce, pudding, oatmeal, Jell-O, etc. to improve its palatability (do not mix in carbonated beverages)
  - Other medications given one hour *before* or four hours *after* cholestyramine or colestipol
- Niacin at bedtime (so flushing reaction can occur while patient is sleeping)
- Fibric acid derivatives: Can be administered with meals to ↓ GI effects
- Statins: IR lovastatin administered with meals; ER lovastatin administered at bedtime
- Most statins administered in the evening (at bedtime)—most hepatic cholesterol production occurs during the night (~2 A.M.); atorvastatin administered in the morning or evening
- After initiating lipid-lowering therapy, lipid profile reassessed in six weeks to determine if any changes in therapy are needed
- LDL-lowering potential of statins: Rosuvastatin >atorvastatin >simvastatin >pravastatin = lovastatin >fluvastatin

Patient Education Pearls

- Fiber/fiber supplements may help minimize GI side effects associated with bile acid resins.
- Any episodes of muscle pain/aches or dark urine should be reported.
- Flushing reaction associated with niacin may be minimized by taking aspirin (325 mg) or an NSAID at least 30 minutes before dose, taking with food, slowly titrating the dose, and avoiding alcohol or hot beverages. Tolerance usually develops.
- Statins should be avoided if the patient is pregnant.

HEART FAILURE

Definition

Heart failure (HF) is a condition in which the heart is unable to pump out enough blood (CO) to meet the metabolic demands of the body. The decrease in CO leads to the activation of numerous compensatory mechanisms, which attempt to improve CO. There are two types of HF: systolic (pumping function/contractility impaired; left ventricular ejection fraction [LVEF] ≤40%) or diastolic (impaired ability to relax, which leads to underfilling; normal LVEF [>40%]). The majority of HF cases are due to either coronary artery disease (CAD) or HTN. A number of drugs can also precipitate or worsen HF by causing negative inotropic effects (e.g., β-blockers, CCBs [except amlodipine and felodipine], antiarrhythmics [except amiodarone and dofetilide], itraconazole, terbinafine), causing Na^+ and water retention (e.g., corticosteroids, NSAIDs, thiazolidinediones), causing vasoconstriction (e.g., sympathomimetics), or acting as a direct cardiotoxin (e.g., anthracyclines, cyclophosphamide, trastuzumab).

Diagnosis

- Diagnosis is primarily based on the patient's physical exam findings in conjunction with the past medical history and results from laboratory and diagnostic tests.
- Echocardiogram provides information regarding LV function and can reflect whether the patient has systolic or diastolic dysfunction.
- B-type natriuretic peptide (BNP) concentration can also be obtained to help differentiate between acute HF and other causes of dyspnea (e.g., pneumonia, bronchitis, COPD, pulmonary embolus) (>500 pg/mL in patients with acute decompensated HF [ADHF]).

Signs and Symptoms

- Signs and symptoms of left-sided HF (reflect pulmonary congestion)
  - Symptoms: Dyspnea, orthopnea, paroxysmal nocturnal dyspnea, cough
  - Signs: Rales (usually bibasilar), pulmonary edema, pleural effusion, S_3 gallop
- Signs and symptoms of right-sided HF (reflect systemic congestion)
  - Symptoms: Anorexia, N/V, constipation, abdominal pain, bloating
  - Signs: Jugular venous distention, (+) hepatojugular reflux, ascites, peripheral edema, hepatomegaly, splenomegaly

Classification of HF

New York Heart Association (NYHA) Functional Classification	American College of Cardiology/ American Heart Association Staging System
• Functional class I = Patients have LV dysfunction but no physical limitations; lack symptoms with ordinary physical activity ("well compensated") • Functional class II = Slight limitation of physical activity; symptoms with ordinary physical activity (e.g., walking two blocks) • Functional class III = Marked limitation of physical activity; minimal activity (e.g., activities of daily living) causes symptoms • Functional class IV = Unable to carry on physical activity without discomfort; symptoms at rest	• Stage A = At high risk for development of HF but have no structural heart disease or symptoms of HF. Includes patients with HTN, DM, and CAD • Stage B = Structural heart disease (e.g., LVH, previous MI, LV systolic dysfunction, or valvular heart disease) but no symptoms of HF (NYHA class I symptoms). • Stage C = Structural heart disease with current or previous symptoms of HF (NYHA class I, II, III, or IV symptoms). • Stage D = Refractory symptoms of HF at rest despite maximal medical therapy (often hospitalized) (end-stage HF) (NYHA class IV symptoms).

Guidelines

Heart Failure Society of America. *J Card Fail* , no. 12 (2006): 12:10–38. www.heartfailureguidelines.com.

Guidelines Summary

The goals of therapy are to relieve symptoms, improve quality of life, improve survival, reduce hospitalizations, and slow the progression of disease.

■ Nonpharmacologic therapy: Regular low-intensity physical activity, ↓ Na$^+$ (≤3 g/day), ↓ fluid intake (<2 L/day), weight loss (if obese), alcohol restriction, and smoking cessation

■ Pharmacologic therapy:

• Stage A: Modify risk factors and control HTN, DM, CAD, and dyslipidemia; ACE-I or ARB in patients with risk factors for vascular disease

• Stage B: ACE-I + β-blocker

• Stage C: ACE-I + β-blocker + diuretic

» Other drugs to be considered:

– Aldosterone receptor antagonist: Current or recent NYHA class IV symptoms who are already receiving ACE-I (or ARB), β-blocker, and diuretic (± digoxin)

– ARBs: Patients who cannot tolerate ACE-Is due to intractable cough; patients who remain symptomatic despite optimal therapy with ACE-I and β-blocker

- Digoxin: Patients who remain symptomatic despite optimal therapy with ACE-I (or ARB), β-blocker, and diuretic
- Hydralazine/isosorbide dinitrate: Patients with intolerance or contraindications (renal insufficiency, hyperkalemia) to ACE-I or ARB; African-American patients who remain symptomatic despite optimal therapy with ACE-I (or ARB) and β-blocker

• Stage D: Chronic positive inotrope therapy (e.g. dobutamine, milrinone), mechanical circulatory support (e.g., LV assist device), heart transplant, end-of-life care/hospice

Medication Charts

Loop Diuretics

Mechanism of action — inhibit Na^+ reabsorption in the ascending limb of loop of Henle; ↓ preload

Generic	Brand	Dose	Contra-indications	Primary Side Effects	Key Monitoring	Pertinent Drug Interactions	Med Pearl	Top 200
Bumetanide	Bumex	0.5–10 mg/day	Sulfa allergy	• Hypocalcemia • Hypokalemia • Hypomagnesemia • Hyponatremia • Hyperglycemia • Hyperuricemia • Metabolic alkalosis • Azotemia	• BP • Electrolytes • BUN/SCr • Blood glucose • Uric acid • Jugular venous pressure • Urine output • Weight (↓ by 0.5–1 kg/day initially)	• May ↑ risk of lithium toxicity • May ↑ risk of ototoxicity with aminoglycosides • May ↓ effect of antidiabetic agents • NSAIDs ↓ effects	• ↓ symptoms; effect on mortality unknown • If initial dose inadequate, double dose, dose 2x daily, add metolazone, or use IV • Similar side effects as thiazides (except loops cause hypocalcemia) • BUN/SCr ratio >20:1 → dehydration (prerenal azotemia)	Yes
Furosemide	Lasix	20–600 mg/day						Yes
Torsemide	Demadex	10–200 mg/day						Yes

ACE Inhibitors (ACE-Is)

- HTN monograph for further details
- Medication pearls specific to their use in HF:
  - ↓ mortality; ↓ preload and afterload
  - Strive to achieve target dose, if possible (titrate dose to symptoms, not BP)

Drug	Initial Dose	Target Dose
Captopril	6.25 mg TID	50 mg TID
Enalapril	2.5 mg BID	10 mg BID
Lisinopril	2.5 mg daily	40 mg daily
Ramipril	1.25 mg daily	10 mg daily
Trandolapril	1 mg daily	4 mg daily
Fosinopril	5 mg daily	40 mg daily
Quinapril	5 mg BID	20 mg BID
Perindopril	2 mg daily	16 mg daily

β-Blockers

Mechanism of action — ↓ activation of the sympathetic nervous system; slows and potentially reverse detrimental effects (e.g., ventricular remodeling) of catecholamines

Generic	Brand	Dose	Contraindications	Primary Side Effects	Key Monitoring	Pertinent Drug Interactions	Med Pearl	Top 200
Bisoprolol	Zebeta	1.25–10 mg/day	• Symptomatic bradycardia • ≥2nd-degree heart block (in absence of pacemaker) • SBP <85 mmHg • Severe asthma • Decompensated HF	See HTN section	• BP • HR • S/S HF • Weight (↓ by 0.5–1 kg/day initially)	Carvedilol may ↑ digoxin levels	• ↓ mortality • Metoprolol succinate (not tartrate) approved for HF • Patient should be fairly euvolemic before starting • Strive to achieve target dose, if possible • Dose can be doubled every 2–4 wks to achieve target dose (unless side effects) • Manage worsening HF by ↑ diuretic dose • If hypotension occurs, may ↓ dose of ACE-I, ARB, or other vasodilator (more common with carvedilol) • If bradycardia occurs, ↓ dose • Abrupt discontinuation may cause worsening HF	No
Carvedilol	Coreg, Coreg CR	IR: 6.25–100 mg/day (in two divided doses) CR: 10–80 mg/day (≥1x daily)						Yes
Metoprolol succinate	Toprol XL	12.5–200 mg/day						Yes

Digoxin

Mechanism of action — inhibits Na+/K+ ATPase pump → ↑ intracellular Ca²⁺ → ↑ myocardial contractility; also ↓ neurohormonal activation

Generic	Brand	Dose	Contra-indications	Primary Side Effects	Key Monitoring	Pertinent Drug Interactions	Med Pearl	Top 200
Digoxin	Digitek, Lanoxin	0.125–0.25 mg/day (loading doses not necessary in HF)	≥2nd-degree heart block (in absence of pacemaker)	• Bradycardia/heart block • S/S digoxin toxicity (visual disturbances, N/V, confusion, anorexia, arrhythmias)	• HR • Electrolytes (predisposed to toxicity if hypokalemia, hypomagnesemia, or hypercalcemia) • BUN/SCr • Digoxin concentrations	• Amiodarone, quinidine, verapamil, and clarithromycin may ↑ levels • Antacids may ↓ levels (separate by 1–2 hours) • Use with other negative chronotropes (e.g., β-blockers, verapamil, diltiazem, or clonidine) may ↑ risk of bradycardia	• Improves symptoms, ↓ hospitalizations; no effect on mortality • Abrupt discontinuation may cause worsening HF • ↓ dose by 50% when starting amiodarone • Adjust dose in patients with renal dysfunction • Target level: 0.5–1 ng/mL (↑ mortality if >1 ng/mL)	Yes

Aldosterone Receptor Antagonists

Mechanism of action – inhibit the effects of aldosterone → ↓ remodeling and Na⁺/water retention

- Spironolactone is nonselective aldosterone receptor antagonist (also blocks androgen and progesterone receptors → associated with endocrine side effects)
- Eplerenone is selective aldosterone receptor antagonist (not associated with endocrinologic side effects)

Generic	Brand	Dose	Contraindications	Primary Side Effects	Key Monitoring	Pertinent Drug Interactions	Med Pearl	Top 200
Eplerenone	Inspra	25–50 mg/day	• K⁺ >5 mEq/L • SCr >2.5 mg/dL (or CrCl ≤30 mL/min) • Concomitant ACE-I **and** ARB use • Also for eplerenone: • Use of strong CYP3A4 inhibitors (e.g., ritonavir, ketoconazole, itraconazole, nefazodone, clarithromycin, nelfinavir)	• Hyperkalemia • Also for spironolactone: • Gynecomastia, breast tenderness, menstrual changes, hirsutism	• BP • K⁺ • BUN/SCr	Use with ACE-Is, ARBs, K⁺ supplements, or NSAIDs may ↑ risk of hyperkalemia	• ↓ mortality • Should consider discontinuing or ↓ dose of K⁺ supplements • Eplerenone tends to be used in patients who develop endocrine side effects with spironolactone	No
Spironolactone	Aldactone	12.5–25 mg/day						Yes

Angiotensin II Receptor Blockers

- HTN monograph for further details
- Medication pearls specific to their use in HF:
  - Only candesartan, losartan, or valsartan recommended for the management of HF (only candesartan and valsartan approved for HF)
  - Should not be considered equivalent or superior to ACE-Is

Hydralazine/Isosorbide Dinitrate

Mechanism of action:
- Hydralazine – causes arterial vasodilation (↓ afterload)
- Isosorbide dinitrate – causes venous vasodilation (↓ preload)

Generic	Brand	Dose	Contra-indications	Primary Side Effects	Key Monitoring	Pertinent Drug Interactions	Med Pearl	Top 200
Hydralazine	Apresoline	40–300 mg/day	None	• Headache • Dizziness • Reflex tachycardia • Peripheral edema (hydralazine) • Lupus-like syndrome (hydralazine)	BP HR	None	• ↓ mortality • Often used in patients who cannot tolerate ACE-Is or ARBs due to renal insufficiency, hyperkalemia, or angioedema • Can alternatively use isosorbide mononitrate (has not been studied in HF) • Do not use hydralazine alone (↑ mortality)	Yes
Isosorbide dinitrate	Isordil	30–120 mg/day						No

Combination product:
Hydralazine/isosorbide dinitrate (BiDil) – approved for African-American patients with NYHA class II, III, or IV HF due to LV systolic dysfunction (LVEF ≤40%) who are receiving an ACE-I (or ARB) and a β-blocker (can also use individual products together if there are financial concerns)

Intravenous Drugs for Treatment of ADHF

Drug	Mechanism of Action	Primary Side Effects	Med Pearl
Vasodilators			
Nitroglycerin	• Venous vasodilation → ↓ preload • Can cause arterial vasodilation at higher doses	Hypotension, tachycardia, headache, tolerance	• Especially useful in patients with myocardial ischemia • Tolerance can develop (overcome by ↑ infusion rate)
Nitroprusside	• Arterial and venous vasodilation → ↓ preload and afterload	Hypotension, N/V, cyanide/ thiocyanate toxicity (risk ↑ if infusion >24 hours)	Avoid in patients with renal dysfunction
Nesiritide (Natrecor)	• B-type natriuretic peptide • Arterial and venous vasodilation → ↓ preload and afterload	Hypotension, headache	Infusion should not be titrated more frequently than every 3 hours
Positive Inotropes			
Dopamine	• 0.5–3 mcg/kg/min → Stimulates dopamine receptors → ↑ urine output • 3–10 mcg/kg/min → Stimulates β_1 receptors → ↑ CO, ↑ HR • >10 mcg/kg/min → Stimulates α_1 receptors → ↑ BP	Arrhythmias, tachycardia, myocardial ischemia, N/V	Avoid in patients with myocardial ischemia
Dobutamine	• β_1 and β_2 receptor agonist and weak α_1 receptor agonist → ↑ CO and vasodilation	Arrhythmias, tachycardia, myocardial ischemia, hypokalemia, tremor	• Avoid in patients with myocardial ischemia • Should not be used in patients receiving chronic β–blocker therapy • Tolerance can develop
Milrinone	• PDE III inhibitor → ↑ CO and vasodilation	Hypotension, arrhythmias	• Can be used in patients receiving chronic β–blocker therapy, or in those not responding/tolerating dobutamine • Tolerance does not develop • Use lower initial dose in patients with renal dysfunction

Storage and Administration Pearls

- Captopril should be administered at least one hour *before* or two hours *after* meals.
- Carvedilol should be administered with food to minimize the risk of orthostatic hypotension.
- Nitroprusside infusions should be protected from light.

Patient Education Pearls

- If a patient is taking >1 dose of diuretic each day, the last dose should be taken before 5 p.m. to minimize nocturia.
- Patients should weigh themselves daily (first thing in the morning after urinating) and should contact their healthcare provider if they gain more than 3–5 lb in a week.
- Patients receiving diuretics should wear sunscreen and protective clothing. Also, they should report any episodes of muscle cramps, as this may be a symptom of hypokalemia or hypomagnesemia.
- A patient who is receiving aldosterone antagonists, ACE-Is, or ARBs should avoid excessive intake of foods high in K^+ (e.g., green leafy vegetables, potatoes, apricots, bananas, dates, oranges, avocados) and K^+-containing salt substitutes.
- A patient who is receiving ACE-Is or ARBs should call 911 immediately if he experiences lip, tongue, or facial swelling or is having difficulty breathing. ACE-Is and ARBs should be avoided in patients who are pregnant.
- Patients should not stop their β-blocker or digoxin therapy abruptly, as this may cause a sudden worsening of HF symptoms.

ANTIARRHYTHMIC DRUGS

Class Ia Antiarrhythmics

Mechanism of action – Na+ channel blockers; slow conduction velocity, prolong refractoriness, ↓ automaticity

Generic	Brand	Dose	Contra-indications	Primary Side Effects	Key Monitoring	Pertinent Drug Interactions	Med Pearl	Top 200
Disopyramide	• Norpace • Norpace CR	400–1,600 mg/day	• HF • ≥2nd-degree heart block (in absence of pacemaker) • Long QT syndrome	• Dry mouth • Urinary retention • Blurred vision • Constipation • HF exacerbation • Hypotension • Torsades de pointes (TdP)	• Electrocardiogram (ECG) (QTc interval, QRS duration) • BP • S/S HF • Electrolytes • Disopyramide concentrations	• CYP3A4 inhibitors and anticholinergics may ↑ risk of side effects • CYP3A4 inducers may ↓ effects • ↑ risk of TdP with other drugs that prolong QT interval	• Used for atrial and ventricular arrhythmias • Therapeutic range: 2–5 mcg/mL • Adjust dose in renal dysfunction	No
Procainamide	Pronestyl	IV: *Loading dose:* 15–17 mg/kg over 25–60 min *Maintenance dose:* 1–4 mg/min continuous infusion	• ≥2nd-degree heart block (in absence of pacemaker) • Long QT syndrome	• Lupus-like syndrome • TdP • Hypotension • Agranulocytosis	• ECG (QTc interval, QRS duration) • BP • S/S lupus (e.g., stabbing chest pain, joint pain, rash) • Procainamide/N-acetylprocainamide (NAPA) concentrations • Complete blood count (CBC) with differential • Electrolytes	• ↑ risk of TdP with other drugs that prolong QT interval	• Used for atrial and ventricular arrhythmias • Therapeutic range: 4–10 mcg/mL (procainamide); 15–25 mcg/mL (NAPA); 10–30 mcg/mL (total) • Use with caution, if at all, in renal insufficiency	No
Quinidine	Quinidex, Quinaglute	• Sulfate: 800–2,400 mg/day • Gluconate: 648–2,916 mg/day	• ≥2nd-degree heart block (in absence of pacemaker) • Long QT syndrome • Use of ritonavir	• Diarrhea • Stomach cramps • TdP • Hypotension • Cinchonism (tinnitus, blurred vision, headache) • Thrombocytopenia	• ECG (QTc interval, QRS duration) • BP • Quinidine concentrations • CBC with differential • LFTs • Electrolytes	• CYP3A4 inhibitors may ↑ risk of side effects • CYP3A4 inducers may ↓ effects • ↑ risk of digoxin toxicity • May ↑ toxicity of CYP3A4 and CYP2D6 substrates • ↑ risk of TdP with other drugs that prolong QT interval	• Used for atrial and ventricular arrhythmias • Therapeutic range: 2–5 mcg/mL • Administer with food to minimize GI effects	No

Class Ib Antiarrhythmics

Mechanism of action – Na⁺ channel blockers; little effect on conduction velocity, shorten refractoriness, ↓ automaticity

Generic	Brand	Dose	Contraindications	Primary Side Effects	Key Monitoring	Pertinent Drug Interactions	Med Pearl	Top 200
Lidocaine	Xylocaine	*Loading dose:* 1–1.5 mg/kg, up to 3 mg/kg (total) *Maintenance dose:* 1–4 mg/min	≥2nd-degree heart block (in absence of pacemaker)	CNS toxicity (dizziness, blurred vision, slurred speech, confusion, paresthesias, seizures)	• ECG (QRS duration) • BP • Neurologic exam • Lidocaine concentrations (if duration >24 hours)	Amiodarone may ↑ risk of toxicity	• Used only for ventricular arrhythmias • Therapeutic range: 1.5–5 mcg/mL • Use lower infusion rate in elderly, HF or hepatic dysfunction	No
Mexiletine	Mexitil	600–1,200 mg/day	≥2nd-degree heart block (in absence of pacemaker)	• CNS toxicity (same as lidocaine) • N/V	• ECG (QRS duration) • BP • LFTs • Neurologic exam	• ↑ risk of theophylline toxicity • CYP1A2 and CYP2D6 inhibitors may ↑ risk of toxicity	• Used only for ventricular arrhythmias • Take with food to minimize GI effects • ↓ dose in HF or hepatic dysfunction	No

KAPLAN) MEDICAL

Class Ic Antiarrhythmics

Mechanism of action — Na$^+$ channel blockers (most potent); markedly slow conduction velocity, no effect on refractoriness, ↓ automaticity; propafenone also has nonselective β-blocking properties

Generic	Brand	Dose	Contraindications	Primary Side Effects	Key Monitoring	Pertinent Drug Interactions	Med Pearl	Top 200
Flecainide	Tambocor	*Loading dose (for conversion of atrial fibrillation [AF]):* 200–300 mg x 1 dose *Maintenance dose:* 100–400 mg/day	• ≥2nd-degree heart block (in absence of pacemaker) • History of MI • HF	• Dizziness • Tremor • HF exacerbation • Ventricular tachycardia (VT)	• ECG (QRS duration) • Echocardiogram (at baseline to evaluation LV function) • Electrolytes	• ↑ risk of digoxin toxicity	• Used for atrial and ventricular arrhythmias • Avoid in patients with structural heart disease • Adjust dose in renal dysfunction	No
Propafenone	Rythmol, Rythmol SR	IR: *Loading dose (for AF conversion):* 450–600 mg x 1 *Maintenance dose:* 450–900 mg/day (in three divided doses) SR: *Maintenance dose:* 450–950 mg/day (in two divided doses)	• ≥2nd-degree heart block (in absence of pacemaker) • Bradycardia • Bronchospastic disorders • HF • History of MI	• Bradycardia/heart block • HF exacerbation • Bronchospasm • Taste disturbances • VT	• ECG (QRS duration, PR interval) • BP • HR • Echocardiogram (at baseline to evaluation LV function)	• ↑ risk of digoxin toxicity • ↑ effects of warfarin • Use with other negative chronotropes (e.g., β-blockers, digoxin, verapamil, diltiazem, or clonidine) may ↑ risk of bradycardia	Same as for flecainide	No

Class II Antiarrhythmics

(See medication chart in HTN section for discussion on β-blockers)

Class III Antiarrhythmics

Mechanism of action – K+ channel blockers; no effect on conduction velocity or automaticity; amiodarone has also Na+-channel blocking, β-blocking, and CCB properties; sotalol also has nonselective β-blocking properties

Generic	Brand	Dose	Contra-indications	Primary Side Effects	Key Monitoring	Pertinent Drug Interactions	Med Pearl	Top 200
Amiodarone	Cordarone, Pacerone	Loading dose (IV): 150 mg over 10 min *Stable VT / Ventricular Fibrillation:* 300 mg IV push *AF:* 5 mg/kg over 30–60 min Loading dose (PO): *Ventricular arrhythmias:* 1,200–1,600 mg/day Maintenance dose: IV: 1 mg/min x 6 hrs, then 0.5 mg/min PO: 100–400 mg/day	≥2nd-degree heart block (in absence of pacemaker)	IV: • Hypotension • Bradycardia/heart block • Phlebitis PO: • Hypo/hyper-thyroidism • Pulmonary fibrosis • Bradycardia/heart block • Corneal microdeposits • Optic neuritis • N/V • ↑LFTs • Ataxia • Paresthesias • Photosensitivity • Blue-gray skin discoloration	• ECG (QTc interval, QRS duration, PR interval) • BP • HR • Chest x-ray (every 12 months) • Pulmonary function tests (if symptoms) • Thyroid function tests (TFTs) (every 6 months) • LFTs (every 6 months) • Ophthalmologic exam (every 12 months)	• Inhibits CYP1A2, CYP2C9, CYP1D6, and CYP3A4 • CYP3A4 substrate • ↑ risk of digoxin toxicity (↓ digoxin dose by 50%) • ↑ effects of warfarin (↓ warfarin dose by 30%) • Use with other negative chronotropes may ↑ risk of bradycardia • May ↑ cyclosporine or phenytoin levels • May ↑ risk of side effects of simvastatin and lovastatin	• Used for atrial and ventricular arrhythmias • Half-life = 40–60 days • If pulmonary fibrosis or blurred vision occur, discontinue therapy • If TFTs abnormal, treat thyroid disorder • If ↑ LFTs occur, ↓ amiodarone dose • Take with food to minimize GI effects	Yes

Class III Antiarrhythmics (cont'd)

Generic	Brand	Dose	Contra-indications	Primary Side Effects	Key Monitoring	Pertinent Drug Interactions	Med Pearl	Top 200
Dofetilide	Tikosyn	• 500 mcg 2x daily (if CrCl >60 mL/min) • Adjust dose if CrCl ≤60 mL/min	• CrCl <20 mL/min • QTc interval >440 msec • Hypokalemia/hypomagnesemia • Use of verapamil, ketoconazole, cimetidine, trimethoprim, prochlorperazine, hydrochlorothiazide, megestrol, or other drugs that prolong QT interval	TdP	• ECG (QTc interval) • SCr • Electrolytes	↑ risk of TdP with other drugs that prolong QT interval	• Used only for atrial arrhythmias • Adjust dose based on renal function and QT interval	No
Ibutilide	Corvert	1 mg over 10 min; repeat x 1, if needed	• QTc interval >440 msec • Hypokalemia/hypomagnesemia • Concurrent use of other drugs that prolong QT interval	TdP	• ECG (QTc interval) • Electrolytes	↑ risk of TdP with other drugs that prolong QT interval	Used only for atrial arrhythmias	No

Class IV Antiarrhythmics

(See medication chart in HTN section for discussion on CCBs)

ISCHEMIC HEART DISEASE

Definitions

Ischemic heart disease (IHD) is characterized by a lack of oxygen resulting from inadequate perfusion of the myocardium, which is often due to narrowing or blockage in a coronary artery. Patients with IHD may present with chronic stable angina, vasospastic angina (variant or Prinzmetal's angina), or an acute coronary syndrome (ACS). ACS can include unstable angina (UA), non–ST-segment-elevation MI (NSTEMI), or ST-segment–elevation MI (STEMI). An ACS is precipitated by rupture of an atherosclerotic plaque, followed by formation of a thrombus at the site of plaque rupture. In NSTEMI, the thrombus tends to contain more platelets than fibrin ("white clot") and does not completely occlude the vessel. In STEMI, the thrombus contains more fibrin and red blood cells than platelets ("red clot") and completely occludes the vessel.

This section reviews the management of NSTEMI and STEMI.

Diagnosis

- If ischemic-like chest pain persists for at least 20 minutes, ACS should be suspected.
  - An ECG should be performed and serial cardiac enzymes (troponin, CK-MB) should be obtained.

Findings	UA	NSTEMI	STEMI
Cardiac enzymes (troponin, CK-MB)	Negative	Positive	Positive
ECG changes	ST-segment depression, T-wave inversion, or no ECG changes (any changes are usually transient)	ST-segment depression, T-wave inversion, or no ECG changes	ST-segment elevation

Signs and Symptoms

- Chest pain/pressure (substernal, crushing) that may radiate to the left arm, jaw, shoulders, and back are common symptoms.
- Other symptoms include dyspnea, diaphoresis, N/V.
- When compared to chronic stable angina, pain in ACS may be more severe, occur at rest, occur more frequently, be precipitated by less exertion, and be refractory to sublingual nitroglycerin (NTG).
- Patients may also present with signs/symptoms of HF or with arrhythmias.

Guidelines

American College of Cardiology/American Heart Association (NSTEMI guidelines), *J Am Coll Cardiol*, no. 50 (2007): 652–76.

American College of Cardiology/American Heart Association (STEMI guidelines), *J Am Coll Cardiol*, no. 51 (2008): 210–47.

Guidelines Summary

Acute Pharmacologic Management of UA/NSTEMI—Anti-Ischemic and Analgesic Therapy

Morphine

- Can be given to patients who continue to have chest discomfort despite the use of NTG or have recurrence of chest pain despite the use of other anti-ischemic therapies
- Dose: 1–5 mg IV every 5–30 minutes as needed for pain

NTG

- Can be given to patients with ongoing chest discomfort (0.4 mg SL every 5 min x 3 doses); following these doses, IV NTG within the initial 48 hours if patients continue to have ischemia, or if they present with HF or are hypertensive
- Dose: 5–10 mcg/min continuous infusion; can be titrated up to 100 mcg/min for relief of symptoms
- Adverse effects: Reflex tachycardia, hypotension, headache

β-Blockers

- Oral β-blockers: Given within the first 24 hours to patients who **do not** have signs/symptoms of HF, risk factors for developing cardiogenic shock (age >70 years, SBP <120 mmHg, HR >110 bpm or <60 bpm, or prolonged duration since presenting with UA/NSTEMI), PR interval >0.24 seconds, ≥2nd-degree heart block, or severe reactive airway disease
- IV β-blockers as an alternative

CCBs

- A non-DHP CCB (verapamil or diltiazem) administered alternatively if the patient has a contraindication to β-blocker therapy and does not have evidence of LV dysfunction
- A long-acting non-DHP CCB in patients who have recurrent ischemia despite being on a β-blocker and nitrate therapy

ACE-Is

- Should be given within the first 24 hours to patients with pulmonary congestion or LVEF ≤40%, provided they are not hypotensive (SBP <100 mmHg) or have contra-indications
- Can also be useful if given within the first 24 hours to patients without pulmonary congestion or LVEF ≤40%, provided they are not hypotensive (SBP <100 mmHg) or have contraindications
- An ARB used alternatively in patients who cannot tolerate ACE-Is

ANTIPLATELET THERAPY

Aspirin

- All patients should receive 162–325 mg (non–enteric-coated) at the onset of chest pain (should be chewed and swallowed).
- Patients should continue to receive 162–325 mg daily for at least 1 month after bare-metal stent implantation, 3 months after sirolimus-eluting stent implantation, and 6 months after paclitaxel-eluting stent implantation, and then continue on 75–162 mg daily indefinitely. If no stent received, the dose of aspirin can be immediately ↓ to 75–162 mg daily and continued indefinitely.

Clopidogrel

- This is an alternative to aspirin in patients who are allergic or have a major GI intolerance to aspirin.
- A loading dose of 300–600 mg, followed by a maintenance dose of 75 mg daily should be given to all patients regardless of whether an invasive (PCI) or conservative treatment strategy is planned (should be given **with** aspirin).
- Clopidogrel should be continued (**with** aspirin) for the following durations of time:
  - Bare-metal stent implantation: At least 1 month, ideally up to 1 year
  - Drug-eluting stents (sirolimus or paclitaxel): At least 1 year
  - No stent: At least 1 month, ideally up to 1 year

Glycoprotein IIb/IIIa Receptor Blockers (GPBs)

- PCI planned: Clopidogrel and/or GPB (eptifibatide or tirofiban) can be initiated prior to angiography; delay to angiography, high-risk features, or recurrent ischemia favor use of both agents prior to angiography. Do not need GPB if bivalirudin + 300 mg loading dose of clopidogrel (given ≥6 hours before angiography) are used.

- Conservative strategy: Adding eptifibatide or tirofiban to clopidogrel can be considered (especially if patient has recurrent ischemia and requires angiography).

Anticoagulant Therapy

- PCI planned: Either unfractionated heparin (UFH) or enoxaparin should be added to antiplatelet therapy; fondaparinux or bivalirudin can be used alternatively.
- Conservative strategy: Either enoxaparin or fondaparinux should be added to antiplatelet therapy; UFH can be used alternatively.

ACUTE PHARMACOLOGIC MANAGEMENT OF STEMI

Anti-Ischemic and Analgesic Therapy

Morphine, NTG, β-Blockers, ACE-Is

- Same recommendations as for UA/NSTEMI

Antiplatelet Therapy

Aspirin

- Same recommendations as for UA/NSTEMI

Clopidogrel

- This is an alternative to aspirin in patients who are allergic or have a major GI intolerance to aspirin.
- Clopidogrel 75 mg daily should be added to aspirin therapy in all patients regardless of whether or not they undergo reperfusion with a fibrinolytic. A loading dose of 300 mg can be considered in patients age <75 years.
- Clopidogrel should be continued (**with** aspirin) for the following durations of time:
  - Bare-metal stent implantation: At least 1 month, ideally up to 1 year
  - Drug-eluting stents (sirolimus or paclitaxel): At least 1 year
  - No stent: At least 14 days (can be considered for up to 1 year)

GPBs

- Can be used if patient's undergoing primary PCI

Fibrinolytic Therapy

- Should be used in patients presenting to a hospital without the capability to perform PCI or cannot perform PCI within 90 minutes of first medical contact ("door-to-balloon" time)
- Should be initiated within 30 minutes of presenting to the hospital ("door-to-needle" time)

Anticoagulant Therapy

- Fibrinolytic administered: UFH, enoxaparin, or fondaparinux should be administered to patients receiving fibrinolytic therapy; should be continued for up to 8 days; UFH should only be used if the treatment duration is <48 hrs because of risk for heparin-induced thrombocytopenia [HIT] with prolonged therapy).
- Primary PCI: UFH, bivalirudin, or enoxaparin can be used.

Secondary Prevention of MI

- **Aspirin:** See recommendation above regarding dosing and duration of therapy.
- **Clopidogrel:** See recommendations above in respective NSTEMI and STEMI sections regarding dosing and duration of therapy.
- **β-blockers:** Continue indefinitely.
- **ACE-Is:** Should be given and continued indefinitely in all patients; ARB can be used in patients intolerant of ACE-Is.
- **Aldosterone receptor antagonist:** Should be given to patients with LVEF ≤40% receiving optimal ACE-I and β-blocker therapy who have DM or HF.
- **Statins:** Should be given and continued indefinitely in all patients (LDL-C goal <100 mg/dL; <70 mg/dL is considered reasonable).

Glycoprotein IIb/IIIa Receptor Blockers

Generic	Brand	Dose	Contra-indications	Primary Side Effects	Key Monitoring	Pertinent Drug Interactions	Med Pearl
Mechanism of action – block the glycoprotein IIb/IIIa receptor on platelets to prevent the binding of fibrinogen → Inhibit platelet aggregation							
Abciximab	ReoPro	*Loading dose:* 0.25 mg/kg IV bolus *Maintenance dose:* 0.125 mcg/kg/min (max of 10 mg/min); continue for 12 hr after PCI	• Active bleeding • Prior stroke within past 30 days or any hemorrhagic stroke • History of intracranial neoplasms or aneurysm • Thrombocytopenia • BP >180/110 mmHg • Dialysis-dependent (for eptifibatide)	• Bleeding • Thrombocytopenia	• CBC • Prothrombin time (PT)/activated partial thromboplastin time (aPTT) • Activated clotting time (ACT) (with PCI) • S/S bleeding	Anticoagulants and other antiplatelets may ↑ risk of bleeding	• Abciximab preferred over others in NSTEMI only if there is no significant delay to PCI (otherwise, eptifibatide or tirofiban preferred) • Adjust maintenance dose infusion of tirofiban and eptifibatide in renal dysfunction
Eptifibatide	Integrilin	*Loading dose:* 180 mcg/kg IV bolus x 2 (given 10 min apart) *Maintenance dose:* 2 mcg/kg/min; continue for 18–24 hr after PCI					
Tirofiban	Aggrastat	*Loading dose:* 0.4 mcg/kg/min x 30 min *Maintenance dose:* 0.1 mcg/kg/min; continue for 18–24 hr after PCI					

Anticoagulants

Mechanism of action
- UFH: Potentiates the action of antithrombin III, which inactivates the clotting factors, IIa (thrombin), IXa, Xa, XIa, and XIIa, and ultimately prevents the conversion of fibrinogen to fibrin
- Low molecular-weight heparins (LMWHs): Similar mechanism as UFH, but primarily inhibits factor Xa
- Fondaparinux: Selective inhibitor of factor Xa
- Bivalirudin: Direct thrombin inhibitor

Generic	Brand	Dose	Contra-indications	Primary Side Effects	Key Monitoring	Pertinent Drug Interactions	Med Pearl
UFH	None	*Loading dose:* 60 units/kg IV bolus (max = 4,000 units) *Maintenance dose:* 12 units/kg/hr (max = 1,000 units/hr)	• Active bleeding • History of HIT • Recent stroke	• Bleeding • Thrombocytopenia (UFH and LMWH)	• PT/aPTT (only for UFH) • CBC • Anti-Xa levels (for LMWHs) (consider in obese or renal dysfunction) • S/S bleeding	Antiplatelets and other anticoagulants may ↑ risk of bleeding	• If platelets <100,000 or ↓ by >50% from baseline, test for HIT; discontinue UFH and start direct thrombin inhibitor (e.g., lepirudin, argatroban) • Protamine can be used to reverse effects of UFH
Enoxaparin	Lovenox	*Loading dose:* 30 mg IV x 1 *Maintenance dose:* 1 mg/kg SC every 12 hr					• ↓ enoxaparin dose to 1 mg/kg every 24 hr if CrCl <30 mL/min • Avoid using dalteparin in renal dysfunction
Dalteparin	Fragmin	120 units/kg (max = 10,000 units) SC every 12 hr					• Should not used in patients with suspected HIT • Protamine only partially reverses effects of LMWHs
Fondaparinux	Arixtra	2.5 mg SC daily	• Active bleeding • CrCl <30 mL/min				• For STEMI, can give initial dose IV
Bivalirudin	Angiomax	*Loading dose:* 0.1 mg/kg IV bolus *Maintenance dose:* 0.25 mg/kg/hr	Active bleeding		PT/aPTT ACT		• Can also be used during PCI in patients with HIT

Fibrinolytic Agents

Mechanism of action – activate and convert plasminogen into plasmin, which then degrades fibrin (lyses the clot) to form fibrin degradation products

Generic	Brand	Dose	Contra-indications	Primary Side Effects	Key Monitoring	Pertinent Drug Interactions	Med Pearl
Reteplase (rPA)	Retavase	10 units IV x 2 doses (separated by 30 min)	• Active bleeding • Any history of intracranial hemorrhage • Known intracranial neoplasm or AV malformation • Suspected aortic dissection • Significant closed head or facial trauma within 3 months	Bleeding	• CBC • ECG (for signs of reperfusion) • S/S bleeding	Antiplatelets and other anticoagulants may ↑ risk of bleeding	tPA also approved for treatment of acute ischemic stroke and pulmonary embolism
Streptokinase (SK)	Streptase	1.5 million units IV over 60 min					
Tenecteplase (TNK)	TNKase	All doses given as IV bolus: • <60 kg: 30 mg • 60–69.9 kg: 35 mg • 70–79.9 kg: 40 mg • 80–89.9 kg: 45 mg • ≥90 kg: 50 mg					
Tissue plasminogen activator (tPA)	Alteplase	15 mg IV bolus, then 0.75 mg/kg (max = 50 mg) over 30 min, then 0.5 mg/kg (max = 35 mg) over 60 min					

LEARNING POINTS

- **HTN**
  - For patients with stage 1 HTN who do not have a compelling indication, a thiazide diuretic should be considered 1st-line therapy. If these patients have stage 2 HTN, two antihypertensives should be started initially, one of which should be a thiazide diuretic. If patients have a compelling indication, antihypertensive agent(s) that can also be used to treat this disease state should be initiated.
  - Patients with DM or CKD have lower BP goals (<130/80 mmHg)!

- **Dyslipidemia**
  - For all patients (except for those with TG >500 mg/dL), the primary objective of therapy is achieving their individualized LDL-C goal.
  - Statins are the most effective drugs for ↓ LDL-C.
  - Niacin is the most effective drug for ↑ HDL-C.
  - Myopathy and ↑ LFTs are potential side effects of niacin, fibric acid derivatives, and statins.

- **Heart Failure**
  - ACE-Is, β-blockers, aldosterone antagonists, and hydralazine/isosorbide dinitrate have been shown to ↓ mortality in patients with systolic HF.
  - β-blockers should not be initiated in patients who have evidence of fluid overload (peripheral or pulmonary); patients should be relatively euvolemic before starting β-blocker therapy.
  - ARBs can be used in patients who develop intolerable cough from ACE-I therapy. Hyperkalemia and renal insufficiency can be associated with both ACE-Is and ARBs. If patients are unable to tolerate ACE-Is or ARBs because of hyperkalemia or renal insufficiency, hydralazine/isosorbide dinitrate can be used as an alternative.

- **Antiarrhythmic Drugs**
  - Dosages of disopyramide, procainamide, flecainide, sotalol, and dofetilide must be adjusted in patients with renal dysfunction.
  - Amiodarone and dofetilide are the antiarrhythmics of choice in patients with AF who have HF.
  - Flecainide and propafenone should be avoided in patients with structural heart disease.
  - Lidocaine and mexiletine are only effective for ventricular arrhythmias.

- Amiodarone has a large volume of distribution and a very long half-life. It can be associated with toxicities that affect just about every organ system in the body. Chest x-ray and ophthalmologic exam should be performed annually while TFTs and LFTs should be evaluated every 6 months. Pulmonary function tests can be performed if patient complains of symptoms, such as shortness of breath or cough.

- **Ischemic Heart Disease**
  - Fibrinolytic drugs should only be used for STEMI.
  - For patients undergoing PCI and receiving a stent, clopidogrel should be administered for at least 1 month (ideally for up to 1 year) for bare metal stents and for at least 1 year for drug-eluting stents.
  - Know examples of GP IIb/IIIa inhibitors, LMWHs, factor Xa inhibitors, direct-thrombin inhibitors, and fibrinolytic drugs.
  - Drugs used for the secondary prevention of MI include aspirin, statins, β-blockers, ACE-Is, clopidogrel, and aldosterone antagonists.

PRACTICE QUESTIONS

1. Which of the following drugs may be associated with bradycardia?

    I. Bisoprolol
    II. Clonidine
    III. Amlodipine

    (A) I only
    (B) III only
    (C) I and II only
    (D) II and III only
    (E) I, II, and III

2. A patient has been on simvastatin 80 mg PO at bedtime for 3 weeks and is now complaining of muscle pain. Which of the following laboratory tests should be obtained?

    (A) Blood glucose
    (B) Creatine kinase
    (C) Complete blood count
    (D) Simvastatin blood concentration
    (E) Thyroid function tests

3. Which of the following are potential side effects of nitroglycerin?

    I. Arrhythmias
    II. Headache
    III. Tachycardia

    (A) I only
    (B) III only
    (C) I and II only
    (D) II and III only
    (E) I, II, and III

4. Which of following drugs are considered positive inotropes?

    I. Nesiritide
    II. Hydralazine
    III. Dobutamine

    (A) I only
    (B) III only
    (C) I and II only
    (D) II and III only
    (E) I, II, and III

ANSWERS

1. C

Both bisoprolol and clonidine decrease atrioventricular (AV) nodal conduction, and therefore may cause bradycardia and/or heart block. Thus, choice (C) is correct. The non-DHP CCBs (i.e., verapamil, diltiazem) also decrease AV nodal conduction and can cause bradycardia. However, the DHP CCBs, including amlodipine, have no effect on AV nodal conduction. Instead, these drugs can actually cause reflex tachycardia.

2. B

For a patient on a statin who complains of muscle pain, a creatine kinase should be obtained. Therefore, choice (B) is correct.

3. D

Nitroglycerin could potentially cause headaches and tachycardia, so choice (D) is correct. Nitroglycerin does not cause cardiac arrhythmias.

4. B

Dobutamine stimulates β_1 receptors in the heart and increases myocardial contractility and is therefore considered a positive inotrope. Nesiritide is an arterial and venous vasodilator, while hydralazine is a direct arterial vasodilator. While these drugs may increase CO, they do so by decreasing afterload and not my increasing myocardial contractility. Therefore, choice (B) is correct.

Infectious Diseases

2

This chapter reviews the various antibiotic agents, including antibacterial, antifungal, and antiviral agents. A brief overview of the recommended pharmacologic treatments of the following infections is also provided:

- **Urinary tract infections (UTIs)**
- **Pneumonia**
- **Meningitis**
- **Sexually transmitted diseases (STDs) (chlamydia, gonorrhea, syphilis)**
- **Human immunodeficiency virus (HIV)**

 Suggested Study Time: **3 hours**

PRINCIPLES OF ANTIBIOTIC THERAPY

Factors to Consider When Selecting Antibiotic Therapy

- Identity/Susceptibility of Bacteria
  - Important to know which bacteria may be causing the infection
    - » Can begin empiric antibiotic therapy without knowing the actual identity (or sensitivities) of the organism; select antibiotic(s) (usually broad-spectrum) based on the organism(s) *most* likely to cause a particular infection
    - » Once organism (and sensitivities) are identified, can adjust/narrow antibiotic therapy, as needed, to cover this organism
- Site of Infection
  - Especially important for meningitis, UTIs, prostatitis, and osteomyelitis
    - » Only certain drugs can penetrate into these areas to target the infection; these drugs may need to be used at higher doses, especially for meningitis, prostatitis, and osteomyelitis

- Patient Allergies
- Concomitant Medications
  - May need to be concerned with potential drug interactions when selecting an antibiotic
- Hepatic and Renal Function
  - May need to adjust antibiotic dosages if hepatic or renal dysfunction present
- Past Medical History
  - Certain antibiotics may need to be avoided in particular disease states (e.g., seizure disorders)
- Patient Age
  - Some antibiotics are contraindicated in pediatric patients
- Pregnancy/Breast Feeding
  - Some antibiotics are contraindicated in these patients

URINARY TRACT INFECTIONS

Common Organisms

Community-Acquired	Nosocomial (Hospital-Acquired)
• *E. coli* • *Staphylococcus saprophyticus* • *Klebsiella pneumoniae* • *Proteus mirabilis*	• *E. coli* • *Pseudomonas aeruginosa* • *Klebsiella pneumoniae* • *Proteus mirabilis* • *Enterobacter* spp. • *Staphylococcus aureus* • Fungus (e.g., *Candida*)

Diagnosis

- Confirmed by urinalysis
  - Bacteruria: > 10^2 cfu/mL
  - Pyuria: > 5–10 white blood cells (WBCs)/mm^3
  - Nitrite-positive
  - Leukocyte esterase–positive
  - Casts (may be present in pyelonephritis)

Signs and Symptoms

- Lower UTI (Cystitis)
  - Dysuria

- Urgency
- Frequency
- Nocturia
- Suprapubic pressure/pain
- Upper UTI (Pyelonephritis)
  - All of the above symptoms, PLUS
  - Flank pain
  - Fever
  - Nausea/vomiting (N/V)
- Complicated UTI factors
  - Male
  - Elderly
  - Pregnancy
  - Children
  - Nosocomial
  - Recent use of antibiotics
  - Diabetes
  - Immunosuppressed
  - Catheterized

Guidelines

Infectious Disease Society of America. *Clin Infect Dis*, no. 29 (1999): 745–58.

Guidelines Summary

Diagnosis	Treatment	Duration
Uncomplicated cystitis	Trimethoprim/sulfamethoxazole (TMP/SMX) **OR** Fluoroquinolone (FQ)	3 days
Uncomplicated pyelonephritis (outpatient therapy)	TMP/SMX **OR** FQ	7–14 days
Complicated UTIs	FQ **OR** Aminoglycoside **OR** Extended-spectrum β-lactam	10–14 days

PNEUMONIA

Common Organisms

Community-Acquired	Hospital-Acquired (occurs ≥48 hours after admission)
• *Mycoplasma pneumoniae* • *Streptococcus pneumoniae* • *Haemophilus influenzae* • *Chlamydia pneumoniae* • *Legionella pneumophila* • *Moraxella catarrhalis* • Viruses	• *Staphylococcus aureus* • *Pseudomonas aeruginosa* • *Klebsiella pneumoniae* • *Enterobacter* • *E. coli* • *Acinetobacter* spp. • *Serratia* spp. • Anaerobes

Diagnosis

■ Symptoms and ausculatory findings consistent with pneumonia, plus an infiltrate on chest x-ray

Signs and Symptoms

■ Fever, chills, dyspnea, cough (may or may not be productive)
■ Physical examination:
  • Tachypnea
  • Tachycardia
  • Dullness to percussion
  • Inspiratory crackles
  • Decreased breath sounds over affected area
■ Laboratory findings
  • ↑ WBCs
■ Infiltrate on chest x-ray

Guidelines

Community-acquired pneumonia, Infectious Disease Society of America/American Thoracic Society. *Clin Infect Dis*, no. 44 (Suppl 2) (2007): S27–72.

Hospital-acquired, ventilator-associated, and healthcare-associated pneumonia, American Thoracic Society/Infectious Disease Society of America. *Am J Respir Crit Care Med*, no. 171 (2005): 388–416.

Guidelines Summary

Diagnosis	Treatment	Duration
Community-acquired (ambulatory)	*Previously healthy and no antibiotic therapy in past 3 months:* Macrolide (clarithromycin or azithromycin) **OR** Doxycycline	≥ 5 days
	With comorbidities (see below)[1] or antibiotic use in past 3 months: FQ (moxifloxacin, gemifloxacin, or levofloxacin) **OR** Macrolide (or doxycycline) *plus* one of the following: • High-dose amoxicillin • Amoxicillin/clavulanate • Cephalosporin (ceftriaxone, cefuroxime, or cefpodoxime)	
Community-acquired (hospitalized)	*Moderate:* FQ (moxifloxacin, gemifloxacin, or levofloxacin) **OR** Macrolide (or doxycycline) *plus* one of the following: • Ampicillin • Ceftriaxone • Cefotaxime	
	Severe: FQ (moxifloxacin, gemifloxacin, or levofloxacin) OR Azithromycin, *plus* one of the following: • Ampicillin/sulbactam • Ceftriaxone • Cefotaxime	
Hospital-acquired	*Hospitalized <5 days and no risk factors for multidrug-resistant (MDR) organisms (select one of the following drugs):[2]* • Third-generation cephalosporin (ceftriaxone or cefotaxime) • FQ (ciprofloxacin, moxifloxacin, or levofloxacin) • Ampicillin/sulbactam • Ertapenem	8 days (14 days if due to *Pseudomonas*)
	Hospitalized ≥5 days or risk factors for MDR organisms:[2] FQ (ciprofloxacin or levofloxacin) OR aminoglycoside, *plus* one of the following: • Ceftazidime or cefepime • Imipenem/cilastatin or meropenem • Piperacillin/tazobactam	

[1] *Comorbidities: Chronic obstructive pulmonary disease (COPD), diabetes, chronic renal failure, chronic liver failure, heart failure (HF), cancer, asplenia, immunosuppressed*

[2] *Risk factors for MDR organisms: Recent antibiotic therapy (in last 90 days), hospitalized ≥5 days, ↑ resistance in environment, nursing home resident, chronic dialysis, home infusion therapy, immunosuppressed*

Meningitis

Common Organisms

Age Group	Most Common Organisms
<1 mo	• *Streptococcus agalactiae* (Group B Strep) • *E. coli* • *Listeria monocytogenes* • *Klebsiella* spp.
1–23 mo	• *Streptococcus pneumoniae* • *Neisseria meningitidis* • Group B Strep • *Haemophilus influenzae* • *E. coli*
2–50 yr	• *Neisseria meningitidis* • *Streptococcus pneumoniae*
>50 yr	• *Streptococcus pneumoniae* • *Neisseria meningitidis* • Group B Strep

Diagnosis

- Confirmed by analysis of cerebrospinal fluid (CSF)
  - Bacterial meningitis: ↓ glucose, ↑ protein, ↑ WBCs
  - Gram stain can help identify organism

Signs and Symptoms

- Symptoms
  - Fever, chills
  - Headache, photophobia
  - Nuchal rigidity
  - N/V
  - Altered mental status
  - Petechiae/purpura (*Neisseria meningitidis*)
- Signs
  - Brudzinski's sign (flexion of hips and knees upon flexing the neck)
  - Kernig's sign (pain develops when the knee is extended after flexing the hip to 90 degrees)
  - Bulging fontanelle (children)

Guidelines

Infectious Disease Society of America. *Clin Infect Dis*, no. 39 (2004): 1267–1284.

Guidelines Summary

Empiric Treatment

Age Group	Treatment
<1 mo	Ampicillin + Aminoglycoside OR Ampicillin + Cefotaxime
1–23 mo	Third-generation cephalosporin (cefotaxime or ceftriaxone) + Vancomycin
2–50 yr	Third-generation cephalosporin (cefotaxime or ceftriaxone) + Vancomycin
>50 yr	Third-generation cephalosporin (cefotaxime or ceftriaxone) + Vancomycin + Ampicillin

SEXUALLY TRANSMITTED DISEASES

Causative Organisms

Disease	Organisms
Chlamydia	*Chlamydia trachomatis*
Gonorrhea	*Neisseria gonorrhoeae*
Syphilis	*Treponema pallidum*

Diagnosis

- Chlamydia: Test performed on urine swab or endocervical/vaginal/male urethral swab
- Gonorrhea: Gram-stained smears or culture (endocervical/vaginal/male urethral/ urine specimen)
- Syphilis: Dark field examination and direct fluorescent antibody stains of exudates
  - Serologic testing
    - » Non treponemal: Venereal Disease Research Laboratory (VDRL) slide test, rapid plasma regain (RPR) test; can be used for screening
    - » Treponemal: Fluorescent treponemal antibody absorbed (FTA-ABS), *T. pallidum* particle agglutination (TP-PA); can be used to confirm diagnosis

Signs and Symptoms

- Chlamydia
  - Penile/vaginal discharge, dysuria
  - May also be asymptomatic
- Gonorrhea
  - Penile/vaginal discharge, dysuria, urinary frequency
  - May also be asymptomatic
- Syphilis
  - Primary (10–90 days after exposure): Presence of chancre
  - Secondary (2–8 wk after development of primary stage): Variety of rashes/lesions, flulike symptoms, and lymphadenopathy
  - Latent (positive serologic test but no clinical manifestations)
  - Tertiary: Cardiovascular (e.g., aortic insufficiency) and neurologic abnormalities (e.g., deafness, blindness, dementia, paresis)

Guidelines

Department of Health and Human Services, Centers for Disease Control and Prevention.

MMWR Recomm Rep, no. 55 (RR-11) (2006): 1–94.

Guidelines Summary

Disease	Treatment
Chlamydia	Azithromycin 1 g PO x 1 dose **OR** Doxycycline 100 mg PO q12h x 7 days
Gonorrhea	Ceftriaxone 125 mg IM x 1 dose, **OR** Cefixime 400 mg PO x 1 dose **PLUS** Treatment for Chlamydia (if not ruled out)
Syphilis	• *Primary, secondary, or early latent syphilis (<1 yr in duration):* • Benzathine penicillin G 2.4 million units IM x 1 dose • *Late latent syphilis (>1 yr in duration), syphilis of unknown duration, or tertiary syphilis (not neurosyphilis):* • Benzathine penicillin G 2.4 million units IM once weekly x 3 weeks • *Neurosyphilis:* • Aqueous penicillin G 3–4 million units IV q4h x 10–14 days

HUMAN IMMUNODEFICIENCY VIRUS

Definitions

Human immunodeficiency virus is a human retrovirus that infects lymphocytes and other cells that bear the CD4 surface protein. Infection leads to lymphopenia and CD4 T-cell depletion, impaired cell-mediated immunity, and polyclonal B-cell activation. Overtime, this immune dysfunction gives rise to acquired immune deficiency syndrome (AIDS), which is characterized by opportunistic infections and malignancies.

Diagnosis

- Persons at high risk for HIV infection should be screened for HIV at least annually.
- An informed consent is required prior to screening.
  - Healthcare workers, IV drug users, homosexual and bisexual men, hemophiliacs, sexual partners with known HIV patients, prostitutes and their partners, persons with STDs, multiple sexual partners with unprotected intercourse, persons who consider themselves at risk
- Screening is performed with an enzyme-linked immunosorbent assay (ELISA).
- A positive screening test is confirmed by a repeat ELISA and a positive Western blot.

Signs and Symptoms

Patients may remain symptom-free for eight or nine years or more. As the virus continues to multiply and destroy immune cells, the patient may develop mild infections or chronic symptoms such as:

- Swollen lymph nodes: often one of the first signs of HIV infection
- Diarrhea, weight loss, fever, cough, and shortness of breath
- Development of opportunistic infections

Guidelines

DHHS Panel on Antiretroviral Guidelines for Adults and Adolescents—2008 Guidelines for the Use of Antiretroviral Agents in HIV-1-Infected Adults and Adolescents. http://aidsinfo.nih.gov/contentfiles/AdultandAdolescentGL.pdf.

Guidelines Summary

For the NAPLEX, you should make learning the names and the drug classes a priority. Below are some helpful learning tips:

- Memorize the non-nucleoside reverse transcriptase inhibitors (NNRTIs)
  - Delavirdine, Efavirenz, Nevirapine
  - Acronym: Never Eat Sushi at Dela Restaurant
- Protease Inhibitors (PIs) "end in" –vir
  - Exception: Darunavir, tenofovir, raltegravir
- Fusion Inhibitors: Enfuvirtide
- Nucleoside reverse transcriptase inhibitors (NRTIs)
  - The remaining agents!

Antiviral therapy should be initiated when viral load >100,000 copies and/or when the patient has a history of AIDS-defining illness or CD4 <350 cells/mm^3.

For the NAPLEX, know the major drug class side effects and learn what to start for treatment-naïve patients.

- Initial regimen for treatment-naïve patients:
  - NNRTI + 2 NRTIs, *or*
  - PI + 2 NRTIs

Medication Charts: Antiretroviral Agents

Non-Nucleoside Reverse Transcriptase Inhibitors (NNRTIs)

Mechanism of action – bind directly to reverse transcriptase, blocking RNA-dependent and DNA-dependent DNA polymerase activities

Generic	Brand	Dose	Contraindications	Primary Side Effects	Key Monitoring	Pertinent Drug Interactions	Med Pearl	Top 200
Nevirapine	Viramune	200 mg PO BID	None	• Dizziness • Impaired concentration • Rash	• Liver function tests (LFTs) • S/S infection	• Inhibits: CYP3A4, CYP2D6, CYP1A2 • Induces: CYP2B6, CYP3A4	• Stop if severe rash and do not rechallenge • Severe hepatotoxicity	No
Efavirenz	Sustiva	600 mg PO QHS	Concurrent use with ergot derivatives, midazolam, triazolam, pimozide, and voriconazole	• N/V • Flu-like symptoms		• Inhibits: CYP2C9, CYP3A4 • Induces: CYP2B6, CYP3A4	Known for causing vivid dreams	No
Delavirdine	Rescriptor	400 mg PO TID	Concurrent use with ergot derivatives, midazolam, triazolam, pimozide	• Rash • Headache, • Stevens-Johnson syndrome • Hepatotoxicity		• Avoid antacids • Inhibits: CYP1A2, CYP2C9, CYP2C19, CYP2D6, CYP3A4	Must swallow 200-mg tablets intact	No

Protease Inhibitors (PIs)

Mechanism of action — inhibit HIV protease and render the enzyme incapable of processing the gag-pol polyprotein precursor which leads to production of noninfectious immature HIV particles.

Generic	Brand	Dose	Contraindications	Primary Side Effects*	Key Monitoring	Pertinent Drug Interactions	Med Pearl	Top 200
Atazanavir	Reyataz	• 400 mg PO daily • 300 mg PO daily with ritonavir	• Concurrent use with ergot derivatives, midazolam, triazolam, pimozide • Hepatic impairment	• Rash • N/V/D • ↑ LFTs • Heart block	• Viral load • CD4 count • Lipid panel • Glucose • LFTs	• CYP3A4 substrate • Inhibits: CYP3A4 and UGT1A1	• Take with meals • Use without ritonavir not recommended in antiretroviral experienced patients with prior virologic failure	No
Darunavir	Prezista	600mg PO BID with ritonavir		↑ LFTs		• CYP3A4 substrate	• Must be given with ritonavir • Take with meals	No
Fosamprenavir	Lexiva	• 1,400 mg PO BID without ritonavir • 700 mg PO BID with ritonavir		• Rash • N/V/D • ↑ LFTs		• CYP3A4 substrate • Inhibits: CYP3A4	• Take suspension with food in children (no food in adults)	No
Indinavir	Crixivan	800 mg PO q8h		• Nephrolithiasis • Nausea		• CYP3A4 substrate • Inhibits: CYP3A4	• Take 1 hour before or 2 hours after meal	No
Lopinavir/ Ritonavir	Kaletra	800 mg lopinavir and 200 mg ritonavir PO daily		• Nausea/ vomiting/ diarrhea (N/V/D) • Pancreatitis		• Ritonavir and lopinavir are CYP3A4 substrates • Ritonavir is a potent CYP3A4 inhibitor and ↑ lopinavir's concentration • Ritonavir also inhibits CYP2D6	• Take with meals • Ritonavir acts as an enhancer to boost the concentration of lopinavir	No
Nelfinavir	Viracept	1,250 mg PO BID		Diarrhea		• CYP3A4 substrate • Inhibits: CYP3A4	• Take with meals	No

Protease Inhibitors (PIs) *(cont'd)*

Generic	Brand	Dose	Contraindications	Primary Side Effects*	Key Monitoring	Pertinent Drug Interactions	Med Pearl	Top 200
Ritonavir	Norvir	600 mg PO BID		• N/V/D • ↑ LFTs • ↑ CPK		• CYP3A4 substrate • Inhibits: CYP3A4 and CYP2D6 • Induces: CYP1A2, CYP2C9, CYP3A4	• Take with meals	No
Saquinavir	Invirase	1,000 mg PO BID with ritonavir		• N/V/D • ↑ LFTs		• CYP3A4 substrate • Inhibits: CYP3A4	• Must be given with ritonavir • Take with meals	No
Tipranavir	Aptivus	500 mg PO BID with ritonavir				• CYP3A4 substrate	• Must be given with ritonavir • Take with a high-fat meal	No

* All PIs may also cause endocrine abnormalities including insulin resistance, body fat redistribution, and hyperlipidemia

NRTIs

Generic	Dose	Contraindications	Primary Side Effects*	Key Monitoring	Pertinent Drug Interactions	Med Pearl	Top 200
Mechanism of action – triphosphate moiety competes with natural substrates for formulation of proviral DNA by reverse transcriptase, thereby inhibiting viral replication							
Emtricitabine	200 mg PO daily	None	• Dizziness • Headache • Fever • Insomnia • Hyperpigmentation • ↑ LFTs	• Viral load • CD4 count • LFTs • Hepatitis B	Ganciclovir or valganciclovir may enhance hematologic toxicity		No
Abacavir	300 mg PO BID or 600 mg daily	Do not challenge patients who have experienced hypersensitivity to abacavir	• Flu-like syndrome • Fever • ↑ LFTs	• Viral load • CD4 count • LFTs		Stop and do not rechallenge if flu-like syndrome ± rash occurs.	No
Didanosine	200 mg PO BID	None	• Peripheral neuropathy • Pancreatitis • Nausea • Diarrhea • ↑ LFTs	• Viral load • CD4 count • Amylase	Avoid antacids, FQs, or tetracyclines by 2 hours	• EC protects drug from inactivation by gastric acid • Should not be chewed or dissolved	No
	400 mg PO daily						No
Stavudine	40 mg PO BID		Peripheral neuropathy ↑ LFTs N/V/D	• Viral load • CD4 count • LFTs	Zidovudine ↓ effects	Activity can be ↑ by concomitant ribavirin	No
Lamivudine	150 mg PO BID or 300 mg PO daily		Nausea Diarrhea ↑ LFTs	• Viral load • CD4 count • LFTs	TMP/SMX ↑ lamivudine levels	Liquid is strawberry-banana flavored	No

NRTIs *(cont'd)*

Generic	Dose	Contraindications	Primary Side Effects*	Key Monitoring	Pertinent Drug Interactions	Med Pearl	Top 200
	300 mg PO BID	None	• Anemia • Neutropenia • Myalgia • ↑LFTs	• Viral load • CD4 count • Complete blood count (CBC) with differential	• ↓ effects of stavudine • Myelosuppressive agents may worsen bone marrow suppression	• First antiviral for HIV called AZT • Resistance is found in many areas	No
	1 tab (zidovudine 300 mg and lamivudine 150 mg) PO BID		See individual drugs			• "The new AZT"	No
	1 cap (abacavir 300 mg, lamivudine 150 mg, and zidovudine 300 mg) PO BID	Do not challenge patients who have experienced hypersensitivity to abacavir				• "The newest AZT"	No
	1 tab (abacavir 600 mg and lamivudine 300 mg) daily					• This combination should only be used in a multidrug regimen for which the individual components are indicated	No
	1 tab (efavirenz 600 mg, emtricitabine 200 mg, and tenofovir 300 mg) daily	See individual drugs					No
	1 tab (emtricitabine 200 mg and tenofovir 300 mg) daily	See individual drugs					No

* All NRTIs may cause also lactic acidosis with hepatic steatosis

CCR5 Antagonist

Mechanism of action – binds to a receptor called CCR5 on WBCs which keeps the HIV virus from entering the cell

Generic	Brand	Dose	Contra-indications	Primary Side Effects	Key Monitoring	Pertinent Drug Interactions	Med Pearl	Top 200
Maraviroc	Selzentry	300 mg PO BID	None	• Hepatotoxicity • Allergic reaction • Orthostatic hypotension	• Viral load • CD4 count • LFTs • Rash • Postural hypotension	• ↓ dose by 50% when used with CYP3A4 inhibitors • *Double* the dose when used with CYP3A4 inducers	• Maraviroc can cause liver damage that may look like an allergic reaction • Educate patients to call their physician if they get an itchy rash, nausea, yellow skin, or dark urine	No

Fusion Inhibitor

Mechanism of action – inhibits the fusion of HIV-1 virus with CD4 cells by blocking the conformational change in gp41 required for membrane fusion and entry to CD4 cells

Generic	Brand	Dose	Contra-indications	Primary Side Effects	Key Monitoring	Pertinent Drug Interactions	Med Pearl	Top 200
Enfuvirtide	Fuzeon	90 mg SC BID	None	• Fatigue • Nausea • Diarrhea • Injection-site reactions	• Viral load • CD4 count	None identified	• Only injectable HIV drug on the market	No

Nucleotide Inhibitor

Mechanism of action – interferes with the HIV viral RNA-dependent DNA polymerase, resulting in inhibition of viral replication

Generic	Brand	Dose	Contra-Indications	Primary Side Effects	Key Monitoring	Pertinent Drug Interactions	Med Pearl	Top 200
Tenofovir	Viread	300 mg PO daily	None	• Nausea • Diarrhea • Depression • ↑ LFTs	• Viral load • CD4 count • LFTs	↑ didanosine levels	• Difference between nucleosides and nucleotides is that the tides require one less phosphorylation step to become active	No

Integrase Inhibitors

Mechanism of action – interferes with the HIV viral RNA-dependent DNA polymerase, resulting in inhibition of viral replication

Generic	Brand	Dose	Contra-indications	Primary Side Effects	Key Monitoring	Pertinent Drug Interactions	Med Pearl	Top 200
Isentress	Raltegravir	400 mg BID	None	• ↑ glucose • ↑ cholesterol • ↑ LFTs	• Viral load • CD4 count • Glucose • LFTs	Rifampin may ↓ levels	• Must be used in combination with other HIV drug therapies • Not 1st-line therapy	No

Storage and Administration Pearls

- Ritonavir capsule and stavudine solution must be refrigerated.
- Delavirdine needs to be protected from humidity.
- Indinavir is sensitive to moisture.
- Lopinavir/ritonavir solution should be stored in the refrigerator.
- Enfuvirtide must be used within 24 hours of reconstitution.

Patient Education Pearls

- Do not take any new prescription, over-the-counter medications, or herbal products during therapy without consulting your prescriber.
- These medications are not a cure for HIV and do not reduce transmission of HIV; use of appropriate precautions to prevent the spread to other persons is important.

Medication Charts: Antibacterial Agents

Penicillins (β-Lactams)

Mechanism of action – inhibit bacterial cell wall synthesis; bactericidal

Generic	Brand	Dose/Dosage Forms	Spectrum of Activity	Contra-indications	Primary Side Effects	Pertinent Drug Interactions	Med Pearl	Top 200
Natural Penicillins								
Penicillin G	Pfizerpen	• 2–4 million units IV q4–6h • Injection	• *Strep. viridans* • *Strep. pyogenes* • *Strep. pneumoniae* (↑ resistance) • Mouth anaerobes	• Allergy to penicillins, cephalosporins, or carbapenems	• Hypersensitivity reaction (rash, hives, dyspnea, throat swelling) • N/V/D • Interstitial nephritis • Hemolytic anemia (with prolonged administration)	• Probenecid may ↑ effects (may be used for this purpose) • May ↓ effects of oral contraceptives	• Adjust dose in renal dysfunction • Penicillin G benzathine or procaine used for syphilis; benzathine also used for Strep throat	No
Penicillin G benzathine	Bicillin LA	• 1.2–2.4 million units IM at specified intervals • Injection						No
Penicillin G procaine	Only available generically	• 1.2–4.8 million units IM/day at specified intervals • Injection					• Take penicillin VK 1 hour before or 2 hours after meals	No
Penicillin VK	Veetids	• 250–500 mg PO q6h • Solution, tabs						Yes
Penicillinase-Resistant Penicillins								
Dicloxacillin	Only available generically	• 125–500 mg PO q6h • Caps	• *Staph aureus* (methicillin-sensitive, MSSA) • *Streptococcus*	Same as natural penicillins	Same as natural penicillins	Same as natural penicillins	• No need to adjust dose in renal dysfunction (cleared by biliary excretion) • Take dicloxacillin 1 hour before or 2 hours after meals	No
Nafcillin	Only available generically	• 500 mg–2 g IV q4–6h • Injection						No
Oxacillin	Only available generically	• 250 mg–2 g IV q4–6h • Injection						No

Penicillins (β-Lactams) *(cont'd)*

Generic	Brand	Dose/Dosage Forms	Spectrum of Activity	Contra-indications	Primary Side Effects	Pertinent Drug Interactions	Med Pearl	Top 200
Aminopenicillins								
Amoxicillin	Amoxil, Trimox	• 250–500 mg PO q8h or 500–875 mg PO q12h • Caps, suspension, tabs	• *Strep pneumoniae* • *H. influenzae* • *E. coli* • *Proteus mirabilis* • *Salmonella* • *Shigella*	Same as natural penicillins	Same as natural penicillins	Same as natural penicillins	• Amoxicillin can be used in three-drug regimen for *H. pylori* • Adjust dose in renal dysfunction	Yes
Ampicillin	Principen	• 250–500 mg PO q6h • 250 mg–2 g IV q4–6h • Caps, injection, suspension					• Take ampicillin 1 hour before or 2 hours after meals	No
Aminopenicillins + β-Lactamase Inhibitors								
Amoxicillin-clavulanic acid	Augmentin	• Immediate-release (IR): 250–500 mg PO q8h or 500–875 mg PO q12h • Extended-release (ER): 2,000 mg PO q12h • Chewable tabs, suspension, tabs (ER and IR)	• β lactamase-producing *Staph. aureus* (MSSA), *H. influenzae, M. catarrhalis, E. coli,* and *K. pneumoniae* • Anaerobes	Same as natural penicillins	Same as natural penicillins	Same as natural penicillins	• Adjust dose in renal dysfunction • Patients on ampicillin sulbactam (IV) can be switched to amoxicillin clavulanate (PO) • Good anaerobic coverage	Yes
Ampicillin-sulbactam	Unasyn	• 1.5–3 g IV q6h • Injection						No
Antipseudomonal Penicillins + β-Lactamase Inhibitors								
Piperacillin-tazobactam	Zosyn	• 3.375 IV q6h or 4.5 g IV q6–8h • Injection	• Same as amoxicillin clavulanic acid and ampicillin-sulbactam	Same as natural penicillins	Same as natural penicillins	Same as natural penicillins	• Adjust dose in renal dysfunction • Primarily used for *Pseudomonas* infections • Good anaerobic coverage • Contain Na+ (use with caution in volume-overloaded patients)	No
Ticarcillin-clavulanic acid	Timentin	• 3.1 g IV q4–6h • Injection	• *Pseudomonas aeruginosa*					No

Cephalosporins (β-Lactams)

Mechanism of action – inhibit bacterial cell wall synthesis; bactericidal
- As it moves from 1st through 4th generation, ↑ activity against Gram (−) organisms and ↓ activity against Gram (+) organisms

Generic	Brand	Dose/Dosage Forms	Spectrum of Activity	Contraindications	Primary Side Effects	Pertinent Drug Interactions	Med Pearl	Top 200
First-Generation								
Cefadroxil	Duricef	• 500 mg–1 g PO q12h • Caps, suspension, tabs	• Staph. aureus • Staph. epidermidis • Strep. pyogenes • Strep. pneumoniae • E. coli • P. mirabilis • K. pneumoniae	Allergy to penicillins, cephalosporins, or carbapenems (up to 10% risk of cross-sensitivity)	Same as natural penicillins	Same as natural penicillins	• Adjust dose in renal dysfunction	No
Cefazolin	Ancef	• 250 mg–1 g IV q8h • Injection						No
Cephalexin	Keflex	• 250–500 mg PO q6h • Caps, suspension, tabs						Yes
Second-Generation								
Cefaclor	Raniclor	• 250–500 mg PO q8h • Caps, chewable tabs, ER tabs, suspension	• Gram (+) activity similar to 1st-generation agents • Same Gram (−) activity as 1st-generation agents, but with added activity against Acinetobacter, Citrobacter, Enterobacter, Neisseria, Serratia, and H. influenzae • Anaerobic activity (cefotetan and cefoxitin only)	Same as 1st-generation agents	• Same as natural penicillins • Bleeding/bruising (with cefotetan and cefoxitin)	• Same as natural penicillins • Disulfiram-like reaction may occur if alcohol is used during treatment with cefotetan • Cefotetan and cefoxitin may ↑ effects of warfarin	• Adjust dose in renal dysfunction • Take cefaclor ER tabs and cefuroxime suspension with food to ↑ absorption	No
Cefotetan	Only available generically	• 1–2 g IV q12h • Injection						No
Cefoxitin	Mefoxin	• 1–2 g IV q6–8h • Injection						No
Cefprozil	Cefzil	• 250–500 mg q12–24h • Suspension, tabs						Yes
Cefuroxime	Ceftin, Zinacef	• 250–500 mg PO q12h • 500 mg–1.5 g IV q8h • Injection, suspension, tabs						Yes

Cephalosporins (β-Lactams) *(cont'd)*

Generic	Brand	Dose/Dosage Forms	Spectrum of Activity	Contraindications	Primary Side Effects	Pertinent Drug Interactions	Med Pearl	Top 200
Third-Generation								
Cefdinir	Omnicef	• 300 mg PO q12h or 600 mg PO daily • Caps, suspension	• Limited Gram (+) activity • More extensive Gram (−) activity vs. 2nd-generation agents • *Pseudomonas aeruginosa* (ceftazidime only)	• Same as 1st-generation agents • Ceftriaxone should be avoided in neonates (↑ risk of hyperbilirubinemia, kernicterus)	• Same as natural penicillins • Bleeding/bruising (with cefoperazone)	• Same as natural penicillins • Antacids and iron may ↓ absorption of cefdinir • Antacids and H₂ antagonists may ↓ absorption of cefpodoxime • Disulfiram-like reaction may occur if alcohol is used during treatment with cefoperazone • Cefoperazone may ↑ effects of warfarin	• Adjust dose for all, except cefoperazone and ceftriaxone, in renal dysfunction • Take cefpodoxime tabs with food to ↑ absorption • Take ceftibuten suspension 2 hours before or 1 hour after meals	Yes
Cefixime	Suprax	• 400 mg PO daily • Suspension						No
Cefoperazone	Cefobid	• 1–2 g IV q12h • Injection						No
Cefpodoxime	Vantin	• 100–400 mg PO q12h • Suspension, tabs						No
Cefotaxime	Claforan	• 1–2 g IV q8h • Injection						No
Ceftazidime	Fortaz, Tazicef	• 1–2 g IV q8–12h • Injection						No
Ceftibuten	Cedax	• 400 mg PO daily • Caps, suspension						No
Ceftizoxime	Cefizox	• 1–2 g IV q8–12h • Injection						No
Ceftriaxone	Rocephin	• 1–2 g IV daily • Injection						No
Fourth-Generation								
Cefepime	Maxipime	• 1–2 g IV q8–12h • Injection	• Gram (+) activity better than 3rd-generation agents • More extensive Gram (−) activity vs. 3rd-generation agents • *Pseudomonas aeruginosa*	Same as 1st-generation agents	Same as natural penicillins	Same as natural penicillins	Adjust dose in renal dysfunction	No

Carbapenems (β-Lactams)

Mechanism of action – inhibit bacterial cell wall synthesis; bactericidal

Generic	Brand	Dose/Dosage Forms	Spectrum of Activity	Contraindications	Primary Side Effects	Pertinent Drug Interactions	Med Pearl	Top 200
Doripenem	Doribax	• 500 mg IV q8h • Injection	• Broad-spectrum (active against Gram (+), Gram (–), and anaerobic organisms) • All, except ertapenem, are active against *Pseudomonas aeruginosa*	Allergy to penicillins, cephalosporins, or carbapenems	• Same as natural penicillins • Seizures (esp. in patients with renal dysfunction or history of seizure disorder)	• Same as natural penicillins • May ↓ valproic acid levels	• Adjust dose in renal dysfunction • Risk of seizures is highest with imipenem/cilastatin	No
Ertapenem	Invanz	• 1 g IV daily • Injection						No
Imipenem-cilastatin	Primaxin	• 250 mg–1 g IV q6–12h • Injection						No
Meropenem	Merrem	• 500 mg–1 g IV q8h • Injection						No

Monobactam (β-Lactam)

Mechanism of action – inhibit bacterial cell wall synthesis; bactericidal

Generic	Brand	Dose/Dosage Forms	Spectrum of Activity	Contra-indications	Primary Side Effects	Pertinent Drug Interactions	Med Pearl	Top 200
Aztreonam	Azactam	• 500 mg–2 g IV q6–12h • Injection	Only effective against Gram (–) organisms, including *Pseudomonas aeruginosa*	None	Same as natural penicillins	None	• Can be used in patients allergic to penicillins, cephalosporins, or carbapenems • Adjust dose in renal dysfunction	No

Aminoglycosides

Mechanism of action – inhibit bacterial protein synthesis by binding to the 30S subunit of the bacterial ribosome; bactericidal

Generic	Brand	Dose/Dosage Forms	Spectrum of Activity	Contra-indications	Primary Side Effects	Pertinent Drug Interactions	Med Pearl	Top 200
Amikacin	Amikin	• 15 mg/kg IV q24h or 5–7.5 mg/kg IV q8h • Injection	• Primarily used for Gram (−) organisms (E. coli, Klebsiella, P. mirabilis, Enterobacter, Acinetobacter, Serratia, Pseudomonas aeruginosa)	None	• Nephrotoxicity • Ototoxicity (both related to dose and duration of therapy; may be reversible)	• May ↑ effects of neuromuscular blocking agents • ↑ risk of nephrotoxicity when used with amphotericin B, loop diuretics, tacrolimus, cyclosporine, or cisplatin	• Bactericidal effect is concentration-dependent • Target serum concentrations (for traditional dosing): • Amikacin: Peak = 20–30 mcg/mL; Trough <6 mcg/mL	No
Gentamicin	Garamycin, Gentak	• 5–7 mg/kg IV q24h or 1–2.5 mg/kg IV q8–12h • Injection, ophthalmic ointment/solution, topical cream	• Provide synergistic activity against Staph., Strep., or Enterococcus when used with penicillins or vancomycin				• Gentamicin and tobramycin: Peak = 4–10 mcg/mL; Trough <1 mcg/mL • Target serum concentrations (for extended-interval dosing) (peaks not routinely monitored):	No
Kanamycin	Kantrex	• 5–7.5 mg/kg IV q8–12h • Injection						No
Neomycin	Neo-Fradin	• 500 mg–2 g PO q6–8h • Powder, solution, tabs						No
Streptomycin	Only available generically	• 15 mg/kg/day IM • Injection	• Streptomycin and amikacin active against Mycobacteria				• Amikacin: Trough <5 mcg/mL • Gentamicin and tobramycin: Trough <1 mcg/mL • TOBI® used for cystic fibrosis patients	No
Tobramycin	TOBI, Tobrex	• 5–7 mg/kg IV q24h or 1–2.5 mg/kg IV q8–12h • Injection, nebulizer solution, ophthalmic ointment/solution	• Neomycin used as prep for bowel surgery or for hepatic encephalopathy					No

Macrolides and Ketolides

Mechanism of action – inhibit bacterial protein synthesis by binding to the 50S subunit of the bacterial ribosome; bacteriostatic

Macrolides

Generic	Brand	Dose/Dosage Forms	Spectrum of Activity	Contraindications	Primary Side Effects	Pertinent Drug Interactions	Med Pearl	Top 200
Azithromycin	Zithromax, Zmax	• 250–500 mg PO/IV q24h • Zmax: 2 g PO x 1 • Injection, ophthalmic solution, suspension (IR and ER), tabs	• Gram (+) organisms (esp. *Streptococcus*); azithromycin and clarithromycin have better activity against *Streptococcus* than erythromycin • Gram (−) organisms	QT interval prolongation or concurrent use with other drugs that prolong QT interval (clarithromycin and erythromycin)	• N/V/D QT interval prolongation (clarithromycin and erythromycin) • Phlebitis (erythromycin IV)	• Clarithromycin and erythromycin are major substrates and inhibitors of CYP3A4 (azithromycin least affected by CYP interactions) • CYP3A4 inhibitors may ↑ risk of side effects of clarithromycin and erythromycin	• ER suspension is not interchangeable with IR formulations • 400 mg erythromycin ethylsuccinate (EES) = 250 mg erythromycin base or stearate	Yes
Clarithromycin	Biaxin	• IR: 250–500 mg PO q12h • ER: 1,000 mg PO q24h • Suspension, tabs (IR and ER)	• Atypical organisms (e.g., *Chlamydia pneumoniae, Legionella, Mycoplasma pneumoniae*)			• CYP3A4 inducers may ↓ effects of clarithromycin and erythromycin	• Good alternative when patients allergic to penicillins • Take with food to ↓ gastrointestinal (GI) effects • Clarithromycin can be used in three-drug regimen for *H. pylori*	Yes
Erythromycin	E.E.S, Eryped, Ery-Tab, Erythrocin, PCE	• 250–500 mg PO q6h • 500 mg–1 g IV q6h • Caps, injection, ophthalmic ointment, suspension, tabs, topical gel/ointment/solution	• Azithromycin and clarithromycin active against *Mycobacteria*			• Clarithromycin and erythromycin may ↑ effect/toxicity of CYP3A4 substrates • ↑ risk of torsade de pointes (TdP) with other drugs that prolong QT interval (clarithromycin and erythromycin) • May ↑ effects of warfarin • May ↑ risk of digoxin toxicity	• Erythromycin can be used for diabetic gastroparesis • Take ER azithromycin suspension 1 hour before or 2 hours after meals • Take ER clarithromycin tabs with food to ↑ absorption • Azithromycin or erythromycin preferred in pregnancy	No

Macrolides and Ketolides *(cont'd)*

Generic	Brand	Dose/Dosage Forms	Spectrum of Activity	Contraindications	Primary Side Effects	Pertinent Drug Interactions	Med Pearl	Top 200
Ketolides								
Telithromycin	Ketek	• 800 mg PO q24h • Tabs	• Greater activity (vs. macrolides) against resistant *Strep. pneumoniae* and *H. influenzae* • Atypical organisms	• History of hepatitis or jaundice with previous use of telithromycin or macrolides • Myasthenia gravis • QT interval prolongation • Concurrent use with other drugs that prolong QT interval	• N/V/D • ↑ LFTs)/ hepatitis • Visual disturbances (double vision, blurred vision, trouble focusing) • Loss of consciousness • QT interval prolongation	• CYP3A4 inhibitors may ↑ risk of side effects • CYP3A4 inducers may ↓ effects • May ↑ effect/toxicity of CYP3A4 substrates • May ↑ effects of warfarin • May ↑ risk of digoxin toxicity • ↑ risk of TdP with other drugs that prolong QT interval	• Monitor LFTs and vision • Adjust dose in renal dysfunction	No

Tetracyclines

Generic	Brand	Dose/Dosage Forms	Spectrum of Activity	Contraindications	Primary Side Effects	Pertinent Drug Interactions	Med Pearl	Top 200
Mechanism of action – inhibit bacterial protein synthesis by binding to the 30S subunit of the bacterial ribosome; bacteriostatic								
Demeclocycline	Declomycin	• 150 mg PO q6h or 300 mg PO q12h • Tabs	• Gram (+) organisms • Gram (–) organisms • Atypical organisms	Children ≤8 yr and pregnant or breast-feeding women (may cause permanent teeth discoloration and impaired teeth/bone growth)	• N/V/D • Photosensitivity • Phlebitis (IV) • Vertigo (minocycline)	• Absorption ↓ with antacids, dairy products, and products containing iron, magnesium, aluminum, calcium, or zinc (separate by 2 hr) • CYP3A4 inhibitors may ↑ risk of side effects • CYP3A4 inducers may ↓ effects • May ↑ effect/toxicity of CYP3A4 substrates • May ↓ effects of warfarin • May ↓ effects of oral contraceptives	• Demeclocycline also used to treat syndrome of inappropriate antidiuretic hormone secretion (SIADH) • Tetracycline can be used in four-drug regimen for *H. pylori* • All except demeclocycline can be used for acne • Doxycycline is drug of choice for Lyme disease • Take demeclocycline and tetracycline 1 hour before or 2 hours after meals • Do not use after expiration date (can cause Fanconi syndrome) • Adjust dose for all, except doxycycline, in renal dysfunction	No
Doxycycline	Doryx, Vibramycin	• 100 mg IV/PO q12h • Caps, delayed-release caps/tabs, injection, suspension, syrup, tabs						Yes
Minocycline	Dynacin, Minocin	• 100 mg PO q12h • Caps, tabs (IR and ER)						Yes
Tetracycline	Sumycin	• 250–500 mg PO q6–12h • Caps, suspension, tabs						Yes

Glycylcyclines

Generic	Brand	Dose/Dosage Forms	Spectrum of Activity	Contraindications	Primary Side Effects	Pertinent Drug Interactions	Med Pearl	Top 200
Mechanism of action – inhibits bacterial protein synthesis by binding to the 30S subunit of the bacterial ribosome (mechanism similar to tetracyclines); bacteriostatic								
Tigecycline	Tygacil	100 mg IV x 1, then 50 mg IV q12h • Injection	Gram (+) organisms (MSSA, methicillin-resistant *Staph. aureus* [MRSA], vancomycin-sensitive *Enterococcus faecalis*)	Children ≤8 yr and pregnant/ breast-feeding women (may cause permanent teeth discoloration and impaired teeth/bone growth)	• N/V/D • Infusion site reaction • Photosensitivity	May ↑ effects of warfarin	Structurally similar to tetracyclines	No

Oxazolidinones

Mechanism of action — inhibits bacterial protein synthesis by binding to bacterial 23S ribosomal RNA of the 50S subunit of the bacterial ribosome; bacteriostatic

Generic	Brand	Dose/Dosage Forms	Spectrum of Activity	Contra-indications	Primary Side Effects	Pertinent Drug Interactions	Med Pearl	Top 200
Linezolid	Zyvox	• 400–600 mg IV/PO q12h • Injection, suspension, tabs	Gram (+) organisms (vancomycin-resistant *Enterococcus faecium* [VRE], methicillin-resistant *Staphylococcus aureus* (MRSA), resistant *Strep. pneumoniae*)	None	• N/V/D • Headache • Myelosuppression (more common if therapy >2 wk) • Peripheral/optic neuropathy (more common if therapy >4 wk) • Seizures	• Avoid taking with foods or beverages with high tyramine content (may ↑ risk of hypertensive crises) • Use with serotonergic agents may ↑ risk of serotonin syndrome; avoid concurrent use • Use with adrenergic agents (e.g., dopamine, epinephrine) may ↑ risk of hypertensive crises • Use with tramadol may ↑ risk of seizures	• Weak monoamine oxidase inhibitor (MAOI) • Monitor CBC weekly if therapy >2 wk	No

Streptogramins

Mechanism of action — inhibits bacterial protein synthesis by binding to the 50S subunit of the bacterial ribosome; bactericidal

Generic	Brand	Dose/Dosage Forms	Spectrum of Activity	Contra-indications	Primary Side Effects	Pertinent Drug Interactions	Med Pearl	Top 200
Quinupristin-dalfopristin	Synercid	• 7.5 mg/kg IV q8–12h • Injection	VRE, MRSA, methicillin-sensitive *Staphylococcus aureus* (MSSA)	None	• N/V/D • Infusion site reactions (pain, phlebitis) • Muscle/join pain • ↑ bilirubin	May ↑ effect/toxicity of CYP3A4 substrates	• Flush line with D5W before and after infusion • If infusion reaction occurs, can ↑ volume of diluent or administer via central line	No

Fluoroquinolones

Mechanism of action – inhibit bacterial DNA topoisomerase and gyrase → inhibit bacterial DNA replication; bactericidal

Generic	Brand	Dose/Dosage Forms	Spectrum of Activity	Contraindications	Primary Side Effects	Pertinent Drug Interactions	Med Pearl	Top 200
Ciprofloxacin	Cipro, Proquin XR	• IR: • 250–750 mg PO q12h • ER: • 500 mg–1 g PO q24h • IV: 200–400 mg IV q8–12h • Injection, ophthalmic ointment/solution, suspension, tabs (ER and IR)	• Gram (+) organisms (levofloxacin, gemifloxacin, and moxifloxacin have greatest activity against *Streptococcus*) • Gram (−) organisms • Ciprofloxacin active against *Pseudomonas aeruginosa*	• Children <18 yr and pregnant/breast-feeding women (may cause impaired bone growth) • Concurrent use with other drugs that prolong QT interval	• Nausea/diarrhea • Photosensitivity • Tendinitis/tendon rupture • Hyper-/hypoglycemia • Peripheral neuropathy • Seizures • QT interval prolongation	• Absorption ↓ with antacids, dairy products, and products containing iron, magnesium, aluminum, calcium, or zinc (separate by 2 hours) • Use with corticosteroids may ↑ risk of tendon rupture • Use with nonsteroidal anti-inflammatory drugs (NSAIDs) may ↑ risk of seizures	• ER and IR tabs are not interchangeable • Adjust dose for all, except moxifloxacin, in renal dysfunction • Take levofloxacin oral solution and lomefloxacin 1 hour before or 2 hours after meals • Patients with diabetes should monitor their blood glucose more frequently	Yes
Gemifloxacin	Factive	• 320 mg PO q24h • Tabs						No
Levofloxacin	Levaquin	• 250–750 mg IV/PO q24h • Injection, ophthalmic solution, solution, tabs	• Atypical organisms			• Ciprofloxacin and ofloxacin may ↑ effects of CYP1A2 substrates • Ciprofloxacin may ↓ phenytoin levels		Yes
Lomefloxacin	Maxaquin	• 400 mg PO q24h • Tabs				• May ↑ effects of warfarin		No
Moxifloxacin	Avelox	• 400 mg IV/PO q24h • Injection, ophthalmic solution, tabs				• May ↑ effects of antidiabetic agents • ↑ risk of TdP with other drugs that prolong QT interval		No
Ofloxacin	Floxin	• 200–400 mg PO q12h • Ophthalmic solution, otic solution, tabs						No

Sulfonamides

Mechanism of action – inhibit incorporation of para-aminobenzoic acid (PABA) into DNA → inhibit folic acid production and bacterial growth; bacteriostatic

Generic	Brand	Dose/Dosage Forms	Spectrum of Activity	Contraindications	Primary Side Effects	Pertinent Drug Interactions	Med Pearl	Top 200
Sulfadiazine	Only available generically	• 500 mg–1.5 g PO q6h • Tabs	• Gram (+) organisms (including MSSA, MRSA) • Gram (−) organisms • SMX/TMP is 1st-line drug to treat/prevent *Pneumocystis jiroveci* pneumonia (PCP) • Sulfadiazine used to treat toxoplasmosis	• Sulfa allergy • Porphyria • Megaloblastic anemia • Infants and pregnant/breast-feeding women (↑ risk of kernicterus) • G6PD deficiency	• N/V/D • Rash • Stevens-Johnson syndrome • Photosensitivity • Folate deficiency • Hypoglycemia (in patients with diabetes)	• May ↑ effects/toxicity of methotrexate • May ↑ effects of warfarin • May ↑ effects of antidiabetic agents	• Instruct patients to take with a full glass of water (to prevent crystalluria) • Adjust dose in renal dysfunction	No
Sulfamethoxazole (SMX)-trimethoprim (TMP)	Bactrim, Septra	• 1 double-strength tab PO q12h • 10–20 mg/kg/day of TMP IV in divided doses • Injection, suspension, tabs						Yes
Sulfisoxazole	Gantrinsin	• 4–8 g/day PO • Suspension, tabs						No

Cyclic Lipopeptides

Mechanism of action – bind to bacterial cell membranes and cause rapid depolarization → inhibit protein, DNA, and RNA synthesis; bactericidal

Generic	Brand	Dose/Dosage Forms	Spectrum of Activity	Contra-indications	Primary Side Effects	Pertinent Drug Interactions	Med Pearl	Top 200
Daptomycin	Cubicin	• 4–6 mg/kg IV q24h • Injection	Gram (+) organisms (MSSA, MRSA, vancomycin-sensitive *Enterococcus faecalis*, VRE)	None	• Nausea/diarrhea • Infusion site reactions • Muscle pain/weakness	Use with statins may ↑ risk of myopathy; consider discontinuing statin therapy throughout treatment	• Monitor creatine kinase levels weekly • Adjust dose in renal dysfunction	No

Miscellaneous Antibacterial Agents

Generic	Brand	Dose/Dosage Forms	Spectrum of Activity	Contra-indications	Primary Side Effects	Pertinent Drug Interactions	Med Pearl	Top 200
Mechanism of action – inhibits bacterial protein synthesis by binding to the 50S subunit of the bacterial ribosome; bacteriostatic								
Chloramphenicol	Only available generically	• 12.5–25 mg/kg IV q6h • Injection	• Gram (+) organisms (VRE) • Gram (−) organisms	Neonates (↑ risk of gray-baby syndrome)	• N/V/D • Myelosuppression (anemia, leukopenia, thrombocytopenia, aplastic anemia) • Gray-baby syndrome (vomiting, lethargy, respiratory depression, death) • Optic neuritis	• Phenobarbital and rifampin may ↓ effects • May ↑ effects of warfarin and phenytoin	• Only used for life-threatening infections • Monitor CBC frequently • Target serum concentrations: Peak = 15–25 mcg/mL • Trough = 5–10 mcg/mL	No
Mechanism of action – inhibits bacterial protein synthesis by binding to the 50S subunit of the bacterial ribosome; bacteriostatic								
Clindamycin	Cleocin, Clindesse, Evoclin	• 150–450 mg PO q6h • 300–900 mg IV q8h • Caps, injection, solution, topical foam/gel/lotion/ pledgets/solution, vaginal cream/ suppository	• Gram (+) organisms • Anaerobes	History of pseudo-membranous colitis or ulcerative colitis	• N/V/D • Pseudomembranous-colitis (highest incidence)	None significant	• Also used for acne (topical) • Patients using intravaginally should avoid intercourse (↓ efficacy of condoms and diaphragms)	Yes
Mechanism of action – interferes with bacterial DNA synthesis; bactericidal								
Metronidazole	Flagyl, Metrogel, Noritate, Vandazole	• 250–500 mg PO q8–12h • 500 mg IV q8–12h • Caps, injection, tabs (ER and IR), topical cream/gel/lotion, vaginal gel	Anaerobes	Pregnancy (1st trimester)	• Nausea/diarrhea • Confusion • Dizziness • Peripheral neuropathy • Metallic taste	• Disulfiram-like reaction may occur if alcohol is used during treatment • May ↑ effects of warfarin and lithium • Phenobarbital and phenytoin may ↓ effects • Cimetidine may ↑ effects	• Can be used in four-drug regimen for *H. pylori* • Drug of choice for *Clostridium difficile* • Take ER tabs 1 hour before or 2 hours after meals	Yes

Miscellaneous Antibacterial Agents *(cont'd)*

Mechanism of action – Inhibits bacterial cell wall synthesis; bactericidal

Generic	Brand	Dose/Dosage Forms	Spectrum of Activity	Contra-indications	Primary Side Effects	Pertinent Drug Interactions	Med Pearl	Top 200
Vancomycin	Vancocin	• 125–250 mg PO q6h • 500 mg–1 g q12h • Caps, injection	• Gram (+) organisms (MSSA, MRSA) • *Clostridium difficile*	None	• Red-man syndrome (flushing, hypotension, erythema, pruritus) • Nephrotoxicity • Ototoxicity	↑ risk of nephrotoxicity when used with amphotericin B, loop diuretics, tacrolimus, cyclosporine, or cisplatin	• Bactericidal effect is time-dependent • Adjust dose in renal dysfunction • Often used in patients with penicillin allergy • Use PO (NOT IV) to treat *Clostridium difficile* (PO not effective for any other type of infection) • If red-man syndrome occurs, ↓ infusion rate • Target serum concentrations (peaks not routinely monitored): • Trough = 5–10 mcg/ml	No

Medication Charts: Antifungal Agents

Azole Antifungals

Mechanism of action – inhibit synthesis of ergosterol (essential component of fungal cell membrane)
- Imidazoles: butoconazole, clotrimazole, econazole, ketoconazole, miconazole, oxiconazole, sulconazole, tioconazole
- Triazoles: fluconazole, itraconazole, terconazole, posaconazole, voriconazole

Generic	Brand	Dose/Dosage Forms	Spectrum of Activity	Contra-indications	Primary Side Effects	Pertinent Drug Interactions	Med Pearl	Top 200
Fluconazole	Diflucan	• 100–800 mg IV/PO q24h • Injection, tabs, suspension	• *Candida* spp. • *Coccidioides* spp. • *Histoplasma* spp. • *Cryptococcus* spp. • *Aspergillus* spp. (not fluconazole or ketoconazole)	None	• Headache • Nausea/vomiting • Diarrhea • Abdominal pain • Rash • ↑ LFTs • Prolonged QT interval	• May ↑ effect/toxicity of CYP2C9, CYP2C19, and CYP3A4 substrates • Rifampin may ↓ effects • ↑ risk of TdP with other drugs that prolong QT interval	• Adjust dose in patients with renal dysfunction • Conversion from IV to PO is 1:1 • Monitor LFTs	Yes
Itraconazole	Sporanox	• 100–400 mg/day PO • Caps, solution		• Concurrent use of dofetilide, ergot alkaloids, lovastatin, midazolam, pimozide, quinidine, simvastatin, or triazolam • HF	• Nausea • Abdominal pain • Rash • ↑ LFTs • Prolonged QT interval	• CYP3A4 inhibitors may ↑ risk of side effects • CYP3A4 inducers may ↓ effects • May ↑ effect/toxicity of CYP3A4 substrates • ↑ risk of digoxin toxicity • Absorption ↓ with antacids, H₂ antagonists, and proton pump inhibitors (acidic environment required for absorption) (separate by 2 hr) • ↑ risk of TdP with other drugs that prolong QT interval	• Caps and solution cannot be used interchangeably (bioavailability of solution > caps) • Potent negative inotrope • Monitor LFTs	No
Ketoconazole	Nizoral	• 200–400 mg PO q24h • Rx: Cream, gel, shampoo, tabs, topical aerosol • OTC: shampoo		Concurrent use of ergot alkaloids	• N/V • Gynecomastia • Sexual dysfunction • ↑ LFTs • Prolonged QT interval	Same as itraconazole	• May ↓ testosterone levels • Can also be used to treat prostate cancer • Monitor LFTs	Yes

KAPLAN MEDICAL

Azole Antifungals *(cont'd)*

Generic	Brand	Dose/Dosage Forms	Spectrum of Activity	Contra-indications	Primary Side Effects	Pertinent Drug Interactions	Med Pearl	Top 200
Posaconazole	Noxafil	• 100–800 mg/day PO • Suspension		Concurrent use of ergot alkaloids, quinidine, or pimozide	• Headache • N/V • Rash • Prolonged QT interval	• May ↑ effect/toxicity of CYP3A4 substrates • ↑ risk of TdP with other drugs that prolong QT interval	• Must be taken with full meal to ↑ absorption • Monitor LFTs	No
Voriconazole	Vfend	• Loading dose: • 6 mg/kg IV q12h for 24 hr • Maintenance dose: • 3–4 mg/kg IV q12h • 100–300 mg PO q12h • Injection, suspension, tabs		Concurrent use of pimozide, quinidine, long-acting barbiturates, carbamazepine, ergot alkaloids, rifampin, rifabutin, ritonavir (≥800 mg/day), St. John's wort, or sirolimus	• Visual disturbances (transient) (blurred vision, photophobia, altered perception of color) • Rash • Photosensitivity • ↑ LFTs • Hallucinations • N/V • Prolonged QT interval	• May ↑ effect/toxicity of CYP2C9, CYP2C19, and CYP3A4 substrates • CYP2C9 and CYP2C19 inducers may ↓ effects • May ↑ efavirenz levels • Efavirenz may ↓ effects • ↑ risk of TdP with other drugs that prolong QT interval	• ↓ dose of cyclosporine by 50% • When using with efavirenz, ↑ voriconazole dose and ↓ efavirenz dose • ↑ dose of voriconazole when using with phenytoin • Use PO when CrCl <50 mL/min (diluent in IV can accumulate) • Take 1 hour before or after meals • Monitor LFTs and vision	No

Echinocandins

Mechanism of action — inhibit synthesis of 1,3-β-d-glucan (essential component of fungal cell wall)

Generic	Brand	Dose/Dosage Forms	Spectrum of Activity	Contra-indications	Primary Side Effects	Pertinent Drug Interactions	Med Pearl	Top 200
Anidulafungin	Eraxis	• 100–200 mg IV on day 1, then 50–100 mg IV q24h • Injection	• *Candida* spp. • *Aspergillus* spp.	None	• N/V • Headache • Hypokalemia • Rash	None	Monitor LFTs	No
Caspofungin	Cancidas	• 70 mg IV on day 1, then 50 mg IV q24h • Injection			• Fever • ↑ LFTs • Phlebitis	• Rifampin, carbamazepine, dexamethasone, efavirenz, nevirapine, and phenytoin may ↓ effects • May ↓ tacrolimus levels • Cyclosporine may ↑ risk of side effects	• ↑ dose of caspofungin to 70 mg/day when used with rifampin, carbamazepine, dexamethasone, efavirenz, nevirapine, or phenytoin • Adjust dose in moderate hepatic dysfunction • Monitor LFTs	No
Micafungin	Mycamine	• 50–150 mg IV q24h • Injection				None	Monitor LFTs	No

Amphotericin B

Mechanism of action – bind to ergosterol in cell membrane → produce a channel in cell membrane ($\uparrow$ permeability) → allow K$^+$ and Mg^{2+} to leak out of cell ("leaky membrane") → cell death

Generic	Brand	Dose/Dosage Forms	Spectrum of Activity	Contra-indications	Primary Side Effects	Pertinent Drug Interactions	Med Pearl	Top 200
Amphotericin B deoxycholate	Fungizone	• Test dose of 1 mg IV should be given over 20–30 min (monitor patient for 2–4 hr before starting infusion) 0.5–1.5 mg/kg/day IV • Injection	• *Candida* spp. • *Coccidioides* spp. • *Blastomyces* spp. • *Histoplasma* spp. • *Cryptococcus* spp. • *Aspergillus* spp.	None	• Nephrotoxicity (less common with lipid-based formulations) • Infusion reactions (fever, chills, hypotension, nausea, tachypnea) • Phlebitis • Electrolyte disturbances (i.e., hypokalemia, hypomagnesemia)	$\uparrow$ risk of nephrotoxicity when used with aminoglycosides, loop diuretics, tacrolimus, cyclosporine, or cisplatin	• May premedicate with acetaminophen, NSAIDs, diphenhydramine and/or corticosteroid to prevent infusion reactions (give 30–60 min before infusion); meperidine may be used for rigors • Infusion reactions less common with lipid-based formulations (amphotericin B deoxycholate > ABCD > ABLC > L-Amb) • Infusion reactions $\downarrow$ after first few doses • Sodium loading (500 mL of 0.9% NaCl before and after infusion) may $\downarrow$ risk of nephrotoxicity with amphotericin B deoxycholate • Monitor blood urea nitrogen (BUN), serum creatinine (SCr), potassium, and magnesium	No
Amphotericin B lipid complex (ABLC)	Abelcet	• 5 mg/kg IV q24h • Injection						No
Liposomal amphotericin B (L-AmB)	AmBisome	• 3–6 mg/kg IV q24h • Injection						No
Amphotericin B colloidal dispersion (ABCD)	Amphotec	• 3–4 mg/kg IV q24h • Injection						No

Other Antifungals

Generic	Brand	Dose/Dosage Forms	Spectrum of Activity	Contra-indications	Primary Side Effects	Pertinent Drug Interactions	Med Pearl	Top 200
Mechanism of action – similar to amphotericin B								
Nystatin	Mycostatin	• Suspension: 400,000–600,000 units 4 times/day • Topical: Apply 2–3 times daily • Cream, ointment, suspension, tabs, topical powder, vaginal tabs	*Candida* spp.	None	• N/V Diarrhea • Abdominal pain	None	Suspension should be swished and swallowed	Yes
Mechanism of action – inhibits squalene epoxidase → inhibits synthesis of ergosterol								
Terbinafine	Lamisil	• PO: 250 mg q24h • Topical: Apply 1–2 times daily • Rx: Granules, tabs, topical solution • OTC: Cream, gel, topical solution	*Trichophyton* spp.	Liver disease CrCl <50 mL/min	• Headache • N/V Diarrhea • ↑ LFTs	• May ↑ effect/toxicity of CYP2D6 substrates • May ↓ cyclosporine levels	• Oral used for onychomycosis or tinea capitis (scalp ringworm); topical used for tinea pedis (athlete's foot), tinea corporis (ringworm), or tinea cruris (jock itch) • Give for 6 wks for fingernail fungal infection; 12 wks for toenail infection • Monitor LFTs	No

Other Antifungals *(cont'd)*

Mechanism of action – enters fungal cell wall → converted into 5-fluorouracil, which interferes with fungal RNA and protein synthesis

Generic	Brand	Dose/Dosage Forms	Spectrum of Activity	Contra-indications	Primary Side Effects	Pertinent Drug Interactions	Med Pearl	Top 200
Flucytosine	Ancobon	• 25–37.5 mg/kg PO q6h (administered with amphotericin B) • Caps	*Candida* spp. *Cryptoccous* spp.	None	• Confusion • Hallucinations • Ataxia • Headache • N/V Diarrhea • ↑ LFTs • Renal dysfunction • Bone marrow depression	None	• Should not be used as monotherapy • Adjust dose in patients with renal dysfunction • Monitor LFTs, BUN/SCr, and CBC • Flucytosine concentrations: Peak: 50–100 mcg/mL • Trough: 25–50 mcg/mL	No

Mechanism of action – inhibits fungal cell mitosis

Generic	Brand	Dose/Dosage Forms	Spectrum of Activity	Contra-indications	Primary Side Effects	Pertinent Drug Interactions	Med Pearl	Top 200
Griseofulvin	Grifulvin V, Gris-PEG, Fulvicin	• Microsize: 500–1,000 mg/day PO • Ultramicrosize: 375 mg/day PO • Microsize: Suspension, tabs • Ultramicrosize: Tabs	*Trichophyton* spp.	• Liver disease • Porphyria	• Rash/hives • N/V Diarrhea • Headache • Confusion • Photosensitivity	• Barbiturates may ↓ effects • May ↓ effects of cyclosporine and warfarin	• Monitor LFTs • Use with alcohol may cause disulfiram reaction • Administer with high-fat meal to ↑ absorption	No

Medication Charts: Antiviral Agents

Drugs for Treatment of Herpes Simplex Virus and Varicella-Zoster Virus

Mechanism of action – inhibit viral DNA polymerase → inhibit replication of viral DNA

Generic	Brand	Dose/Dosage Forms	Spectrum of Activity	Contra-indications	Primary Side Effects	Pertinent Drug Interactions	Med Pearl	Top 200
Acyclovir	Zovirax	• *Genital herpes (initial episode):* 200 mg PO 5 times/day x 7–10 days 5 mg/kg IV q8h x 5–7 days • *Herpes labialis (cold sores):* 400 mg PO 5 times/day x 5 days • *Varicella (chickenpox):* 800 mg PO q6h • *Herpes zoster (shingles):* 800 mg PO 5 times/day x 7–10 days 10 mg/kg IV q8h x 7 days • Caps, injection, suspension, tabs, topical cream/ointment	• Herpes simplex virus (HSV)-1 (herpes labialis) and HSV-2 (genital herpes) • Varicella zoster virus (causes chickenpox and shingles)	None	• N/V/D Headache • Phlebitis (IV acyclovir) • Renal dysfunction (IV acyclovir) • Seizures (esp. in patients with renal dysfunction)	None	• Adjust dose for all, except penciclovir, in renal dysfunction • To avoid renal damage with IV (can crystallize), infuse slowly and keep patient hydrated	Yes
Famciclovir (prodrug of penciclovir)	Famvir	• *Genital herpes (initial episode):* 250 mg PO q8h x 7–10 days • *Cold sores:* 1,500 mg PO x 1 • *Herpes zoster:* 500 mg PO q8h x 7 days • Tabs						No
Penciclovir	Denavir	*Cold sores:* • Apply q2h while awake x 4 days • Topical cream						No
Valacyclovir (prodrug of acyclovir)	Valtrex	• *Genital herpes (initial episode):* 1 g PO q12h x 7–10 days • *Cold sores:* 2 g PO q12h x 1 day • *Herpes zoster:* 1 g PO q8h x 7 days • Caps						Yes

Drugs for Treatment of Cytomegalovirus

Generic	Brand	Dose/Dosage Forms	Spectrum of Activity	Contra-indications	Primary Side Effects	Pertinent Drug Interactions	Med Pearl	Top 200
Mechanism of action – inhibit replication of viral DNA								
Cidofovir	Vistide	• 5 mg/kg IV once weekly x 2 wk, then q2 wk • Injection	• Cytomegalovirus • HSV (foscarnet)	• SCr >1.5 mg/dL, CrCl ≤55 mL/min, or proteinuria • Use of other nephrotoxic drugs within 7 days	• Nephrotoxicity • Neutropenia • Metabolic acidosis • ↓ intraocular pressure • Uveitis/iritis	Use of antiretroviral drugs may ↑ risk of side effects	• Monitor BUN/SCr • To minimize renal damage, administer 1 L of 0.9% NaCl before and after each infusion; also give 2 g of probenecid 3 hr before each infusion and then 1 g at 2 hr and 8 hr after each infusion • If SCr ↑ by 0.3–0.4 mg/dL above baseline, ↓ dose to 3 mg/kg; if SCr ↑ by ≥0.5 mg/dL, discontinue • Advise patients to use effective contraception	No
Foscarnet	Foscavir	• 60 mg/kg IV q8h or 90 mg/kg IV q12h x 14–21 days, then 90–120 mg/kg IV q24h • Injection		None	• Nephrotoxicity • N/V Anemia • Electrolyte disturbances • Genital sores • Seizures	• ↑ risk of renal dysfunction when used with other nephrotoxic drugs • Zidovudine may ↑ risk of anemia	• Adjust dose in renal dysfunction • Monitor BUN/SCr • To minimize renal damage, administer 1 L of 0.9% NaCl with each infusion • Rapid infusion associated with seizures and arrhythmias	No
Ganciclovir	Cytovene, Vitrasert	• 1 g PO q8h • 5 mg/kg IV q12h x 14–21 days, then either 5 mg/kg/day IV 7 times/wk or 6 mg/kg/day IV 5 times/wk • 4.5 mg intraocularly q5–8 months • Caps, injection, intravitreal implant		• Neutropenia • Thrombocytopenia • Anemia	• Myelosuppression • Fever • Rash • Phlebitis (IV) • ↑ LFTs • Nephrotoxicity • Seizures • N/V/D	• ↑ risk of myelosuppression when used with other immunosuppressive drugs • ↑ risk of renal dysfunction when used with other nephrotoxic drugs • May ↑ effects/toxicity of zidovudine	• For ganciclovir, IV route preferred (PO has poor bioavailability) • Adjust dose in renal dysfunction • Advise patients to use effective contraception during treatment and for at least 90 days after treatment	No
Valganciclovir (prodrug of ganciclovir)	Valcyte	• 900 mg PO q12h x 21 days, then 900 mg PO q24h • Tabs					• Take PO ganciclovir and valganciclovir with food	No

Drugs for Treatment of Influenza

Mechanism of action – inhibit the enzyme (neuraminidase) responsible for releasing the newly formed mature virus from the host cell

Generic	Brand	Dose/Dosage Forms	Spectrum of Activity	Contra-indications	Primary Side Effects	Pertinent Drug Interactions	Med Pearl	Top 200
Oseltamivir	Tamiflu	*Prophylaxis:* 75 mg PO q24h × 10 days (6 wk for community outbreak) *Treatment:* 75 mg PO q12h × 5 days • Caps, suspension	Influenza A and B	None	• N/V/D • Headache • Neuropsychiatric events (e.g., confusion, delirium, hallucinations, self-injury)	None	• For prophylaxis, initiate therapy within 2 days of contact with infected person • For treatment, initiate therapy within 2 days of onset of symptoms • Adjust dose in renal dysfunction • ↓ flu severity and duration by ∼ 1 day • Can be used in children ≥1 yr	Yes
Zanamivir	Relenza	*Prophylaxis:* 2 inhalations q24h × 10 days (28 days for community outbreak) *Treatment:* 2 inhalations q12h × 5 days • Powder for oral inhalation		Asthma/chronic obstructive pulmonary disease	• Bronchospasm • Cough • Headache • Nausea/diarrhea • Neuropsychiatric events (e.g., confusion, delirium, hallucinations, self-injury)		• For prophylaxis, initiate therapy within 1.5 days (5 days in community setting) of contact with infected person • For treatment, initiate therapy within 2 days of onset of symptoms • ↓ flu severity and duration by ∼ 1 day • Can be used in children ≥5 yr (prophylaxis) or ≥7 yr (treatment)	No

LEARNING POINTS

- Compliance is a must with antiretroviral therapy. If a patient is going to stop the prescribed regimen, all the antiretrovirals must be stopped at the same time to prevent resistance.

- Patients receiving antibiotics should complete the entire course of therapy.

- Be aware of the patient's allergies when selecting antibiotic therapy (especially penicillin and sulfa allergies).

- Know agents to treat unique organisms:
  - MRSA: Vancomycin, linezolid, quinupristin/dalfopristin, tigecycline, daptomycin
  - Pseudomonas aeruginosa: Piperacillin/tazobactam, ticarcillin/clavulanic acid, aztreonam, aminoglycosides, ciprofloxacin, ceftazidime, cefepime, carbapenems (except ertapenem)
  - Anaerobes: Metronidazole, clindamycin, piperacillin/tazobactam, ticarcillin/clavulanic acid, cefoxitin, cefotetan, carbapenems

- Know important/notable side effects and drug interactions of antibiotics:
  - Which ones cause nephrotoxicity?
  - Which ones are associated with QT interval prolongation?
  - Which ones cause myelosuppression?
  - Which ones are associated with a disulfiram reaction?
  - Which ones should be avoided with antacids or products containing di-/trivalent cations?
  - Which ones cause photosensitivity?

PRACTICE QUESTIONS

1. Which of the following medications should NOT be given to a 1-year-old child?

    (A) Amoxicillin
    (B) Cefuroxime
    (C) Clindamycin
    (D) Penicillin
    (E) Tetracycline

2. Which of the following medications would be appropriate for the treatment of *Pseudomonas aeruginosa*?

    (A) Ampicillin
    (B) Cefepime
    (C) Ceftriaxone
    (D) Erythromycin
    (E) Clindamycin

3. A patient admitted to the hospital is diagnosed with Aspergillosis. Which of the following antimicrobial agents would be most appropriate to initiate in this patient?

    (A) Nystatin
    (B) Tigecycline
    (C) Chloramphenicol
    (D) Acyclovir
    (E) Caspofungin

4. Patients taking which of the following antimicrobial agents should be counseled to wear sunscreen because of the risk of photosensitivity?

    I.   Cleocin
    II. Biaxin
    III. Factive

    (A) I only
    (B) III only
    (C) I and II only
    (D) II and III only
    (E) I, II, and III

ANSWERS

1. E

Tetracycline should not be given to children younger than 9 years of age, as it can cause enamel hypoplasia or permanent tooth discoloration; therefore choice (E) is correct. The other medications can be administered safely to children.

2. B

Cefepime, a fourth-generation cephalosporin, is the only antibiotic listed that would treat an infection caused by *Pseudomonas aeruginosa*; therefore, choice (B) is correct.

3. E

Aspergillosis is a serious fungal infection. Both caspofungin and nystatin (A) are considered antifungal agents; however, nystatin is used topically (as an oral suspension for thrush or as topical cream/ointment/powder) for local infections caused by *Candida* spp. Caspofungin is administered intravenously and can be used for the treatment of Aspergillosis; thus, choice (E) is correct. Tigecycline (B) and chloramphenicol (C) are used for bacterial infections. Acyclovir (D) is an antiviral agent.

4. B

Fluoroquinolones are associated with an increased risk of photosensitivity. Therefore, patients receiving Factive (gemifloxacin) should be counseled to wear sunscreen during the course of therapy. Neither Cleocin (clindamycin) nor Biaxin (clarithromycin) is associated with photosensitivity.

Pulmonary Disorders

3

This chapter covers the following diseases:

- **Asthma**
- **Chronic obstructive pulmonary disease (COPD)**
- **Tuberculosis (TB)**

 Suggested Study Time: **30 minutes**

ASTHMA

Definitions

Asthma is a disease of the airways characterized by airway inflammation and broncho-constriction of the smooth muscles. This hyperactivity is due to a wide variety of stimuli or triggers. The hyperactivity and inflammation lead to obstruction of the airways, cough, dyspnea, chest tightness, and wheezing. The inflammatory cell infiltration mainly consists of neutrophils (especially in sudden-onset, fatal asthma exacerbations, and in patients who smoke), eosinophils, lymphocytes, mast cell activation, and epithelial cell injury and is called remodeling.

Diagnosis

- Pulmonary function tests (PFTs) provide an objective means to diagnose asthma.
- PFTs are measured using spirometry and demonstrate an obstructive pattern of decreases in expiratory flow rates.
- FEV1 means Forced expiratory volume over 1 second.
- FVC means Forced vital capacity.

- The guidelines recommend that spirometry measurements of FEV1, FVC, and FEV1/FEV are used before and after the patient inhales a short-acting bronchodilator to assess bronchodilation. Improvements are defined as an increase of FEV1 by more than 12%, which is diagnostic of asthma.

Signs and Symptoms

- Shortness of breath and wheezing that lasts for hours
- May be completely symptom-free between attacks
- Triggered by acute exposure to irritants: pollen, dust, chemicals, changes in weather, perfumes, smoke, heartburn, mold
- Nasal polyps
- Excessive mucus and even mucus plugs

Guidelines

National Heart, Lung and Blood Institute, National Asthma Education and Prevention Program, Expert Panel Report 3: Guidelines for the Diagnosis and Management of Asthma—Full Report, 2007. http://nhlbi.nih.gov/guidelines/asthma/asthsumm.pdf.

Guidelines Summary

There are four components to asthma management:

- Measurement of assessment and monitoring
- Controlling environmental factors and comorbid conditions
- Education for asthma care
- Pharmacologic therapy

The goals of therapy are:

- Patient education is a must.
- Daily usage of peak flow meter will provide an objective FEV1.
- Implementation of an action plan:
  - Green zone ("I feel good"), yellow zone ("I do not feel good"), red zone ("I feel awful")
  - Green zone = FEV1 >80% of personal best
  - Yellow zone = FEV1 >50–80% of personal best
  - Red zone = FEV1 <50% of personal best

- Attempt to identify triggers:
  - Consider subcutaneous allergen immunotherapy.
  - Management of GERD can greatly improve symptoms.
  - Avoid aspirin therapy due to prostaglandin inhibition; can cause bronchoconstriction.
  - Smoking cessation is recommended.
  - Consider clean home, dust, plastic case over mattress.
    - » Patient needs to be classified into mild, moderate, severe, or life threatening.
  - Identify frequency of symptoms and nighttime awakenings.
  - Identify use of short-acting beta-2 agonists and lung function.
    - » Ensure compliance with medications.
    - » Ensure proper inhaler technique.
    - » Use a stepwise approach to treatment.
    - » Long-term medications should include anti-inflammatory mechanism.

Asthma

Generic	Brand	Dose	Contra-indications	Primary Side Effects	Key Monitoring	Pertinent Drug Interactions	Med Pearl	Top 200
Mechanism of action — glucocorticoid receptor agonist with an affinity for the receptor resulting in anti-inflammatory and immunosuppressive properties, and antiproliferative actions								
Fluticasone	• Flovent • Flovent HFA	44–440 mcg BID	Primary treatment for acute bronchospasm	• Throat irritation • Cough • Oral candidiasis • Lower respiratory tract infection	• FEV1 • Peak flow • Other pulmonary function tests • HPA axis suppression	None that are pertinent, due to topical administration at the lung tissue	• HFA formulation • Most potent corticosteroid	Yes
Budesonide	• Pulmicort • Respules	200–800 mcg BID					Respules are the only nebulized corticosteroid	Yes
Mometasone	Asmanex	220–440 mcg/day					• True once daily	Yes
Beclomethasone	QVAR	40–320 mcg BID					• HFA formulation	No
Flunisolide	AeroBid	500–2,000 mcg BID					AeroBid(M)has a mint flavor	No
Triamcinolone	Azmacort	150–400 mcg/day QID					• Built in spacer • Least potent corticosteroid	No
Mechanism of action — long-acting beta-2 agonists								
Salmeterol	Serevent	• *Diskus:* 50 mcg/puff • *Max:* 2 puffs/day	• Use as an acute bronchodilator • Presence of tachyarrhythmias	• Headache • Hypertension • Dizziness • Chest pain	• FEV1 • Peak flow • Other pulmonary function tests	None	• Long-acting beta-2 agonists may increase the risk of asthma-related deaths; should be used only in adjunct therapy with inhaled corticosteroids	Yes
Formoterol	Foradil	• *DPI:* 12 mcg/capsule • *Max:* 2 puffs/day				None		No
Mechanism of action — prevents the mass cells from releasing histamine and leukotrienes								
Cromolyn neb & inhaler	Intal	20–80 mg/day	Primary treatment for acute bronchospasms	• Cough and irritation • Unpleasant taste • Increase in sneezing	Pulmonary function tests	None	• Safety is the primary advantage of this drug class	No
Nedocromil neb & inhaler	Tilade	1.75–14 mg/day					• May take 4–6 weeks for full benefit • Approved to <2 yr of age	No

Asthma *(cont'd)*

Generic	Brand	Dose	Contra-indications	Primary Side Effects	Key Monitoring	Pertinent Drug Interactions	Med Pearl	Top 200
Mechanism of action – IgG monoclonal antibody which inhibits IgE receptor on mast cells and basophils.								
Omalizumab	Xolair	SQ 150–375 mg every 2–4 wk, based on weight and serum IgE	Acute bronchospasms	• Pain and bruising of injection sites • Anaphylaxis has been reported	Be prepared for anaphylaxis	None	• Do not administer more than 150 mg per injection site	No
Mechanism of action – selective leukotriene-receptor antagonist of leukotrienes D4 and E4								
Montelukast	Singular	4–10 mg/HS	Hypersensitivity	Rare Churg-Strauss syndrome		CYP450 inhibitor: 2C8 and 2C9	• Approved as young as 1 year of age	Yes
Zafirlukast	Accolate	10–40 mg/day		Increase in LFTs	Must be taken on empty stomach	• CYP450: 1A2 • Warfarin		No
Mechanism of action – 5-lipoxygenase inhibitor limits neutrophil and monocyte aggregation								
Zileuton	Zyflo Zyflo CR	600–2,400 mg/day	Acute liver disease	• Elevations in • LFTs	• LFT baseline every 2 months • Peak flow	CYP450 inhibitor: 1A2	• QID dose is disadvantage	No
Mechanism of action – methylxanthine causes bronchodilation by increasing tissue concentrations of cyclic adenine monophosphate								
• Theophylline • Liquid, sustained-release tabs & caps	Theo-24, Uniphyl	10 mg/kg/day up to 800 mg/day	Allergy to corn-derived dextrose	• Tachycardia • Nausea/vomiting • CNS stimulation • Theophylline toxicity: persistent, repetitive vomiting	• Serum range: 5–15 mcg/mL • Serum levels <20 mcg/mL have few side effects	CYP450: inhibits 1A2, 3A4	• Dosage adjustments should be in small increments (maximum: 25%); elderly patients should be started on 25% reduction in the adult dose	No

Asthma *(cont'd)*

Mechanism of action – relaxes bronchial smooth muscle by acting on beta-2 receptors

Generic	Brand	Dose	Contra-indications	Primary Side Effects	Key Monitoring	Pertinent Drug Interactions	Med Pearl	Top 200
Albuterol	Ventolin Proventil	MDI: 90 mcg/puff Neb: 2.5 mg³/mL	Patients with tachyarrhythmia risk	• Dose-dependent • Angina, atrial fibrillation, arrhythmias, chest discomfort, cough, tremor	• FEV1 • Peak flow • Blood pressure • Heart rate	Nonselective beta-adrenergic blockers decrease albuterol's effect	Excessive use can increase risk of death; nebulizer is compatible with budesonide, cromolyn, ipratropium	Yes
Levalbuterol	Xopenex Xopenex HFA	MDI: 45 mcg/puff 200 puffs/canister Neb: 0.63/3 mL	Less cardiac side effects	Less cardiac side effects			Prime the inhaler by releasing 4 actuations prior to use	Yes
Pirbuterol	Autoinhaler	Autoinhaler: 200 mcg/puff NMT: 12 inhalations/day	Patients with tachyarrhythmia risk	• Dose-dependent • Angina, atrial fibrillation, arrhythmias, chest discomfort, cough, tremor			Autoinhaler is breath-actuated; child <4 years of age may not generate sufficient inspiratory flow	No

Combination

Generic	Brand	Dose	Contra-indications	Primary Side Effects	Key Monitoring	Pertinent Drug Interactions	Med Pearl	Top 200
Fluticasone/ salmeterol	Advair							Yes
Formoterol/ budesonide	Symbicort							No

- See above for individual interactions
- Synergistic effects are likely with combination products
- Maximum dose of Advair is 1 puff BID; dosages: 100/50, 200/50, 500/50

Storage and Administration Pearls

- Metered-dose inhaler (MDI) requires hand coordination and proper technique.
- Dry powder inhaler (DPI) is breath-actuated and requires less coordination.
- Spacer with non breath-actuated MDIs and mouth washing and spitting after inhalation decrease local side effects.
- Chlorofluorocarbons (CFCs) have been found to have an effect on the ozone layer in the earth's stratosphere.
- Hydrofluoroalkane (HFA) is an earth-friendly alternative to CFCs.
- Theophylline is incompatible with phenytoin.

Patient Education Pearls

- Patient should always use a spacer with inhaled corticosteroids for better deposition into the lungs and to prevent thrush.
- Patient should rinse and spit to avoid thrush from inhaled corticosteroids.
- Compliance is a must with all asthma medications.

CHRONIC OBSTRUCTIVE PULMONARY DISEASE (COPD)

Definitions

COPD is characterized by persistent and largely irreversible airflow obstruction causing dyspnea, which does not fluctuate like asthma. Airflow obstruction is generally progressive and associated with abnormal inflammatory responses of lungs to noxious particles and gases. It is a disease entity with a spectrum of manifestation depending on the lung region affected. Chronic bronchitis affects the larger airways; emphysema affects the smaller airways, called alveolar sacs.

Diagnosis

- History of cigarette smoking is a factor.
- Alpha1-antitrypsin deficiency in nonsmokers is a factor.
- Nocturnal symptoms are unusual.
- Chest x-ray often shows low and flattened diaphragms.
- FEV1 and all measurements of expiration airflow are reduced.
- FEV1 is the standard way to assess clinical course for response to therapy.
- In smokers, the rate of decline in the FEV1 is approximately 60 mL/year.

Signs and Symptoms

- Tachypnea – rapid breathing
- Pursed lips when breathing
- Cough and phlegm
- Wheeze and rhonchi
- Hyperinflation
- Use of accessory muscles to assist with respiration
- One or two acute exacerbations per year
- Blue bloater = chronic bronchitis
- Pink puffer = emphysema

Guidelines

American College of Physicians 2008; www.acp.com.

National Heart, Lung and Blood Institute, Expert Panel Report 3: Global Initiative for Chronic Obstructive Lung Disease (GOLD). www.goldcopd.org.

Guidelines Summary

- American College of Physicians – 2008
  - Spirometry should be used to diagnose airway obstruction only in symptomatic patients.
  - In patients with stable COPD, treatment should be reserved for those who are symptomatic with FEV1.
- Global Initiative for Chronic Obstructive Lung Disease (GOLD)
- Educate the patient in avoidance of risk factors (especially tobacco smoke) and start preventive efforts.
  - Smoking cessation for more than a year led to an improvement in lung function, with an FEV1 decline equal to that of nonsmokers (20–30 mL/year).
  - Consider flu and pneumonia vaccinations.
- Add a short-acting bronchodilator when needed.
- Add regular treatment with one or more long-acting bronchodilators and begin rehabilitation.
- Add inhaled glucocorticoids if the patient has repeated acute exacerbations.
- Start long-acting oxygen therapy if the patient is hypoxemic, and consider surgical treatments.

COPD

Generic	Brand	Dose	Contra-indications	Primary Side Effects	Key Monitoring	Pertinent Drug Interactions	Med Pearl	Top 200
Mechanism of action – partial alpha4B2 nicotinic receptor agonist; prevents nicotine stimulation of mesolimbic dopamine system								
Varenicline	Chantix	0.5–2 mg/day	Hypersensitivity	• Insomnia • Headache • Abnormal dreams • Nausea		None	Start 1 week prior to target stop day with 0.5 mg/day	Yes
Mechanism of action – inhibits neuronal uptake of norepinephrine and dopamine								
Bupropion	Zyban	150–300 mg/day	• Seizure disorder • Anorexia/bulimia • Use of MAO inhibitor within 14 days	• Tachycardia • Headache • Insomnia	• Body weight • Mental status for depression • Suicidal ideation	• CYP450 inhibitor • 2D6 • MAO inhibitor	Can be co-administered with nicotine replacement patches	Yes
Mechanism of action – supplements nicotine which exhibits primary effects via autonomic ganglia stimulation								
Nicotine	• Commit, NicoDerm, Nicorette	• Gum: max 24 pieces/day • Inhaler: max 16 cartridges/day • Patch: 1 patch per day • Lozenge: 2–4 mg; max 9/day • Spray: 80 sprays/day	• Smoking or chewing tobacco • Post-myocardial infarction • Life-threatening arrhythmias • Worsening angina	• Headache • Mouth or throat irritation • Dyspepsia • Cough	• Heart rate • Blood pressure • Nicotine toxicity (severe headache, dizziness, mental confusion)	CYP450 inhibits 2A4 and 2E1	Antidepressant medications may increase suicidal behavior in young adults	No
Mechanism of action – blocks acetylcholine at the parasympathetic sites in bronchial smooth muscle, causing bronchodilation								
Ipratropium	• Atrovent • Atrovent HFA • Combivent (ipratropium & albuterol)	• MDI: 17 mcg/puff; max: 12 puffs/24 hours • Neb: 0.25 mg/mL	Hypersensitivity	• Upper respiratory tract infection • Palpitation • Xerostomia • Pharyngeal irritation	• FEV1 • Peak flow • Other pulmonary function tests	CYP450 – substrate 2D6, 3A4	• Not recommended for initial treatment of acute episode of bronchospasm • Anticholinergic side effects are possible. Be careful in BPH, narrow-angle glaucoma, and myasthenia gravis	Yes
Tiotropium	Spiriva	DPI: 18 mcg/puff; max: 1 puff/day	Contains lactose					Yes
Mechanism of action – long-acting beta-2 agonists								
Formoterol	Perforomist	Neb: 20 mcg/2mL	Same as above in asthma					Yes

STORAGE AND ADMINISTRATION PEARLS

- Nicotrol inhaler: Protect from light.
- Tiotropium: Do not store capsules in Handihaler device. Capsules should be used within 2 days of removal from blister pack.

Patient Education Pearls

- For improved outcomes, it is important to have consistent and regular interventions with the patient regarding smoking cessation education.
- When working with patient to stop smoking, it is recommended to use the 5 As: Ask, Advise, Assess, Assist, Arrange.

TUBERCULOSIS

Definitions

Tuberculosis (TB) is a communicable infection disease caused by *Mycobacterium tuberculosis*. It can produce a silent, latent infection, as well as an active disease state. Although TB is far less common today in the United States, it remains the most prevalent infection on the planet. Effective therapy for *Mycobacterium tuberculosis* infections require combination chemotherapy designed to prevent the emergence of resistant organisms. Increased resistance to the conventional antituberculous agents has led to the use of more complex regimens.

Diagnosis

- Diagnosis relies on skin testing with the tuberculin purified protein derivative (PPD).
- PPD should be performed on high-risk patients.
  - High-risk patients include HIV-infected, hospital employees, nursing home staff and residents, workers in prisons, immigrants, and healthcare students.
- The intracutaneous PPD injection should produce a small, raised, blanched wheal. This test should be read by an experienced professional in 48 to 72 hours.
  - Area >5 mm is considered positive for HIV.
  - Area >10 mm is considered positive for immunocompetent patients.
- After a positive PPD skin test, a diagnostic test must be performed to rule out active disease.
  - Confirmatory diagnosis is performed with chest radiographs and microbiologic examination or sputum.

Signs and Symptoms

TB can present with generalized symptoms of weight loss, malaise, fever, and night sweats. As the disease progresses the patient may develop a persistent cough, which is often productive of sputum. Frequently, the onset of TB is insidious; and the diagnosis may not be considered until a chest radiograph is performed.

Guidelines

Currently, there are two sets of guidelines from two national associations. Overall, there are minor differences and the information has been combined for clarity.

American College of Chest Physicians, Medical Specialty Society. (January 2006). NGC:004834. http://guidelines.gov/browse/browsemode.aspx?node=27945&type=1.

American Thoracic Society, Medical Specialty Society Centers for Disease Control and Prevention–Federal Government Agency [U.S.] Infectious Diseases Society of America–Medical Specialty Society. (June 20, 2003). http://guidelines.gov/browse/browsemode.aspx?node=27945&type=1.

Guidelines Summary

The overall goals for treatment of tuberculosis are: (*1*) To cure the individual patient, and (*2*) to minimize the transmission of *Mycobacterium tuberculosis* to other persons.

- Risk factors
  - Location of birth (New York, New Jersey, California, Florida, and Texas account for 92% of cases)
  - Close contact (>40 hours per week) with TB patients
  - Increase in age
  - Race and ethnicity: Hispanics, African American, and Asian Pacific Islanders
- Successful treatment of tuberculosis has benefits for both the individual patient and the community in which the patient resides.
- Prescribing physician responsibility for treatment completion is a fundamental principle in tuberculosis control.
- Treatment of patients with tuberculosis is most successful within a comprehensive framework that addresses both clinical and social issues of relevance to the patient.
- It is strongly recommended that patient-centered care be the initial management strategy, regardless of the source of supervision. This strategy should always include an adherence plan that emphasizes directly observed therapy (DOT).
- There are four recommended regimens for treating patients with tuberculosis caused by drug-susceptible organisms following a continuation phase:
  - Drugs: Isoniazid (INH); Rifampin (RIF); Pyrazinamide (PZA); Ethambutol (EMB)

Tuberculosis

Generic	Brand	Dose	Contra-indications	Primary Side Effects	Key Monitoring	Pertinent Drug Interactions	Med Pearl	Top 200
Mechanism of action – inhibition of mycolic acid synthesis resulting in disruption of the bacterial cell wall								
Isoniazid (INH)	Isotamine	• Latent: 300 mg/day for 9 months • Active: multiple scenarios	• Acute liver disease • Previous severe reactions (drug fever, chills, arthritis)	• Hypertension • Depression • Flushing • Jaundice, increased LFTs	• Baseline LFTs • Sputum cultures, until two consecutive negatives • Hepatitis	• CYP3A4 inhibitor: 1A2, 2A6, 2C19, 2D6, 2E1, 3A4 • Inducers: 2E1	• Severe and sometimes fatal hepatitis may occur within 3 months of treatment • Drinking alcohol is not recommended during treatment • Empty stomach	No
Mechanism of action – inhibits bacterial RNA synthesis by binding to the beta subunit of DNA-dependent RNA polymerase, blocking RNA transcription								
Rifampin (RIF)	Rifadin	• Oral/IV: 10 mg/kg/day • Max: 600 mg/day	• Concurrent use of amprenavir, saquinivir/ ritonivir	• Numbness • Flulike syndrome	• Baseline LFT • CBC • Sputum cultures • Chest x-ray 23 months into treatment	CYP450 inducers: 1A2, 2A6, 2B6, 2C8, 2C9, 2C19, 3A4	Rifabutin often will be used with drug interaction	No
Mechanism of action – kills mycobacteria replicating in macrophages; exact mechanism is not known								
Pyrazinamide (PZA)	Tebrazid	• Tab: 15–30 mg/kg/day • Max: 2 g/day	• Acute gout • Severe hepatic damage	• Malaise • Anorexia • Hepatotoxicity	• LFTs • Uric acid levels • Sputum culture • Chest x-rays	Rifampin and pyrazinamide have been associated with hepatotoxicity	Typically used for the first 2 months of therapy	No
Mechanism of action – suppresses mycobacteria multiplication by interfering with RNA synthesis								
Ethambutol (EMB)	Myambutol	• Tab: 15–25 mg/kg/day • Max: 2.5 g/dose	Optic neuritis	• Myocarditis • Headache • Gout, abnormal LFTs	• Baseline and periodic (monthly) visual testing • Renal, hepatic, hematopoietic tests	• Decreased absorption with aluminum hydroxide. • Avoid antacids by 4 hours	Optic neuritis manifests as decreased red-green color perception, decreased visual field	No
Mechanism of action – inhibits bacterial protein synthesis by binding directly to the 30S ribosomal subunit, causing faulty peptide sequence to form in the protein chain								
Streptomycin		• Inj: 15 mg/ kg/day • Max: 1 g/day	Pregnancy	May cause neurotoxicity, nephrotoxicity	• Hearing (audiogram) • Scr and BUN • Serum concentration	Increased effect with depolarizing neuromuscular blockade agents	• Used as a substitute for ethambutol and for drug-resistant MTB • Does not penetrate the CNS and cannot be used for TB meningitis	No

Storage and Administration Pearls

- Isoniazid: Tablets and oral solution must be protected from light

Patient Education Pearls

- A patient who is taking Rifampin should report any tingling or numbness in the hands or feet.
- A patient who is taking Streptomycin must maintain adequate hydration.

LEARNING POINTS

- Inhaled corticosteroids are the drug of choice when treating asthma. They prevent remodeling, improve symptoms, and prevent exacerbations as compared to the other medications.
- Although peak flow meters are rarely dispensed in pharmacy, they are crucial to the maintenance of asthma. Peak flow meters should be used to determine a patient's personal best and used every morning to identify an early exacerbation.
- Smoking cessation will help slow the progression of COPD and is the most important intervention when dealing with patients who have COPD.
- Given an active case of tuberculosis, the clinician must ensure directly observed therapy to reduce bacterial resistance and exposure to other patients.
- Isoniazid is currently the drug of choice for a positive PPD and in combination-treatments for tuberculosis.

PRACTICE QUESTIONS

1. Which of the following medications is/are used to treat latent tuberculosis?

    I. Pyrazinamide
    II. Rifampin
    III. Ethambutol

(A) I only
(B) III only
(C) I and II
(D) II and III
(E) I, II, and III

2. The device used to measure forced vital capacity is called a

(A) tonometer.
(B) optomyometer.
(C) sphygmomanometer.
(D) spirometer.
(E) gonioscope.

3. QVAR is indicated for which of the following scenarios?

    I. Asthma
    II. COPD
    III. Smoking cessation

(A) I only
(B) III only
(C) I and II only
(D) II and III only
(E) I, II, and III

4. Which of the following have the same active ingredient?

    I. Flonase
    II. Flovent
    III. Veramyst

(A) I only
(B) III only
(C) I and II only
(D) II and III only
(E) I, II, and III

ANSWERS

1. **C**

Pyrazinamide and Rifampin are used to treat active and latent TB. Ethambutol is used only to treat active TB infection.

2. **D**

A spirometer is a gasometer used for measuring respiratory gases, so (D) is correct. A tonometer (A) determines pressure or tension within the eye. An optomyometer (B) is an instrument for determining the relative power of the extrinsic muscles of the eye. A sphygmomanometer (C) measures arterial blood pressure. A gonioscope (E) measures the lens angle in relationship to the eye.

3. **A**

QVAR is an inhaled corticosteroid that is indicated only for the maintenance and pro-phylactic treatment of asthma, so (A) is the only correct answer.

4. **E**

Flonase, Flovent, and Veramyst all have the same active ingredient—fluticasone—so (E) is correct.

Endocrine Disorders

4

This chapter covers the following diseases:

- **Diabetes mellitus (DM) Type 1**
- **Diabetes mellitus (DM) Type 2**
- **Hypothyroidism**
- **Hyperthyroidism**
- **Polycystic ovarian syndrome (PCOS)**

 Suggested Study Time: **40 minutes**

DIABETES MELLITUS (DM) TYPE 1

Definitions

Diabetes mellitus type 1 accounts for fewer than 10% of all cases of diabetes, occurs in younger persons, and is caused by severe insulin deficiency that results from an immune-mediated destruction of the pancreatic-islet beta cells. Exogenous insulin is required to control blood glucose, prevent diabetic ketoacidosis (DKA), and preserve life. A transient period of insulin independence ("honeymoon phase") or reduced insulin requirement may occur early in the course of type 1 DM. When studying for the NAPLEX, be sure to recognize that DKA typically occurs in type 1 diabetes patients.

Diagnosis

- Impaired fasting glucose (IFG) is defined by a fasting plasma glucose between 100 and 125 mg/dL and is indicative of prediabetes.
- Impaired glucose tolerance (IGT) is defined by a 2-hour oral glucose tolerance test plasma glucose between 140 and 200 mg/dL and is indicative of prediabetes.

- A plasma glucose of 126 mg/dL or greater after an overnight fast (and/or)
- Symptoms of diabetes and a random plasma glucose greater than 200 mg/dL (and/or)
- Oral glucose tolerance test indicating a plasma glucose of 200 mg/dL that is greater 2 hours after a 75-g glucose load.

Signs and Symptoms

- Polyuria is a sign, which is characterized by excessive excretion of urine
- Polyphagia is a sign, which is characterized by excessive eating
- Polydipsia is a sign, which is characterized by excessive thirst that is relatively prolonged
- Weight loss is due to excretion of glucose in the urine when blood sugars exceed 180 mg/dL. The excretion of glucose results in loss of calorie retention. In addition, the excessive polyuria leads to polyphagia and polydipsia.

Guidelines

American Diabetes Association, *Diabetes Care*, no. 31 (Suppl 1): S4 (2008). www.diabetes.org

American Association of Clinical Endocrinologists, Endocrine Practice, no. 13 (Suppl 1) (May/June 2007). http://aace.com/pub/guidelines.

Guidelines Summary

- American Diabetes Association (ADA)
  - Goal blood glucose values between 80–120 mg/dL
  - A1c (average blood sugar for 3 months)
    » Less than 7% (average blood sugar of 150 mg/dL)
      – 6% = 120 mg/dL; 7% = 150 mg/dL; 8% = 180 mg/dL
    » A1c as close to 6% as possible without side effects of hypoglycemia
    » LDL-C ≤100 mg/dL; TG ≤200 mg/dL
- American Association of Clinical Endocrinologists (AACE)
  - A1c (test that measures how much glucose has been sticking during the past 3–4 months to hemoglobin)
    » Less than 6.5% (average blood sugar of 135 mg/dL)
  - Guidelines are more strict than ADA in glucose goals and triglycerides; goals: ≤150 mg/dL; LDL-C ≤100 mg/dL

Patient education is integral to successful management of diabetes. Diabetes education should be conducted through an interdisciplinary approach involving a provider, pharmacist, dietician, and nurse.

Dietary modifications should include education and instruction on carbohydrate counting. Men and women should limit carbohydrate intake between 45–60 g of carbohydrates per meal; 15 g of carbohydrates = 1 choice.

Exercise improves insulin sensitivity; reduces fasting and postprandial blood glucose; and offers numerous metabolic, cardiovascular, and psychological benefits. Exercise should consist of moderately intense cardio 30 min/day, 5 days a week; or vigorously intense cardio 20 min/day, 3 days a week, along with 8–10 strength-training exercise with 8–10 repetitions each, 2 day/week. These recommendations come from the American College of Sports Medicine.

DIABETES MELLITUS TYPE 2

Definitions

Diabetes mellitus type 2 accounts for more than 90% of all cases of DM. Usually a disease of adults, type 2 DM is increasingly being diagnosed in younger age groups. Obesity, insulin resistance, and relative insulin deficiency are characteristic findings. Insulin secretion may be sufficient to prevent ketosis under basal conditions, but DKA can develop during severe stress. When studying for the NAPLEX, be sure to understand the mechanism of actions of the medications. This will help with identifying duplications of drug therapy.

Diagnosis

- Impaired fasting glucose (IFG) is defined by a fasting plasma glucose between 100 and 125 mg/dL and is indicative of pre-diabetes.
- Impaired glucose tolerance (IGT) is defined by a 2-hour oral glucose tolerance test plasma glucose between 140 and 200 mg/dL and is indicative of prediabetes.
- Plasma glucose of 126 mg/dL or greater after an overnight fast (and/or)
- Symptoms of diabetes and a random plasma glucose greater than 200 mg/dL (and/or)
- Oral glucose tolerance test indicating a plasma glucose of 200 mg/dL greater 2 hours after a 75-g glucose load.

Signs and Symptoms

- Polyuria is a sign, which is characterized by excessive excretion of urine
- Polyphagia is a sign, which is characterized by excessive eating
- Polydipsia is a sign, which is characterized by excessive thirst that is relatively prolonged
- Weight loss is due to excretion of glucose in the urine with blood sugars exceeding 180 mg/dL. The excretion of glucose results in loss of calorie retention. In addition, the excessive polyuria leads to polyphagia and polydipsia.

Guidelines

See Guidelines for Diabetes Mellitus Type 1.

Guidelines Summary

See Guidelines Summary for Diabetes Mellitus Type 1.

Drugs for Diabetes (Insulin)

Generic	Brand	Onset	Peak	Duration	Comments	Top 200
Rapid Acting					• Hypoglycemia is the most common side effect. It is defined as blood sugar <70 mg/dL and must be treated as soon as recognized.	
Aspart	NovoLog	5–15 min	30–90 min	<5 hrs		Yes
Lispro	Humalog	5–15 min	30–90 min	<5 hrs	• Insulin dosage is individually based due to sensitivity; 0.51.0 units/kg/day for the average non-obese patient.	Yes
Glulisine	Apridra	5–15 min	30–90 min	<5 hrs	• Duration of action is prolonged in renal failure.	No
Insulin human rDNA Inhalation powder	Exubera*	5–15 min	30–90 min	5–8 hrs	• Pulmonary function test required with inhaled insulin. Precaution with asthma, COPD, and smokers.	No
Short-Acting						
Regular	Humulin R (OTC)	30–60 min	2–3 hrs	5–8 hrs		No
Intermediate, Basal						
NPH (Neutral Protamine Hagedorn)	Humulin N (OTC)	2–4 hrs	4–10 hrs	10–16 hrs		Yes
Long-Acting, Basal						
Glargine	Lantus	2–4 hrs	No peak	20–24 hrs		Yes
Detemir	Levemir	3–8 hrs	No peak	6–24 hrs		No
Premixed						
75% Lispro protamine/25% lispro	Humalog Mix 75/25	5–15 min	Dual	10–16 hrs		Yes
50% Lispro protamine / 50% lispro	Humalog Mix 50/50	5–15 min	Dual	10–16 hrs		Yes
70% Insulin aspart protamine / 30% aspart	NovoLog Mix 70/30	5–15 min	Dual	10–16 hrs		Yes
70% NPH / 30% regular	70/30 (OTC)	30–60 min	Dual	10–16 hrs		Yes

• OTC insulin is available without a prescription.
• Rapid-acting insulin should be given at time of meal ingestion, no more than 15 minutes from eating.
• Regular insulin should be given 30 minutes prior to meal due to delayed onset of action.

*(Might be pulled off market)

Drugs for Diabetes (Oral)

Generic	Brand	Dose & Max	Contra-indications	Primary Side Effects	Key Monitoring	Pertinent Drug Interactions	Med Pearl	Top 200
Sulfonylureas, first generation – stimulate insulin release from the pancreatic beta cells								
Tolbutamide	Apo-tolbutamide	0.5–2 g	• Type 1 DM • Sulfa allergy	• Hypoglycemia • Weight gain	Fasting plasma glucose and A1c at 3 months	• Cimetidine may increase hypoglycemia effects (CYP450) • Chronic ethanol ingestion may decrease hypoglycemic effect	• Response plateaus after half maximum dose	No
Acetohexamide		0.25 mg–1.5 g						No
Tolazamide	Tolinase	0.1–1 g						No
Chlorpropamide	Diabinese	0.1–0.5 g						No
Sulfonylureas, second generation – stimulate insulin release from the pancreatic beta cells								
Glyburide	Micronase	1.25–20 mg	• Type 1 DM • Sulfa allergy	• Hypoglycemia • Weight gain	Fasting plasma glucose and A1c at 3 months	• Cimetidine may increase hypoglycemia effects (CYP450) • Chronic ethanol ingestion may decrease hypoglycemic effect	• Response plateaus after half maximum dose	Yes
Glipizide	• Glucotrol • Glucotrol XL	2.5–40 mg						Yes
Glimepiride	Amaryl	1–8 mg						No
Meglitinides – stimulates insulin release from the pancreatic beta cells								
Repaglinide	Prandin	1–16 mg	Type 1 DM	• Hypoglycemia • Weight gain	Postprandial plasma glucose and A1c	• Decrease effect by CYP3A4, 2C8/9 inducers • Increase effect by CYP3A4 inhibitors	• Faster acting and shorter duration than the traditional sulfonylureas, and recommended for postprandial blood sugars	No
Amino acid derivative – stimulates insulin release from the pancreatic beta cells								
Nateglinide	Starlix	180–360 mg	Type 1 DM	• Hypoglycemia • Weight gain	Postprandial plasma glucose and A1c	• Decrease effect by CYP3A4, 2C8/9 inducers • Increase effect by CYP3A4 inhibitors	• Faster acting than the traditional sulfonylureas, and recommended for postprandial blood sugars	No

Drugs for Diabetes (Oral) *(cont'd)*

Biguanide – decreases hepatic glucose production, decreases intestinal absorption of glucose, improves insulin sensitivity

Generic	Brand	Dose & Max	Contra-indications	Primary Side Effects	Key Monitoring	Pertinent Drug Interactions	Med Pearl	Top 200
Metformin	• Glucophage • Glucophage XR	500 mg–2.550 g	• Scr ≥1.5 male • Scr ≥1.4 female • Lactic acidosis	GI intolerance (flatulence and diarrhea); lactic acidosis	• Serum creatinine • Fasting plasma glucose • A1c every 3 months	• Cimetidine increases peak metformin plasma and whole blood concentration by 60%	• Lactic acidosis black box warning. Contraindicated in severe heart failure, renal failure, radiographic dyes	Yes

Alpha-glucosidase inhibitors – inhibit pancreatic alpha-amylase and alpha-glucosidases, block carbohydrate hydrolysis to glucose

Generic	Brand	Dose & Max	Contra-indications	Primary Side Effects	Key Monitoring	Pertinent Drug Interactions	Med Pearl	Top 200
Acarbose	Precose	75–300 mg	• Cirrhosis • Inflammatory bowel disease • Intestinal obstruction	• Abdominal pain and diarrhea • Flatulence	• LFTs q3 months x 1 year • Postprandial blood sugars and A1c	• Hypoglycemia risk when given with sulfonylureas or insulin	• Must treat hypoglycemia with simple carbohydrate such as glucose	No
Miglitol	Glyset	75–300 mg			• Postprandial blood sugars and A1c			No

Thiazolidinediones – PPAR-gamma activator, which improves insulin sensitivity

Generic	Brand	Dose & Max	Contra-indications	Primary Side Effects	Key Monitoring	Pertinent Drug Interactions	Med Pearl	Top 200
Rosiglitazone	Avandia	2–8 mg	History of liver disease	Fluid retention and hepatotoxicity	Monitor LFTs, baseline and periodically	• Decrease effect by CYP3A4, 2C8 inducers • Decrease effect by 2C8 inhibitors	• Rosi: potential link to an increase in cardiovascular events; however, very controversial	Yes
Pioglitazone	Actos	15–45 mg				• Decrease effect by CYP3A4, 2C8 inducers	• Pio: thought to have a better lipid profile	Yes

Amylinomimetic – Amylin cosecreted with insulin reduces post-prandial blood sugars, prolonging gastric emptying, reducing postprandial glucagon secretion, and caloric intake through centrally-mediated appetite suppression

Generic	Brand	Dose & Max	Contra-indications	Primary Side Effects	Key Monitoring	Pertinent Drug Interactions	Med Pearl	Top 200
Pramlintide	Symlin	15–120 mcg	• Gastroparesis • Hypoglycemia unawareness	• Nausea from delayed gastric emptying • Severe hypoglycemia	• Hypoglycemia • Blood sugars and A1c	• May delay absorption of other drugs due to increased gastric emptying time • Pramlintide: must reduce dose of insulin by 50% when starting	• Administer medications 1 hour prior to the use of pramlintide and exanatide • Exenatide: black box warning for acute pancreatitis	No

Drugs for Diabetes (Oral) *(cont'd)*

GLP-1 Inhibitors – glucagon-like peptide which increases insulin secretion, increases B-cell growth/replication, slows gastric emptying, decreases food intake

Generic	Brand	Dose & Max	Contra-indications	Primary Side Effects	Key Monitoring	Pertinent Drug Interactions	Med Pearl	Top 200
Exenatide	Byetta	5–20 mcg	• Type 1 diabetes • Pancreatitis • Diabetic ketoacidosis	• Nausea • Hypoglycemia • Decreased appetite	• Renal function • Blood sugars and A1c			Yes

Dipeptidyl-peptidase 4 inhibitors – prolong the active incretin levels of GLP and GIP

Generic	Brand	Dose & Max	Contra-indications	Primary Side Effects	Key Monitoring	Pertinent Drug Interactions	Med Pearl	Top 200
Sitagliptin	Januvia	25–100 mg	Type 1 diabetes	Headache	• Renal function • Blood sugars and A1c	May increase digoxin concentration	100 mg dose is preferred unless patient has renal impairment	Yes

Combination

Generic	Brand	Dose & Max						Top 200
Sitagliptin/ metformin	Janumet	• See above for individual interactions. • Synergistic effects are likely with combination products. • Maximum dose of metformin is 2,000 mg in combination products. • Maximum dose for immediate release is 2,550 mg per day.						No
Glyburide/ metformin	Glucovance							Yes
Rosiglitazone/ metformin	Avandamet							Yes
Rosiglitazone/ glimepiride	Avandaryl							No
Pioglitazone/ metformin	Actos Plus							No
Glipizide/ metformin	Metaglip							No

Storage and Administration Pearls

- Unopened containers of insulin should be stored in the refrigerator.
- If not refrigerated, use within 28 days and protect from heat and light.
- Do not freeze insulin.
- Once opened or in use, vials may be stored in refrigerator or at room temperature for up to 28 days.
- IV infusion: Must be kept stable for 24 hours at room temperature.
- Detemir's Mechanism of Action (MOA) is slightly different than the other insulin. It binds to albumin to extend its half-life.

Patient Education Pearls

- A patient who is on alpha-glycosidase inhibitors must use a simple sugar to treat hypoglycemia anytime.
- Rotate insulin injection sites.
- Mixing rule: "Clear, then cloudy" is the rule. It still applies to NPH (cloudy), regular (clear), fast-acting (clear).
- The exceptions: Never mix Detemir or glargine (clear) with anything.

HYPOTHYROIDISM

Definitions

Primary hypothyroidism accounts for more than 90% of cases. It is due to actual disease of the thyroid itself and not from a feedback or hypothalamus issue. Hashimoto's disease is the most common cause and may be associated with Addison's disease (chronic adrenocortical insufficiency) and other endocrine deficits.

Diagnosis

Plasma thyroid-stimulating hormone (TSH) is the best initial diagnostic test. A TSH that is markedly elevated (>20 mcgU/mL) confirms the diagnosis.

Signs and Symptoms

- Most symptoms are nonspecific and develop gradually.
- Typical symptoms are cold intolerance, fatigue, somnolence, poor memory, and depression.
- Atypical symptoms are constipation, menorrhagia, myalgias, and hoarseness.
- Physical exam will often show slow tendon reflexes, bradycardia, and facial and periorbital edema.

Guidelines

American Association of Clinical Endocrinologists, *Arch Intern Med*, no. 160 (2000): 1573–1575. http://aace.com/pub/guidelines.

Guidelines Summary

The treatment and management of chronic thyroiditis and clinical hypothyroidism must be tailored to the individual patient. Many clinical endocrinologists treat the goiter of chronic thyroiditis with levothyroxine, even in patients with normal levels of TSH, and all physicians will treat clinical hypothyroidism with levothyroxine replacement therapy.

Drugs for Hypothyroidism

Generic	Brand	Dose	Contra-indications	Primary Side Effects	Key Monitoring	Pertinent Drug Interactions	Med Pearl	Top 200
Mechanism of action – T4 is converted to T3 and exerts many metabolic effects through control of DNA transcription and protein synthesis								
Levothyroxine (T4)	• Synthroid • Levoxyl • Levothroid • Unithroid	• Inj. powder: 0.2 and 0.5 mg • Tab: 25–300 mcg	• Recent myocardial infarction or thyrotoxicosis • Uncorrected adrenal insufficiency	• Angina • Anxiety • Alopecia • LFTs increased • Tachycardia	• TSH • T3 • T4 • Free T4 • Heart rate • Blood pressure • Weight	• Some drugs will decrease absorption: cholestyramine, aluminum-containing, sucralfate, Kayexalate, Phenytoin, carbamazepine, rifampin may decrease levothyroxine levels	• T4: not the active compound; must be converted to T3 to become active • Thyroid treatment: used to augment depression treatment	Yes
Liothyronine (T3)	Cytomel	• Inj. powder: 10 mcg/mL • Tab: 5–100 mcg					• Narrow therapeutic index drug • Often involved in drug errors	No
Desiccated thyroid T4 (80%) T3 (20%)	• Armour • Thyroid	Tab: 15–120 mg per day	• Hypersensitivity to beef or pork • Recent myocardial infarction or thyrotoxicosis • Uncorrected adrenal insufficiency				• Same as above • Origin: hog, beef, sheep • 80% T4 and 20% T3 is to mimic natural physiologic production	Yes

Storage and Administration Pearls

- Levothyroxine: Administered on an empty stomach
- Levothyroxine tabs: Protect from light and moisture
- Levothyroxine injection at room temperature (59–86°F)
- IV solution not mixed with other IV infusion solutions
- Dilute vial with 5 mL of normal saline and inject immediately

Patient Education Pearls

- Thyroid supplementation is ineffective and potentially toxic for weight reduction.

HYPERTHYROIDISM

Definitions

Hyperthyroidism includes Graves' disease, which causes most cases of hyperthyroidism, especially in young patients. This autoimmune disorder may cause exophthalmos (protrusion of the eyes) and pretibial myxedema (nodules and plaques on skin). Toxic multinodular goiter is a common cause. Other causes can be drug-induced by amiodarone or radiographic contrast media and thyroid adenomas.

Diagnosis

- Plasma TSH is the best initial diagnostic test. The TSH will be markedly suppressed (<0.1 mcg/mL).

Signs and Symptoms

- Typical symptoms: Heat intolerance, insomnia, weight loss, weakness, palpitations, oligomenorrhea, and anxiety
- Sinus tachycardia, atrial fibrillation, and exacerbation of coronary artery disease
- Brisk tendon reflexes, fine tremor, proximal weakness, stare, and eyelid lag

Guidelines

American Association of Clinical Endocrinologists, *Arch Intern Med*, no. 160 (2000): 1573–75. http://aace.com/pub/guidelines.

Guidelines Summary

Three types of therapy are available for Graves' disease: (*1*) Surgical intervention, (*2*) antithyroid drugs, and (*3*) radioactive iodine.

- In the United States, radioactive iodine is currently the treatment of choice for Graves' disease. Many clinical endocrinologists prefer an ablative dose of radioactive iodine, but some prefer use of a smaller dose in an attempt to render the patient euthyroid. Ablative therapy with radioactive iodine yields quicker resolution of the hyperthyroidism than does small-dose therapy, and thereby minimizes potential hyperthyroid-related morbidity.

- Although thyroidectomy for Graves' disease was frequently used in the past, it is now uncommonly performed in the United States unless coexistent thyroid cancer is suspected.

- Antithyroid medications methimazole and propylthiouracil have been used since the 1940s and are prescribed in an attempt to achieve a remission. The remission rates are variable, and relapses are frequent. Patients in whom remission is most likely to be achieved are those with mild hyperthyroidism and small goiters. Antithyroid drug treatment is not without the risk of adverse reactions, including minor rashes and, in rare instances, agranulocytosis and hepatitis.

Drugs for Hyperthyroidism

Mechanism of action – inhibits synthesis of thyroid hormones by blocking the oxidation of iodine in the thyroid gland

Generic	Brand	Dose	Contra-indications	Primary Side Effects	Key Monitoring	Pertinent Drug Interactions	Med Pearl	Top 200
Propylthiouracil	PTU	• Initial: 300–600 mg daily divided by TID or QID • Maintenance: 50–300 mg daily • Maximum: 1,200 mg daily	Breastfeeding	• Minor: therapy may still continue • Benign transient leukopenia (WBC <4,000/mm³, most common) • Pruritic maculopapular rashes, arthralgias, fevers	• WBC with differential • Granulocyte <250/mm³ (most severe) • LFT • TSH	Increase activity of anticoagulants	• Clinical improvement approx. 4–8 weeks • PTU is an error-prone abbreviation • Tapering doses may start once clinical improvement seen	No
Methimazole (MMI)	Tapazole	• Initial: 30–60 mg TID • Maintenance: 5–30 mg daily • Maximum: 129 mg daily	• Breastfeeding • Category D	• Greater frequency in higher doses and in children • Rashes may be treated with antihistamines • Severe side effect require discontinuation • Fever, malaise, gingivitis, sore throat, oropharyngeal infections • Aplastic anemia, lupus-like syndrome, polymyositis (rhabdomyolysis), GI intolerance, hepatotoxicity, hepatitis, hypoprothrombinemia, death	• T3 • T4	• CYP450 inhibitor • Moderate: 2D6 • Weak: 3A4, 1A2	• Alternate thioamide may be used, but cross-sensitivity is 50% • Correction of hyperthyroidism may alter disposition of beta-blockers, digoxin, and theophylline • PTU preferred in pregnancy	No

Storage and Administration Pearls

- Methimazole: Protect from light.
- On the NAPLEX and in the work force, PTU is an error-prone abbreviation and is not recommended for use on prescription pads, verbally, or within your computer system.

Patient Education Pearls

- If the patient is pregnant or is thinking about getting pregnant, it is recommended that she avoid taking Propylthiouracil and Methimazole; it crosses the placenta and is found in breast milk. PTU is preferred in pregnancy.

POLYCYSTIC OVARIAN SYNDROME (PCOS)

Definitions

Polycystic ovarian syndrome (PCOS) is a metabolic disorder involving infertility, hirsutism, obesity, and amenorrhea. The fundamental defect of PCOS is unknown but is thought to be from adrenal androgen excess of obesity, which results in enhanced extraglandular formation of estrogen. The dysfunctional uterine bleeding is usually due to estrogen excess.

Diagnosis

- History and physical examination, including the onset and duration of various signs of androgen excess; menstrual history; family history of diabetes and cardiovascular disease; lifestyle factors; evaluation of blood pressure, body mass index, and waist-hip ratio; and presence of acne, hirsutism, androgenic alopecia, and acanthosis nigricans
- Laboratory tests, including documentation of biochemical hyperandrogenemia (total testosterone and/or bioavailable or free testosterone); exclusion of other causes of hyperandrogenism, such as thyroid dysfunction, hyperprolactinemia, nonclassical congenital adrenal hyperplasia, and Cushing's syndrome; evaluation for metabolic abnormalities; and fasting lipid and lipoprotein level
- Optional tests to consider:
  - Ultrasound evaluation of ovaries
  - Gonadotropin determinations
  - Fasting insulin levels
  - 24-hour urine test

Signs & Symptoms

- Infertility: Inability to become pregnant
- Hirsutism: Caused by excess androgen levels
- Obesity: BMI >29
- Anovulation: Lack of ovulation; however, the woman may experience withdrawal bleeding after progestogen administration

Guidelines

American College of Obstetricians and Gynecologists, Medical Specialty Society. (December 2002). www.acog.org

Guidelines Summary

Treatment is based on a symptoms approach for anovulation, amenorrhea, ovulation induction, and hirsutism.

Anovulation and Amenorrhea

- Combination oral contraceptives are often used to regulate or restore irregular or absent menses.
- Weight-reduction programs are important, and they affect and improve insulin resistance.
- Progestin, including medroxyprogesterone acetate, is often used to induce menses.
- Insulin-sensitizing agents, including metformin, pioglitazone, and rosiglitazone, are used to reduce insulin resistance.

Ovulation Induction

- Lifestyle modifications, especially weight loss, will assist with ovulation induction.
- Clomiphene citrate is used to induce ovulation for up to six months.
- Ovarian drilling with laser or diathermy can be considered but is not recommended.
- Insulin-sensitizing agents, such as metformin and thiazolidinediones, can induce ovulation.

Hirsutism

- Oral contraceptives can reduce hair growth.
- Antiandrogens, including spironolactone, flutamide, and insulin-sensitizing agents, and Eflornithine can be used to reduce hair growth.
- Mechanical hair removal, such as shaving, plucking, waxing, depilatory creams, electrolysis, and laser vaporization, can also be used.

Drugs for Polycystic Ovarian Syndrome

Generic	Brand	Dose	Contraindications	Primary Side Effects	Key Monitoring	Pertinent Drug Interactions	Med Pearl	Top 200
Mechanism of action – inhibits secretion of pituitary gonadotropins, which prevents follicular maturation and ovulation; causes endometrial thinning								
Medroxyprogesterone	Provera	Amenorrhea: 5–10 mg x 10 days	• History of deep venous thrombosis, pulmonary embolism • Pregnancy	• Headaches • Weight changes • Edema • Menstrual irregularities	• Pregnancy should be ruled out • Symptoms of migraine	• CYP450 • Induces 3A4	Long-term use can lead to loss of bone mineral density	No
Mechanism of action – Enclomiphene is less potent in inducing ovulation; however, it is rapidly absorbed to be metabolized, allowing for the more potent zuclomiphene to act. Zuclomiphene – inhibits normal estrogen negative feedback, which results in release of LH and FSH. More potent than enclomiphene								
Clomiphene citrate* – zuclomiphene (38%) – enclomiphene (62%)	Clomid	50–100 mg	• Liver disease • Abnormal uterine bleeding • Ovarian cysts • Uncontrolled thyroid or adrenal dysfunction • Pregnancy Category X	• Ovarian enlargement • Hot flashes • Breast discomfort • Nausea • Bloating	• Pregnancy test • Menstrual cycle		Dosages of 150 mg or greater do not improve symptoms for PCOS	No
Mechanism of action – competes with aldosterone receptor sites in the distal tubules								
Spironolactone	Aldactone	50–200 mg	• Acute renal failure • Hyperkalemia • Pregnancy C/D	• Gynecomastia (men) • Hyperkalemia • Nausea, cramping	• Blood pressure • Renal function • Potassium	May reduce the inotropic (contraction) effect of digoxin and mitotane.	• Needs to be renally adjusted • RALES study showed 25 mg decreased heart failure events	Yes
Mechanism of action – nonsteroidal antiandrogen that inhibits androgen uptake or inhibits binding to androgen in target tissue								
Flutamide	Eulexin	125–250 mg	• Severe hepatic impairment • Pregnancy D	• Gynecomastia • Hot flashes • Breast tenderness • Galactorrhea • Libido decreased	LFTs monthly for 4 months, then periodically	• CYP450 • inhibits 1A2	• Black Box warning – Liver failure within 3 months of taking flutamide	No

*Racemic mixture

Drugs for Polycystic Ovarian Syndrome *(cont'd)*

Generic	Brand	Dose	Contraindications	Primary Side Effects	Key Monitoring	Pertinent Drug Interactions	Med Pearl	Top 200
Mechanism of action – inhibitor of 5-alpha reductase which results in the inhibition of the conversion of testosterone to dihydrotestosterone								
Finasteride	• Proscar • Propecia	1–5 mg/day	Pregnancy X Hirsutism	• Impotence • Ejaculation disturbances • Testicular pain	Absolute need for dual forms of birth control	• CYP450 • substrate 3A4	• Category X in pregnancy (abnormalities of external male genitalia were reported in animal studies) • High-alert medication	Yes
Mechanism of action – inhibits ornithine decarboxylase (ODC), the rate-limiting enzyme in biosynthesis of putrescine, spermin, and spermidine (rapid dividing cell most susceptible)								
Eflornithine	Vaniqa	Cream (facial hair)	Hypersensitivity	• Acne • Pruritus • Alopecia	CBC and platelets (systemic only)	• Cream could interact with other creams		No

Storage and Administration Pearls

- Finasteride needs to be protected from light.
- Spironolactone needs to be protected from light.

Patient Education Pearls

- Prolonged use of medroxyprogesterone contraception injection may result in a loss of bone mineral density (BMD).

LEARNING POINTS

- The basic diagnoses for type 1 and type 2 diabetes are identical. However, patients with type 2 will go undiagnosed for as long as 10 years; whereas type 1 is usually diagnosed within 6 months. As a result, it is important to consider and assess risk factors for type 2 diabetes.
- For the NAPLEX, it is important that you understand the different mechanisms of action of the diabetes medications to ensure you can catch duplication of actions within the patient's drug profile.
- Hypothyroidism and hyperthyroidism have opposite side effects (i.e., somnolence with hypothyroid; insomnia with hyperthyroidism).
- PCOS has become more common as obesity rates have risen and as more women want to become pregnant.
- Remember, many women with diabetes may have PCOS and may be placed on an insulin sensitizer such as a glitazone. As a result, it is important to counsel the patient on an increased risk for ovulation if her uterus is still intact.

PRACTICE QUESTIONS

1. All of the following are used to treat conditions of hyperthyroidism EXCEPT

   (A) Propylthiouracil (PTU).
   (B) Methimazole (MMI).
   (C) Propranolol.
   (D) Lugol's solution.
   (E) Cytomel.

2. Patients with overactive thyroid may present with which of the following symptoms?

   (A) Weight loss
   (B) Heat intolerance
   (C) Heart palpitations
   (D) Goiter
   (E) All of the above

3. Which of the following statements is/are TRUE?

   I. T3 = Triiodothyronine = active form
   II. T4 = Thyroxine = converted to T3
   III. Thyroid peridoxase, tyrosine, and iodine all play a role in the thyroid hormone system.

   (A) I only
   (B) III only
   (C) I and II
   (D) II and III
   (E) I, II, and III

4. Which of the following conditions is/are associated with elevated thyroid hormone levels?

   I. Thyrotoxicosis
   II. Graves' disease
   III. Hashimoto's disease

   (A) I only
   (B) III only
   (C) I and II
   (D) II and III
   (E) I, II, and III

5. A patient comes to the pharmacy and tells you that her blood sugars were 126 and 127 mg/dL fasting on two occasions. She wants some advice because her doctor didn't have time to talk with her. What is the main point you will be addressing with this woman?

    (A) This patient does not have diabetes because the doctor did the same test.
    (B) This patient has diabetes but it's not bad and will not need medication.
    (C) This patient has diabetes but does not need education; she should just watch what she eats and exercise more.
    (D) This patient doesn't have diabetes but might develop it soon.
    (E) This patient has diabetes, needs a formal diabetes education class, and is likely a candidate for a medication called metformin.

6. How many days can a Humalog stay out of the refrigerator and be considered safe to administer?

    (A) 1 day
    (B) 28 days
    (C) 56 days
    (D) 90 days
    (E) 180 days

ANSWERS

1. **E**

Cytomel, or T3, is the active form of thyroid hormone and should not be used if the patient has an overactive thyroid. It is used in hypothyroidism to stimulate thyroid hormone production. The other answer choices are all used in the treatment of hyperthyroidism.

2. **E**

Weight loss, heat intolerance, heart palpitations, and goiter are all commonly seen symptoms with hyperthyroid disorders. Other common symptoms include nervousness, emotional lability, bowel frequency, irregular menses, and increased appetite.

3. **E**

T3, or triiodothyronine, is the active form of thyroid hormone. T4, or thyroxine, is the bound form of thyroid hormone and must be converted into triiodothyronine to be active. Iodide + tyrosine + thyroid peroxidase is converted to iodotyrosine, which in turn forms triiodothyronine and thyroxine.

4. **C**

Thyrotoxicosis, or hyperthyroidism, is caused by excessive levels of T3 or T4 or both. Graves' disease is an autoimmune disorder in which TSH (thyroid-stimulating hormone) is stimulated in the body. Hashimoto's disease (III), however, is the most common form of spontaneous hypothyroidism.

5. **E**

This patient has diabetes and needs a formal diabetes education class. The newest guidelines suggest starting all eligible patients on metformin at the time of diagnosis. Choice (A) is not correct because this woman does have diabetes—her fasting blood sugar was verified and was ≥126 mg/dL. Although the doctor caught the disease early, the patient still needs to seek formal education as this will lead to the best management.

6. **B**

Most unopened insulin preparations are stable at normal temperatures for 28 days. They should not be used if frozen or exposed to temperature greater than 98.6°F. Once opened (in use), vials may be stored in the refrigerator or for up to 28 days at room temperature.

Neurological Disorders

5

This chapter covers the following disease states:

- **Multiple sclerosis**
- **Epilepsy**
- **Parkinson's disease**
- **Migraine headache**

 Suggested Study Time: **45 minutes**

MULTIPLE SCLEROSIS

Definitions

Multiple sclerosis (MS) is a disease of the central nervous system (CNS) characterized by inflammation within the brain and spinal cord that results in areas of plaque formation and sclerosis and leads to neurological symptoms. The basic pathophysiological defect in MS is the demyelinization of the sheath surrounding the neurons in the CNS.

Diagnosis

The diagnosis of MS is primarily based on clinical presentation and requires two or more episodes of neurologic symptoms that: (*1*) Cannot be attributed to another cause, (*2*) represent distinct areas of CNS involvement, and (*3*) occur at least three months apart. The McDonald criteria are often used to diagnose MS. These criteria do require two lesions separated by three months but allow for the use of magnetic resonance imaging (MRI) and cerebrospinal fluid analysis to be used as identification of a second attack. The MRI is a useful tool for confirming diagnosis of MS because it is highly selective for MS lesions.

Signs and Symptoms

- The most common symptoms of early MS include weakness/numbness of limbs and visual disturbances. The clinical presentation of MS varies among patients and is classified as relapsing-remitting, primary progressive, or secondary progressive.

- Relapsing-remitting MS is most common (85%) and is characterized by frequent symptomatic episodes of ≥24 hours' duration followed by periods of remission of at least 30 days. During remission, residual symptoms and increasing clinical deficit are common.

- Primary progressive MS occurs in ~10% of patients and consists of persistently progressive disease from the time of disease onset that does not include remissions or relapses. This classification is associated with a poor prognosis.

- Secondary progressive MS occurs in about 5% of patients and consists of few exacerbations, no permanent disability, and gradual worsening of neurological symptoms. Many patients originally classified as relapsing-remitting may be reclassified as secondary progressive during the course of illness.

Guidelines

Medical Advisory Board of the National Multiple Sclerosis Society 2005. Disease Management Consensus Statement Expert Opinion Paper. www.nationalmssociety.org.

Guidelines Summary

The clinical management of MS should include consideration of treatment for acute exacerbations, retarding disease process, and alleviating ongoing symptoms related to the disease.

Disease-modifying drugs (DMDs) are used to alter the disease process and should be initiated as soon as possible after diagnosis. Therapies should be continued indefinitely except in the case of intolerable side effects, clear lack of benefit, or new therapy considerations.

Acute exacerbations — The cornerstone of therapy for acute exacerbations is IV corticosteroids. Methylprednisolone is most commonly used at 50–100 mg/day for three to ten days. Oral prednisone may also be considered, but there is not strong evidence for this route. Although corticosteroids have been shown to be very effective in the treatment of acute exacerbations, they do not alter the disease process.

Altering disease process — DMDs are the therapy of choice in altering the MS disease process. There are currently five approved DMDs: interferon-β1a (Avonex and Rebif), interferon-β1b (Betaseron), glatiramer acetate (Copaxone), natalizumab (Tysabri), and mitoxantrone (Novantrone).

- The interferon agents and glatiramer acetate are considered first-line DMDs, while natalizumab is reserved for patients who do not respond to those therapies.
- Mitoxantrone is the only available agent that is approved to treat worsening relapsing-remitting MS and progressive MS.
- Patients are generally treated with one DMD at a time, but worsening disease can be treated with combination DMD + mitoxantrone pulse therapy.

Disease-Modifying Drugs

Disease-Modifying Drugs

Mechanism of action – Interferon β: anti-inflammatory and immunomodulatory effects are exerted through binding of interferon to human cell-surface receptors and subsequent decreased T-cell production of pro-inflammatory cytokines, decreased production of pro-inflammatory lymphocytes, and increased production of anti-inflammatory lymphocytes.

Generic	Brand	Dose & Max	Contra-indications	Primary Side Effects	Key Monitoring Parameters	Pertinent Drug Interactions	Med Pearls	Top 200
Interferon-β1a	• Avonex intramuscular injection • Rebif subcutaneous injection	30 mcg IM 1 x week 8.8 mcg SC TIW–44 mcg SC TIW	• Hypersensitivity • Severe depression	Influenza-like symptoms (fever, chills, fatigue, muscle aches); injection site reactions; mild anemia; thrombocyto-penia; liver damage; depression	• Liver transaminases periodically; response to therapy; presence of adverse effects; periodic complete blood count (CBC)	May decrease efficacy of vaccinations	• Acetaminophen or NSAIDs can decrease influenza-like symptoms • Neutralizing antibodies may develop, rendering the drug less efficacious	No
Interferon-β1b	• Betaseron subcutaneous injection	0.25 mg SC QOD	• Hypersensitivity • Severe depression	Influenza-like symptoms (fever, chills, fatigue, muscle aches); injection site reactions; mild anemia; thrombocyto-penia; liver damage; depression	• Liver transaminases periodically; response to therapy; presence of adverse effects; periodic complete blood count (CBC)	May decrease efficacy of vaccinations	• Acetaminophen or NSAIDs can decrease influenza-like symptoms • Neutralizing antibodies may develop, rendering the drug less efficacious	No

Mechanism of action – Glatiramer acetate: influences immature CD4 cells to become less inflammatory, thereby suppressing demyelination and preventing nerve fiber damage

Generic	Brand	Dose & Max	Contra-indications	Primary Side Effects	Key Monitoring Parameters	Pertinent Drug Interactions	Med Pearls	Top 200
Glatiramer acetate	Copaxone subcutaneous injection	20 mg SC daily	Hypersensitivity to the drug or to mannitol	Injection site reactions; post-injection reaction (chest pain, palpitations)	• Response to therapy	None known	Does not produce neutralizing antibodies	No

Disease-Modifying Drugs *(cont'd)*

Mechanism of action – Natalizumab: monoclonal antibody inhibits pro-inflammatory interactions within vascular endothelial cells and parenchymal brain cells.

Generic	Brand	Dose & Max	Contra-indications	Primary Side Effects	Key Monitoring Parameters	Pertinent Drug Interactions	Med Pearls	Top 200
Natalizumab	Tysabri intravenous infusion	300 mg IV infusion every 4 wks	Hypersensitivity	Infusion reactions are common (rash, drowsiness, fever, chills, hypotension, nausea, shortness of breath); headache, fatigue, urinary tract infection, joint pain, abdominal discomfort Rare, potentially fatal ADE – progressive multifocal leukoencephalopathy (PML)	• MRI at baseline, 3 mos, 6 mos, liver enzymes periodically	Interferon β products decrease natalizumab clearance; other DMDs increase risk of PML	• Reserved for patients who have not responded to other DMDs; should be used as monotherapy *only*; combining with other DMDs increases risk of PML • Available only through a restrictive prescribing program – TOUCH	No

Mechanism of action – Mitoxantrone decreases migration of T cells into the CNS by arresting the cell cycle and interfering with DNA repair and RNA synthesis

Generic	Brand	Dose & Max	Contra-indications	Primary Side Effects	Key Monitoring Parameters	Pertinent Drug Interactions	Med Pearls	Top 200
Mitoxantrone	Novantrone IV infusion	12 mg/m² IV infusion every 3 mos; max cumulative dose of 140 mg/m²	LVEF <50%; hypersensitivity	Cardiac toxicity (heart failure, decreased LVEF); nausea; leukopenia; alopecia; menstrual irregularities; urinary and respiratory infections	• LVEF at baseline and prior to each IV infusion • Periodic CBC	Natalizumab (combination increases risk of PML)	Black Box warning on cardiac risks and need for frequent LVEF monitoring	No

Storage and Administration Pearls

- Interferon β1a, Interferon β1b, glatiramer acetate, natalizumab, and mitoxantrone should be refrigerated to 2–8°C (36° to 46°F). These products should not be frozen and should be protected from light.

- Interferon β1 products and glatiramer acetate are available in prefilled syringes.

- Interferon β1 products and glatiramer acetate can be self-administered. Natalizumab and mitoxantrone are administered via IV infusion by qualified healthcare professionals.

Patient Education Pearls

- For self-injectable therapies:
  - Use the auto-injector supplied by the manufacturer (when available).
  - Apply ice to the injection site prior to injection.
  - Allow the medication to reach room temperature prior to injection.
  - Rotate injection sites.
- For those newly initiated on therapy, a Natalizumab medication guide should be provided. Both patient and provider must be enrolled in TOUCH prescribing program.

EPILEPSY

Definitions

Epilepsy is a symptom of disturbed electrical activity within the brain. Epilepsy is a general term that encompasses a wide variety of symptomatic presentations that include periodic and recurrent seizures with or without convulsions. Seizures are classified as partial, generalized, or status epilepticus.

Partial seizures begin in one hemisphere of the brain and result in symptoms that are asymmetrical. Partial seizures can be classified as simple (no impairment of consciousness), complex (with impaired consciousness), or secondarily generalized (partial onset which becomes generalized).

Generalized seizures are bilateral/symmetrical in symptoms and can be classified as absence, myoclonic, clonic, tonic, tonic-clonic, atonic, or infantile spasms. The most common types are absence and tonic-clonic.

Diagnosis

The diagnosis of epilepsy is based on comprehensive history and physical, electroencephalography (EEG), and brain imaging by CT scan or MRI. Differential diagnosis is important with exclusion of potential underlying causes of seizure including metabolic abnormalities (ruled out with evaluation of routine laboratory chemistries), traumatic head injury (determined by history), and presence of underlying structural abnormalities such as tumor (ruled out through brain imaging studies).

Signs and Symptoms

The clinical presentation of epilepsy is dependent upon the classification of seizure type.

- Partial seizures result in asymmetrical alterations in motor function and in sensory or somato-sensory symptoms, and may or may not involve a loss of consciousness. Nervous ticks, aberrations of normal behavior, and memory loss are also possible.
- Generalized seizures have symptoms that indicate involvement of both hemispheres of the brain. Motor symptoms are bilateral and there is a loss of consciousness.
- Absence seizures manifest as sudden interruption of ongoing activities, a blank stare, or an upward rotation of the eyes. Tonic-clonic seizures consist of sharp tonic muscle contractions, rigidity, and clonic movement that are accompanied by a loss of consciousness and may be preceded by an aura.

Guidelines

Efficacy and tolerability of the new antiepileptic drugs I: treatment of new onset epilepsy: report of the Therapeutics and Technology Assessment Subcommittee and Quality Standards Subcommittee of the American Academy of Neurology and the American Epilepsy Society. Neurology, no. 62 (8) (2004): 1252–60. www.guideline.gov/summary/summary.aspx?ss=15&doc_id=5183&nbr=3565.

Guidelines Summary

- Goals of treatment include a lack of seizure activity, minimal medication side effects of treatment, and improved quality of life.
- Treatment with anti-epileptic drugs (AEDs) is warranted for patients that experience multiple seizures or have significantly affected quality of life. AED choice is based on the specific seizure type, the patient's age, comorbidities, ability to adhere to the regimen, and insurance coverage.
- AED monotherapy is preferred, but some patients do require combination therapy.

- First-line AEDs for partial seizures include carbamazepine, phenytoin, lamotrigine, valproic acid, and oxcarbazepine.

- First-line AEDs for generalized absence seizures include valproic acid and ethosuximide.

- First-line AEDs for tonic-clonic seizures include phenytoin, carbamazepine, and valproic acid.

- Alternative AEDs include gabapentin, topiramate, levetiracetam, zonisamide, tiagabine, primidone, felbamate, lamotrigine, and phenobarbital.

Anti-Epileptic Drugs

Generic	Brand	Dose & Max mg (frequency)	Contra-indications	Primary Side Effects	Key Monitoring Parameters	Med Pearls	Top 200
Mechanism of action – Carbamazepine inhibits voltage-gated sodium channels, thereby depressing electrical transmission in the nucleus ventralis anterior of the thalamus							
Carbamazepine	Tegretol	200–1,200 mg daily (BID)	Bone marrow suppression, porphyria, hypersensitivity	• Dizziness, drowsiness, unsteadiness, nausea, vomiting • Rare: aplastic anemia, agranulocytosis	CBC periodically	First line for partial seizures and generalized tonic-clonic seizures.	Yes
Mechanism of action – valproic acid: not fully understood, thought to increase gamma amino butyric acid (GABA) concentrations in the brain							
Valproic acid (divalproex sodium)	• Depakote, • Depakote ER • Depakene • Depacon	10–60 mg/kg/day	• Hepatic dysfunction • Hypersensitivity • Urea cycle disorders	• Hepatic impairment • Thrombocytopenia • Hyperammonemia • Weight gain • Pancreatitis	• Serum drug concentrations (50–100 mcg/mL) • Liver function tests at baseline and periodically • Periodic CBC and serum ammonia levels	• First line for partial, generalized, tonic-clonic, and absence seizures. • Highly teratogenic • Available in oral capsules, tablets, extended-release tablets, sprinkle caps, oral syrup, and IV solution	Yes
Mechanism of action – Phenytoin: promotes neuronal sodium efflux, thereby stabilizing the threshold against hyperexcitability							
Phenytoin	Dilantin	300–600 mg daily (divided TID)	Hypersensitivity	• Nystagmus, ataxia, slurred speech, dizziness, insomnia, headache, tremor, gingival hyperplasia • Rare: Stevens-Johnson rash	Serum drug concentrations (10–20 mcg/mL)	• First line option for partial and generalized tonic-clonic seizures • Abrupt discontinuation should be avoided. This may precipitate status epilepticus • Takes 7–10 days to reach steady state	Yes
Mechanism of action – depresses motor cortex and elevates the threshold of the CNS to convulsive stimuli							
Ethosuximide	Zarontin	250–1,500 mg daily	Hypersensitivity	• Ataxia • Drowsiness • GI upset • Blood dyscrasias • Rash (Stevens-Johnson possible)	• Periodic CBC • Response to therapy • Presence of adverse effects	Available as capsules or syrup; used *only* for absence seizure	No

Anti-Epileptic Drugs *(cont'd)*

Generic	Brand	Dose & Max mg (frequency)	Contra-indications	Primary Side Effects	Key Monitoring Parameters	Med Pearls	Top 200
Mechanism of action – blocks voltage-sensitive sodium channels, resulting in stabilization of hyperexcitable neuronal membranes							
Oxcarbazepine	Trileptal tablets and oral suspension	600–2,400 mg daily (BID)	Hypersensitivity	Sedation, dizziness, ataxia, nausea, rash (Stevens Johnson possible), hyponatremia,	Periodic Na, renal function; serum concentrations 12–30 mcg/ml	CrCl < 30 ml/min requires half of initial dose	Yes
Felbamate	Felbatol	1,200–3,600 mg daily (TID-QID)	• Hypersensitivity • Blood dyscrasias • Liver dysfunction	• Aplastic anemia • Acute lever failure • Anorexia • Nausea, vomiting • Insomnia • Headache	• Frequent CBC • Frequent liver transaminases	• AST or ALT >2 x ULN requires discontinuation • Not a first-line agent; reserved for refractory cases	No
Mechanism of action – although structurally similar to GABA, pharmacological effects in epilepsy are not fully understood							
Gabapentin	• Neurontin • Tablets, capsules, oral solution	900–3,600 mg daily (TID)	Hypersensitivity	• Dizziness • Fatigue • Somnolence • Ataxia • Weight gain	Response to therapy; presence of adverse effects	• No known drug interactions • Renal dose adjustment necessary when CrCl <60 mL/min	Yes
Mechanism of action – inhibition of voltage-sensitive sodium channels, thereby stabilizing neuronal membranes and decreasing hyperexcitability to convulsive stimuli							
Lamotrigine	• Lamictal • Oral tablets, chewable tablets	25–700 mg daily (once to BID)	Hypersensitivity, history of Stevens-Johnson rash	Stevens-Johnson rash, other rash, diplopia, dizziness, headache	Response to therapy, presence of side effects	• Risk of rash increased when combined with VPA • First-line option for partial seizures • Slow dose titration necessary	Yes
Mechanism of action – blocks voltage-dependent sodium channels, augments GABA activity, antagonizes glutamate receptors							
Topiramate	• Topamax • Tablets and sprinkle caps	25–400 mg daily (BID)	Hypersensitivity	Difficulty concentrating, psychomotor slowing, speech problems, somnolence, fatigue, dizziness, headache, weight loss, kidney stones	Response to therapy, presence of side effects	Adjunctive therapy in patients with partial seizures Slow titration necessary to avoid adverse effects	Yes

Anti-Epileptic Drugs *(cont'd)*

Generic	Brand	Dose & Max mg (frequency)	Contra-indications	Primary Side Effects	Key Monitoring Parameters	Med Pearls	Top 200
Mechanism of action – not well understood							
Levetiracetam	• Keppra • Tablets, oral solution, parenteral solution	1,000–3,000 mg daily (BID)	Hypersensitivity	Dizziness, asthenia, behavioral disturbances (hostility, nervousness); somnolence, infection	Response to therapy, presence of side effects, renal function	• No known drug interactions • Dose adjustment required in renal impairment (CrCl <80 mL/min) • Adjunctive therapy for partial seizures and for generalized tonic-clonic seizures	Yes
Mechanism of action – elevates seizure threshold by decreasing postsynaptic excitability through stimulation of postsynaptic GABA inhibitory responses							
Phenobarbital	• Solfoton • Tablets, capsules, elixir • Luminal intravenous injection	60–600 mg daily	Severe liver impairment, hypersensitivity, porphyria	Sedation, nystagmus, ataxia, hyperactivity, headache, nausea, blood dyscrasias (agranulocytosis, granulocytopenia), rash, behavior changes, intellectual blunting, mood change	Serum concentrations, 10–40 mcg/mL; periodic CBC; periodic LFTs	• Drug of choice for neonatal seizures; otherwise, adjunctive therapy for partial and generalized (other than absence) seizures. • Frequency of side effects limits use • Titrate dose slowly to minimize adverse effects. • Avoid abrupt discontinuation • Takes 3–4 wks to reach steady-state	Yes
Primidone	Mysoline	125–2,000 mg daily (TID-QID)			Serum concentrations, 5–10 mcg/mL; periodic CBC; periodic LFTs	• Metabolized to Phenobarbital • Avoid abrupt discontinuation	No
Mechanism of action – potent and specific inhibitor of GABA uptake into neuronal elements, thereby enhances GABA activity by decreasing its removal from the neuronal space							
Tiagabine	Gabitril	4–80 mg daily (BID–QID)	Hypersensitivity	Dizziness, fatigue, difficulty concentrating, nervousness, tremor, blurred vision, depression, weakness	Response to therapy, presence of adverse effects	• Adjunctive therapy in partial seizures. • Do not abruptly discontinue; taper dose	No

Anti-Epileptic Drugs *(cont'd)*

Generic	Brand	Dose & Max mg (frequency)	Contra-indications	Primary Side Effects	Key Monitoring Parameters	Med Pearls	Top 200
Mechanism of action – blocks voltage-dependent sodium and calcium channels, thereby reducing repetitive neuronal firing							
Zonisamide	Zonegran	100–600 mg daily	Hypersensitivity to zonisamide or sulfonamides	Sedation, dizziness, cognitive impairment, nausea, rash (Stevens-Johnson possible), oligohidrosis	Serum drug concentrations 10–40 mcg/mL (not routine)	• Adjunctive therapy in partial seizures • Takes up to 2 wks to achieve steady-state	No

AED Drug Interactions

AED	Interacting Medication	Effect
Carbamazepine	Felbamate	↓ Carbamazepine
	Phenobarbital	↓ Carbamazepine
	Phenytoin	↓ Carbamazepine
	Cimetidine	↑ Carbamazepine
	Erythromycin	↑ Carbamazepine
	Fluoxetine	↑ Carbamazepine
	Isoniazid	↑ Carbamazepine
	Propoxyphene	↑ Carbamazepine
	Oral contraceptives	↓ Contraceptives
	Doxycycline	↓ Doxycycline
	Theophylline	↓ Theophylline
	Warfarin	↓ Warfarin
VPA	Carbamazepine	↓ VPA
	Lamotrigine	↓ VPA
	Phenobarbital	↓ VPA
	Primidone	↓ VPA
	Phenytoin	↓ VPA
	Cimetidine	↑ VPA
	Salicylates	↑ VPA
	Oral contraceptives	↓ Contraceptives
Phenytoin	Carbamazepine	↓ Phenytoin
	Felbamate	↑ Phenytoin
	Phenobarbital	↑ or ↓ Phenytoin
	VPA	↓ Phenytoin
	Antacids	↓ Phenytoin
	Cimetidine	↑ Phenytoin
	Chloramphenicol	↑ Phenytoin
	Disulfiram	↑ Phenytoin
	Ethanol (acute)	↑ Phenytoin
	Ethanol (chronic)	↑ Phenytoin
	Warfarin	↑ Phenytoin
	Propoxyphene	↑ Phenytoin
	Fluconazole	↑ Phenytoin
	Isoniazid	↑ Phenytoin
	Oral contraceptives	↓ Contraceptives
	Folic acid	↓ Folic acid
	Quinidine	↓ Quinidine
Oxcarbazepine	Carbamazepine	↓ Oxcarbazepine
	Phenytoin	↓ Oxcarbazepine
	Phenobarbital	↓ Oxcarbazepine
	Oral contraceptives	↓ Contraceptives
Felbamate	Carbamazepine	↓ Felbamate
	Phenytoin	↓ Felbamate
	VPA	↑ Felbamate

AED Drug Interactions *(cont'd)*

AED	Interacting Medication	Effect
Lamotrigine	Carbamazepine Phenobarbital Phenytoin Primidone VPA	↓ Lamotrigine ↓ Lamotrigine ↓ Lamotrigine ↓ Lamotrigine ↑ Lamotrigine
Topiramate	Carbamazepine Phenytoin VPA Oral contraceptives	↓ Topiramate ↓ Topiramate ↓ Topiramate ↓ Contraceptives
Phenobarbital	Felbamate Phenytoin VPA Acetazolamide Oral contraceptives	↑ Phenobarbital ↑ Phenobarbital ↑ Phenobarbital ↑ Phenobarbital ↓ Contraceptives
Primidone	Carbamazepine Phenytoin VPA Isoniazid Nicotinamide Chlorpromazine Corticosteroids Quinidine Tricyclics	↓ Primidone, ↑ Phenobarbital ↓ Primidone, ↑ Phenobarbital ↑ Primidone, ↓ Phenobarbital ↑ Primidone, ↓ Phenobarbital ↑ Primidone, ↓ Phenobarbital ↓ Chlorpromazine ↓ Corticosteroids ↓ Quinidine ↓ Tricyclics
Tiagabine	Carbamazepine Phenytoin	↓ Tiagabine ↓ Tiagabine
Zonisamide	Carbamazepine Phenytoin Phenobarbital	↓ Zonisamide ↓ Zonisamide ↓ Zonisamide

Storage and Administration Pearls

- Valproic acid: Extended-release divalproex sodium should be swallowed whole and should not be chewed, crushed, or split. Divalproex sodium sprinkle caps may be swallowed whole or may be opened and sprinkled on a small amount (~ teaspoon) of soft food, such as pudding or applesauce.

- Phenytoin: Available in chewable tablets, capsules, extended-release capsules, oral suspension and parenteral solution (IM or IV).

- Oxcarbazepine oral suspension should be shaken well before administration and should be used within 7 weeks of opening the bottle.

Patient Education Pearls

- Anti-epileptic medication should not be abruptly discontinued, as this may result in increased and emergent seizure activity.

- Any skin rash that develops should be reported to a healthcare provider immediately.

- When taking any new medications, patients should consult with their pharmacist, as multiple drug interactions are possible.

PARKINSON'S DISEASE

Definitions

Parkinson's disease (PD) is a syndrome characterized by tremor, rigidity, bradykinesia, and/or postural instability caused by a progressive depletion of dopamine neurons in the substantia nigra of the basal ganglia. Symptoms are a result of the dopamine deficiency and subsequent relative acetylcholine excess.

Diagnosis

Diagnosis of PD is based on careful clinical history and physical exam. There are no agreed-upon objective or definitive lab or imaging criteria for diagnosis.

Signs and Symptoms

PD has an insidious onset and begins with nonspecific symptoms such as malaise and fatigue. Tremor is generally the first of the cardinal signs and is generally unilateral and occurring at rest rather than upon intention. Rigidity of the limbs manifests as resistance to passive movement of the joints, and bradykinesia as slow movements or difficulty moving. Symptoms generally begin unilaterally and progress asymmetrically.

Summary of Treatment Recommendations

- Initial therapy generally consists of either a dopamine agonist or carbidopa/levodopa.
  - Patients ≥65 years of age or those with significant disability due to their PD should receive carbidopa/levodopa as initial therapy.
  - Patients <65 years of age should receive a dopamine agonist as initial therapy.
  - Inadequate response to maximum tolerable doses of initial therapy with a dopamine agonist or levodopa should result in the addition of the alternate medication.
  - Subsequently, COMT inhibitors may be added to ongoing levodopa therapy, and adjunctive therapies such as amantadine or anticholinergics may be utilized.
  - Anticholinergic agents are primarily useful for the treatment of tremor- predominant PD but should be used with caution in elderly patients and avoided in patients with pre-existing cognitive impairment.
  - Because dopamine agonists and levodopa therapies are aimed at increasing the available dopamine in the CNS, side effects such as hallucinations and delusions are possible. Psychiatric side effects which occur at the lowest effective doses of these drugs may be treated with antipsychotic medications such as clozapine or quetiapine.

Drugs for Parkinson's Disease

Generic	Brand	Dose & Max	Contra-indications	Primary Side Effects	Key Monitoring Parameters	Pertinent Drug Interactions	Med Pearls	Top 200
Mechanism of action – antiviral that blocks the uncoating of influenza A virus, preventing penetration of virus into host								
Amantadine	Symmetrel	200–300 mg daily	Hypersensitivity	• Confusion, nightmares, hallucinations, insomnia, nervousness, irritability	Response to therapy, presence of adverse effects	• Quinidine and triamterene increase plasma amantadine concentrations	Renal dose adjustment necessary for CrCl <30 mL/min	No
Mechanism of action – monoamine-oxidase (MAO) B inhibitors: inhibit the catabolism of dopamine by selectively inhibiting the monoamine oxidase B enzyme								
Selegiline	• Eldepryl: Tablets • Emsam: transdermal patch • Zelapar: disintegrating tablets	5–10 mg daily (once to BID)	Hypersensitivity; use of meperidine or other opioids	Nausea, hallucinations, insomnia, depression, orthostasis, arrhythmia Rare: hypertensive crisis (if high-tyramine foods are ingested)		• Avoid use with meperide, other opioid analgesics, or dextromethorphan; may result in fatal increased activity of analgesics. • Co-administration with other serotonergic agents risk of serotonin syndrome	• Avoid tyramine-containing foods. • Discontinue 14 days prior to surgery if possible; should not be taken with general anesthesia	No
Rasagiline	Azilect	0.5–1 mg daily						
Mechanism of action – Levodopa is a direct precursor to dopamine and is converted to dopamine once it crosses the blood-brain barrier; Carbidopa is a dopa decarboxylase inhibitor, and it is necessary to combine this with levodopa in order to prevent the peripheral degradation of levodopa prior to entry into the blood-brain barrier.								
Carbidopa/ levodopa	• Sinemet • Sinemet CR • Parcopa: Orally disintegrating tablets	• Carbidopa 75–300 mg daily (75 mg required, side effects if >300 mg day) • Levodopa 100–2,000 mg daily (individualized)	Hypersensitivity, narrow-angle glaucoma	Nausea, vomiting, orthostasis, confusion, hallucinations, wearing-off fluctuations, dyskinesias	Response to therapy, presence of side effects	• Nonselective MAO inhibitors should be avoided; may cause hypertensive crisis • Pyridoxine (vitamin B6) decreases effectiveness of levodopa	• Immediate-release and controlled-release tabs often used simultaneously; IR tabs can treat wearing-off symptoms of CR tabs; CR is less bioavailable (~30% less) than IR	Yes

Drugs for Parkinson's Disease *(cont'd)*

Generic	Brand	Dose & Max	Contra-indications	Primary Side Effects	Key Monitoring Parameters	Pertinent Drug Interactions	Med Pearls	Top 200
L-Dopa	Larodopa	Individualized (not more than 8 g/day)	Hypersensitivity; narrow-angle glaucoma	Nausea, vomiting, orthostasis, confusion, hallucinations, wearing-off fluctuations, dyskinesias	Response to therapy, presence of side effects	• Nonselective MAO inhibitors should be avoided; may cause hypertensive crisis • Pyridoxine (vitamin B6) decreases effectiveness of levodopa	• Only used to supplement carbidopa/levodopa therapy in patients that need a larger dose of levodopa than can be achieved with combination tablets	No
Mechanism of action – dopamine agonists: direct stimulation of striatal dopamine receptors								
Bromocriptine (Ergot-derivative)	Parlodel	1.25–40 mg daily (divided TID)	Uncontrolled hypertension, sensitivity to ergot alkaloids	• Cardiac valve fibrosis • Nausea, hallucinations, dizziness, drowsiness	Response to therapy, presence of adverse effects	• Decrease levodopa dose by 20–30% when initiating	• Cardiac side effects decrease clinical use; nonergot derivatives used much more commonly	No
Pramipexole (Nonergot derivative)	Mirapex	1.5–4.5 mg daily	Dementia; hypersensitivity	Nausea, vomiting, constipation, orthostasis, hypersexuality, hallucinations, syncope	Renal function periodically, response to therapy, presence of adverse effects	• Decrease levodopa dose by 20–30% when initiating; metoclopramide and phenothiazines decrease efficacy	• Renal dose adjustment required when CrCl <60 mL/min (pramipexole only) • Titrate dose slowly and taper upon discontinuation	Yes
Ropinirole (Nonergot derivative)	Requip	0.75–12 mg daily (divided TID)						Yes

Drugs for Parkinson's Disease *(cont'd)*

Generic	Brand	Dose & Max	Contra-indications	Primary Side Effects	Key Monitoring Parameters	Pertinent Drug Interactions	Med Pearls	Top 200
Rotigotine	Neupro transdermal delivery system	2–8 mg daily (apply one patch daily)	Dementia; hypersensitivity	Application site reactions, nausea, vomiting, somnolence, insomnia, hallucinations, abnormal dreams	Response to therapy, presence of adverse effects	• Decrease levodopa dose by 20–30% when initiating; metoclopramide and phenothiazines decrease efficacy	• Transdermal patch • Taper dose upon discontinuation	No

Mechanism of action – COMT inhibitors: inhibit the degradation of dopamine through inhibition of the catechol-0-methyltransferase enzyme

Generic	Brand	Dose & Max	Contra-indications	Primary Side Effects	Key Monitoring Parameters	Pertinent Drug Interactions	Med Pearls	Top 200
Tolcapone	Tasmar	300–600 mg daily (divided TID)	AST or ALT >2 x ULN, known liver disease, history or nontraumatic rhabdomyolysis	Liver failure; dyskinesias, nausea, vomiting, hallucinations	Frequent LFT monitoring,	• Nonselective MOA inhibitors; increased activity of drugs known to be metabolized by COMT (dopamine, dobutamine, isoproterenol, methyldopa)	• Reserved for third-line therapy in patients that do not respond adequately to levodopa and dopamine agonists • Only used as adjunct therapy with levodopa	No
Entacapone	Comtan	200–1,600 mg daily (divided up to 8x daily; administered with carbidopa/levodopa tablets)	Hypersensitivity	Dyskinesias, nausea, vomiting, hallucinations, urine discoloration	• Response to therapy, presence of adverse effects, periodic LFTs	• Increased activity of drugs known to be metabolized by COMT (dopamine, dobutamine, isoproterenol, methyldopa)	• Reserved for third-line therapy in patients that do not respond adequately to levodopa and dopamine agonists • Preferred over tolcapone, as no fatal liver injury has been reported with this agent	No

Drugs for Parkinson's Disease *(cont'd)*

Mechanism of action – anticholinergics: through diminished activity of acetylcholine, help to decrease the relative increase in activity compared to dopamine, thereby decreasing tremor

Generic	Brand	Dose & Max	Contra-indications	Primary Side Effects	Key Monitoring Parameters	Pertinent Drug Interactions	Med Pearls	Top 200
Benztropine	Cogentin	0.5–6 mg daily (BID)	Avoid in patients with cognitive impairment and in elderly (>75 years of age)	Dry mouth, blurred vision, constipation, urinary retention, confusion, memory impairment, hallucinations	• Response to therapy, presence of adverse effects	• Additive anticholinergic side effects when co-administered with other anticholinergic medications	• Caution use in elderly patients who are at risk for mental status changes with anticholinergic medications; Primarily used for tremor and/or drooling	Yes
Trihexyphenidyl	Artane	1–15 mg daily (BID–TID)						No

Storage and Administration Pearls

- Selegiline is available as a tablet, capsule, transdermal patch, and oral disintegrating tablet. Oral disintegrating tablets should be taken in the morning before any food or water. Tablets dissolve on the tongue, and food/drink should be avoided for 5 minutes after dose.

- Carbidopa/levodopa extended-release tablets can be taken as whole tablets or half tablets but should not be chewed or crushed. Extended-release tablets are less bio-available than immediate-release tablets and patients may require up to a 30% dose increase to attain similar efficacy.

- Rotigotine patch should be worn continuously for 24 hours. Heat may increase absorption.

Patient Education Pearls

- Avoid concomitant alcohol with any antiparkinsonian agent.

- Rotigotine patch should be worn continuously for 24 hours. Heat may increase absorption. Patients should not take a hot bath or sauna or apply a heated pad while wearing patch.

- Hallucinations, delusions, or strange dreams should be immediately reported to a physician.

MIGRAINE HEADACHE

Definitions

Migraine headaches are defined as recurring headaches of moderate to severe intensity and are associated with gastrointestinal, neurological, and autonomic symptoms. Migraine headaches may or may not be preceded by an aura.

Diagnosis

Diagnostic criteria are established by the International Headache Society (IHS) and consist of distinct criteria for migraine with aura and migraine without aura.

Migraine with aura:

- At least two attacks
- Aura symptoms that do not last more than 60 minutes
- Organic disorder ruled out or headaches do not relate temporally to organic disorder

Migraine without aura:

- At least five attacks
- Headache lasts 4–72 hours
- Unilateral, pulsating, moderate/severe intensity, or aggravated by physical activity
- Nausea/vomiting, photophobia, or phonophobia
- Organic disorder ruled out or headaches do not relate temporally to organic disorder

Signs and Symptoms

Pain is the primary symptom of migraine headache. The pain is generally gradual in onset, peaks in intensity over minutes to hours, and lasts 4–72 hours if untreated. Intensity is often described as moderate to severe and generally stated as a 5 or greater on a 0–10 pain scale. Most commonly, pain occurs in the fronto-temporal region and is most often unilateral and pulsating. Other symptoms that may accompany the pain include gastrointestinal symptoms of nausea/vomiting and neurological symptoms of photo- or phonophobia.

Guidelines

Treatment of primary headache: acute migraine treatment. Standards of care for headache diagnosis and treatment. National Headache Foundation; Chicago, IL. (2004): p 27–39. www.guideline.gov/summary/summary.aspx?ss=15&doc_id=6579&nbr=4139.

Guidelines Summary

- Migraine treatment is divided into abortive treatment, rescue treatment, and prophylactic treatment. The majority of patients will respond to abortive treatment and can be controlled without the addition of rescue or prophylactic therapy.
- Abortive treatment options include analgesics (over-the-counter and prescription), NSAIDs (detailed in bone and joint chapter), ergotamine and dihydroergotamine, serotonin agonists, and butorphanol. Over-the-counter analgesics, prescription non-opioid analgesics and NSAIDs are reserved for patients with mild symptoms.
- The serotonin agonists are the mainstay of abortive therapy options for patients with moderate to severe symptoms. Various dosage forms are available and there is only slight variability between the efficacy and safety of available agents. Patients may respond to one agent in this class and not to another; therefore, trial and error is often the approach taken.
- For patients who have >2 headaches/week or >8 headaches/month, or who do not have an adequate response to abortive therapy, prophylactic therapy may be warranted.

- Available prophylactic agents include antihypertensive medications such as propranolol, atenolol, and metoprolol (detailed in cardiovascular chapter); antidepressant medications such as amitriptyline, paroxetine, fluoxetine, and sertraline (detailed in psychiatric disorders chapter); and anticonvulsant medications such valproic acid, gabapentin, tiagabine, and topiramate (detailed earlier in this chapter). In general, migraine prophylactic doses are low compared to normal doses of these medications.

Drugs for Migraine

Generic	Brand	Dose & Max	Contra-indications	Primary Side Effects	Key Monitoring Parameters	Pertinent Drug Interactions	Med Pearls	Top 200
Analgesics								
Acetaminophen 250 mg/aspirin 250 mg/caffeine 65 mg	Excedrin Migraine	2 tablets PO at onset, then q6 hrs PRN	Hypersensitivity to any component	Minimal	Response to therapy, presence of adverse effects	Other acetaminophen-containing meds	Available OTC	No
Aspirin or acetaminophen with butalbital and caffeine	• Fiorinal • Fioricet	1–2 tabs PO q4–6 hrs PRN	Hypersensitivity to any component	Tachycardia, dizziness, drowsiness or insomnia, orthostatic hypotension	Response to therapy, presence of adverse effects	• Alcohol • Additive CNS depression with butalbital	• Limit to 4 tablets/day and use max of 2 days/week • Dependence may develop with continued use	No
Isometheptene 65 mg/dichloral-phenazone 100 mg/ APAP 325 mg	Midrin	2 caps PO at onset, 1 cap q hour PRN	Glaucoma, severe renal or heart disease, hypertension	Dizziness, skin rash	Response to therapy, presence of adverse effects	MAOIs: potential for hypertensive crisis	Max 6 caps/day; 20 caps/month	No
Mechanism of action — ergotamine tartrate: exerts serotonergic agonist activity, resulting in vasoconstriction								
Ergotamine tartrate	Ergomar sublingual tablet	• 1 tab at onset and 1 tab q30 min PRN • Not to exceed 3 tabs/day	Peripheral vascular disease, heart disease, hypertension, impaired hepatic or renal function, hypersensitivity	Chest pain, hypertension, tachycardia, nausea, edema	Response to therapy, presence of adverse effects	Other meds with potential to increase blood pressure	Potential for dependence with long-term use	No
Mechanism of action — dihydroergotamine: serotonin agonistic activity, results in cerebral vasoconstriction								
Dihydroergotamine	DHE 45 SC, IM or IV injection 1 mg/mL	1 mg at onset, repeated at 1-hr intervals (max = 2 mg/day IV or 3 mg/day SC or IM)	• Ischemic heart disease • Uncontrolled hypertension • Peripheral arterial disease	Hypertension, vasospasm, myocardial infarction, tachycardia	Blood pressure, heart rate, response to therapy, presence of side effects	Potent inhibitors of CYP3A4, including protease inhibitors and macrolide antibiotics	Use significantly limited by adverse effects	No
	Migranal nasal spray	1 spray (0.5 mg) in each nostril followed by repeat spray in each nostril >15 minutes (max = 3 mg/day)						

Drugs for Migraine *(cont'd)*

Mechanism of action — serotonin agonists (triptans): serotonin 5HT receptor agonists, resulting in vasoconstriction in the cerebral vasculature

Generic	Brand	Dose & Max	Contra-indications	Primary Side Effects	Key Monitoring Parameters	Pertinent Drug Interactions	Med Pearls	Top 200
Sumatriptan	Imitrex oral tablets	25–100 mg PO at onset, then q2 hrs PRN up to 200 mg/day	Ischemic cardiac disease, peripheral vascular disease, cerebrovascular disease	Fatigue, dizziness, flushing, neck/throat pressure	Response to therapy, presence of side effects	MAO – A inhibitors – increased Triptan levels can lead to serotonin syndrome and cardiac side effects; sibutramine and SSRI coadministration – increased risk of serotonin syndrome	First approved serotonin agonist for migraine	Yes
	Imitrex SC injection	4–6 mg subcutaneously; may repeat in 1 hour. Max: 2 doses /day						
	Imitrex nasal spray	10–20 mg spray intranasally at onset; may repeat after 2 hrs. • Max: 40 mg/day						
Zolmitriptan	• Zomig • Oral tabs; rapid disintegrating tabs; nasal spray	1–5 mg at onset, redose >2 hrs if needed (max 10 mg/day)					Rapidly disintegrating tablets offer quicker-onset option	No
Naratriptan	Amerge oral tablets	1–2.5 mg at onset; may re-dose >4 hrs if needed (max 5 mg/day)						No

Drugs for Migraine *(cont'd)*

Generic	Brand	Dose & Max	Contra-indications	Primary Side Effects	Key Monitoring Parameters	Pertinent Drug Interactions	Med Pearls	Top 200
Rizatriptan	Maxalt oral tabs	5–10 mg PO at onset; redose >2 hrs (max 30 mg/day)	Ischemic cardiac disease, peripheral vascular disease, cerebrovascular disease	Fatigue, dizziness, flushing, neck/throat pressure	Response to therapy, presence of side effects	MAO – A inhibitors – increased Triptan levels can lead to serotonin syndrome and cardiac side effects; sibutramine and SSRI coadministration – increased risk of serotonin syndrome	Rapidly disintegrating tablets offer quicker-onset option	No
	• Maxalt • MLT rapid disintegrating tablets	5–10 mg dissolved followed by redose after 2 hrs if needed (max 30 mg/day)						
Almotriptan	Axert oral tablets	6.25–12.5 mg PO at onset; redose >2 hrs if needed (max 25 mg/day)						No
Eletriptan	Relpax oral tablets	20–40 mg PO at onset; redose >2 hrs if needed (max 80 mg/day)					• Metabolized by CYP3A4 • Dosage form is hydro-bromide salt 24.2 mg (= 20-mg base) and 42.5 mg (= 40-mg base)	Yes
Frovatriptan	Frova oral tablets	2.5 mg PO at onset; redose >2 hrs if needed (max 7.5 mg/day)						No
Mechanism of action – butorphanol: mixed opioid agonist/antagonist with opioid analgesic properties								
Butorphanol	Stadol nasal spray	1 mg (one spray) intranasally at onset; may repeat after 1 hour and then q3–4 hrs PRN.	• Hypersensitivity, CrCl <30 mL/min • Patients with a history of narcotic dependence	Somnolence, dizziness, nausea, nasal congestion, insomnia	Response to therapy, presence of adverse effects	Concurrent use of other CNS depressants will have additive adverse effects and should be avoided	• Pharmacist often assembles nasal spray prior to patient use • Not routinely used for migraine • High addiction potential; controlled substance	No

Storage and Administration Pearls

- Store all preparations between 2–30°C (36–86°F). Protect from light.
- Place rapid disintegrating tablets directly on tongue and allow them to dissolve.
- Sumatriptan and zolmitran nasal sprays are sprayed into one nostril only.
- Sumatriptan injection is self-administered subcutaneously using prefilled syringes and an autoinjector.

Patient Education Pearls

- Rapid disintegrating tablets should be placed directly on the tongue and allowed to dissolve.
- Follow dosing recommendations carefully to decrease risk of adverse effects or dependence.

LEARNING POINTS

- Disease-modifying drugs are the agents of choice in treating multiple sclerosis.
- First-line choice of antiepileptic drug is based on seizure classification. Options include carbamazepine, phenytoin, lamotrigine, valproic acid, and oxcarbazepine.
- Antiepileptic drugs have a significant number of drug-drug interactions due to their impact on and metabolism by the cytochrome P450 enzyme system.
- Carbidopa/levodopa is the mainstay of therapy for Parkinson's disease and is available in numerous dosage forms. Controlled- and immediate-release tablets are often prescribed simultaneously.
- Anticholinergic agents should be avoided in elderly patients.
- Agents affecting dopamine, including dopamine agonists and carbidopa/levodopa, may elicit psychiatric side effects.
- Serotonin agonists are the mainstay of treatment for migraine headache and are available in numerous dosage forms.

PRACTICE QUESTIONS

1. What is recommended first-line for newly diagnosed multiple sclerosis?

    (A) Oral prednisone 50 mg PO daily for 1 week, then slowly tapered over 1 month
    (B) Betaseron
    (C) Methylprednisolone 100–500 mg/day for 3–10 days
    (D) Natalizumab
    (E) Rebif + mitoxantrone

2. What patient counseling should be provided when dispensing an interferon injectable prescription for multiple sclerosis?

    (A) If the medication cannot be used within 1 month, freeze the syringe to allow beyond-date use.
    (B) Apply heat to the injection site before and after the injection.
    (C) Try to use the same injection site each time.
    (D) If the medication reaches room temperature, it is no longer usable and must be discarded.
    (E) NSAIDs may decrease the flulike symptoms.

3. Which of the following is NOT a first-line agent for treatment of generalized tonic-clonic seizures?

    (A) Tegretol
    (B) Topiramate
    (C) Depakote
    (D) Dilantin
    (E) Carbamazepine

ANSWERS

1. **B**

Interferon agents (such as Betaseron, Avonex, and Rebif) and glatiramer acetate (Copax-one) are considered first-line disease-modifying drugs (DMDs) for the treatment of MS. Therefore, (B) is correct. Natalizumab (D) is reserved for patients who do not respond to traditional therapy. Treatment is usually initiated one agent at a time; and as the disease progresses, treatment with DMD + mitoxantrone pulse therapy (E) may be used. Corti-costeroids (A and C) are the cornerstone of acute exacerbations but will play no role in treating the disease itself.

2. **E**

Acetaminophen or NSAIDs can reduce the flulike symptoms associated with the Inter-feron injections. The injectables for multiple sclerosis should never be frozen (A) and should always be protected from light. To ease the discomfort of the injections, ice—not heat (B)—can be applied to the injection site prior to the injection, and the injection site should be rotated each time (making choice C incorrect). It is perfectly fine and recom-mended to allow the injectable to reach room temperature prior to the injection (D), but it should otherwise be stored in the refrigerator.

3. **B**

First-line treatment for tonic-clonic seizures includes phenytoin (D), valproic acid (C), and carbamazepine (E). Tegretol (A) is the generic for carbamazepine so it is also cor-rect. Topiramate (B) is considered an alternate anti-epileptic agent; it can be used as adjunctive therapy in partial seizures.

Gastrointestinal Disorders

6

This chapter covers the following diseases:

- **Gastroesophageal reflux disease/peptic ulcer disease**
- **Inflammatory bowel disease**

 Suggested Study Time: **45 minutes**

GASTROESOPHAGEAL REFLUX DISEASE/ PEPTIC ULCER DISEASE

Definitions

Gastroesophageal reflux disease (GERD) is a condition in which patients have symptoms or mucosal damage resulting from the abnormal reflux of stomach contents into the esophagus. If the esophagus is chronically exposed to these contents, inflammation of the esophagus can develop which is termed reflux esophagitis, and/or the esophageal mucosa can become ulcerated, leading to erosive esophagitis. Often, GERD results because of reduced lower esophageal sphincter (LES) pressures; however, this condition may also arise because of a delay in gastric emptying, use of certain medications or foods, or a hiatal hernia. Various medications may precipitate GERD symptoms either by decreasing LES pressure (e.g., anticholinergics, benzodiazepines, β-agonists, calcium channel blockers, dopamine agonists, estrogen, opioid narcotics, nicotine, nitrates, progesterone, theophylline) or by irritating the esophageal mucosa (e.g., nonsteroidal anti-inflammatory drugs [NSAIDs], bisphosphonates, salicylates, iron, potassium chloride).

Peptic ulcer disease (PUD) refers to the development of duodenal or gastric ulcers. The majority of PUD cases are caused by either *Helicobacter pylori* (*H. pylori*) infection or the use of NSAIDs, but can also be induced by stress. A number of risk factors exist that may predispose patients to NSAID-induced ulcers, including a prior gastrointestinal (GI) ulcer or hemorrhage; age >60 years; and concurrent use of corticosteroids, antiplatelets, or anticoagulants.

Diagnosis

Gastroesophageal Reflux Disease

- Diagnosis for uncomplicated cases is based primarily on description of symptoms and potential risk factors. Response to treatment can also be used as a diagnostic strategy.
- Endoscopy is recommended for the following patients:
  - Age >45 years
  - Presenting with atypical or alarm symptoms (see below)
  - Refractory to initial treatment
- Ambulatory pH testing can also be used if patients continue to have symptoms despite either normal endoscopic findings or appropriate therapy.

Peptic Ulcer Disease

- Clinical history (including symptoms and history of medication use) can be helpful in arriving at a preliminary diagnosis (not important to differentiate between duodenal and gastric ulcers).
- All patients with a suspected diagnosis of PUD should be tested for *H. pylori*.
  - Invasive tests (endoscopy): rapid urease tests (80–95% sensitive, 95–100% specific; false negatives can occur if patients previously on proton pump inhibitors [PPIs], H_2 receptor antagonist, or bismuth therapy; patient needs to be off these drugs for at least 1 week before performing this test)
  - Noninvasive tests:
    » Serological: 85% sensitive, 79% specific; not influenced by prior acid-suppressive therapy; can be used to confirm diagnosis but will not be helpful in determining eradication of infection
    » Urea breath test: 97% sensitive, 95% specific; influenced by prior acid-suppressive and antibiotic therapy ($\uparrow$ risk of false negative); can be used to confirm diagnosis and eradication
    » Stool antigen test: 88–92% sensitive, 87% specific; influenced by prior acid-suppressive therapy; can be used to confirm diagnosis and eradication

Signs and Symptoms

Gastroesophageal Reflux Disease:

- Typical symptoms: heartburn (pyrosis), regurgitation, belching, water brash (↑ salivation)
- Atypical symptoms: Noncardiac chest pain, hoarseness, nausea, asthma-like symptoms, chronic cough, sore throat, dental erosions
- Alarm symptoms (indicate need for immediate evaluation): Dysphagia (difficulty swallowing), odynophagia (painful swallowing), bleeding, weight loss
- Long-term complications: Esophageal strictures, Barrett's esophagus, esophageal cancer

Peptic Ulcer Disease:

- Abdominal pain (usually epigastric): The most common symptom
  - Can be described as burning, discomfort, or fullness
  - Duodenal ulcer: Pain often occurs 1–3 hours after a meal and is relieved with food
  - Gastric ulcer: Pain brought on by food
- Other symptoms: Heartburn, belching, bloating, nausea, anorexia
- Long-term complications: Upper GI bleeding, perforation

Guidelines

Gastroesophageal Reflux Disease

American College of Gastroenterology. *Am J Gastroenterol*, no. 100 (2005): 190–200.

Peptic Ulcer Disease

Guidelines for the treatment of Helicobacter pylori infection (American College of Gastroenterology). *Am J Gastroenterol*, no. 93 (1998): 2330–2338.

Guidelines for treatment and prevention of NSAID-induced ulcers (American College of Gastroenterology). *Am J Gastroenterol*, no. 93 (1998): 2037–2046.

Guidelines Summary

Gastroesophageal Reflux Disease

The goals of therapy are to relieve symptoms, promote healing of esophageal mucosa, prevent recurrence, and prevent complications.

- **Lifestyle modifications**
  - Unlikely to control symptoms, when used alone, in most patients
  - Dietary changes: Avoid foods that can worsen symptoms (alcohol, caffeine, chocolate, citrus juices, peppermint/spearmint, coffee, spicy foods, tomatoes, high-fatty meals, garlic, onions); avoid eating before bedtime; remain upright after meals
  - Weight loss
  - Smoking cessation
  - Head elevated off the bed by 6–8 inches
  - No tight-fitting clothes
  - No medications that can worsen symptoms
- **Pharmacological therapy**
  - Step 1: Antacids and over-the-counter (OTC) acid suppressants (H_2 receptor antagonists, omeprazole) can be used initially on an as-needed basis for intermittent or mild symptoms. If symptoms persist after 2 weeks, proceed to Step 2.
  - Step 2: PPI or H_2 receptor antagonist (can be used at higher prescription doses).
    - » PPIs are considered more effective than H_2 receptor antagonists.
  - A promotility agent (e.g., metoclopramide) can be used as adjunctive therapy, if needed.

Peptic Ulcer Disease

The goals of therapy are to relieve symptoms, promote healing of the ulcer, prevent recurrence, and prevent complications.

- **Lifestyle modifications:** reduce stress, smoking cessation, discontinue NSAIDs use, avoid foods that can worsen symptoms
- **Pharmacological therapy**
  - *H. pylori*-associated ulcers: PPI + two antibiotics (usually clarithromycin and amoxicillin); duration = 10–14 days. If this therapy fails, four-drug therapy should be used (PPI + bismuth + metronidazole + tetracycline); duration = 14 days.
  - NSAID-induced ulcers
    - » Treatment:
      - 1st-line therapy: PPI (duration of therapy = 6–8 weeks; may be longer if recurrent symptoms, heavy smoker, or continued NSAID use)
      - 2nd-line therapies: Misoprostol or H_2 receptor antagonist
    - » Primary prevention
      - If patients have any of the risk factors described above (see Definitions), can use PPI + NSAID, a cyclooxygenase-2 inhibitor (alone), or misoprostol + NSAID.
      - PPI + NSAID regimen is preferred in patients with cardiovascular risk factors who require chronic NSAID use.
      - H_2 receptor antagonists is not effective for primary prevention.

Antacids

Mechanism of action – neutralize stomach acid and ↑ gastric pH

Generic	Brand	Dose	Contra-indications	Primary Side Effects	Key Monitoring	Pertinent Drug Interactions	Med Pearl	Top 200
Magnesium hydroxide/aluminum hydroxide	Maalox, Mylanta	15 mL with meals and at bedtime	None	• Diarrhea (from magnesium [Mg2+]) • Constipation (from aluminum [Al3+] or calcium [Ca2+])	S/S GERD	May bind to numerous drugs (separate from other drugs by at least 2 hrs)	Use Mg^{2+}-and Al^{3+}-containing products with caution in patients with renal dysfunction	No
Calcium carbonate	Tums, Rolaids, Maalox Chewables	1-2 tablets every 2 hrs as needed						No

H₂ Receptor Antagonists

Mechanism of action – reversibly inhibit histamine (H₂) receptors in the gastric parietal cells, which inhibits secretion of gastric acid

Generic	Brand	Dose	Dosage Forms	Primary Side Effects	Key Monitoring	Pertinent Drug Interactions	Med Pearl	Top 200
Cimetidine	Tagamet	200–1,600 mg/day	• Rx: Tabs, solution, injection • OTC: Tabs	• Headache • Fatigue • Dizziness • Confusion • Gynecomastia (cimetidine)	S/S GERD/PUD	• Cimetidine inhibits CYP enzymes to greater extent than the other drugs (inhibits CYP1A2, CYP2C19, CYP2D6, and CYP3A4) • May ↑ effects of warfarin, theophylline, phenytoin	• Dosage adjustment required for all drugs in renal insufficiency • Pepcid Complete also contains calcium carbonate + magnesium hydroxide	No
Famotidine	Pepcid	20–80 mg/day	• Rx: Tabs, suspension, injection • OTC: Tabs, gelcaps					Yes
Nizatidine	Axid	150–300 mg/day	• Rx: Caps, solution • OTC: Tabs					No
Ranitidine	Zantac	75–300 mg/day	• Rx: Tabs, effervescent tabs, syrup, injection • OTC: Tabs					Yes

Proton Pump Inhibitors

Mechanism of action – irreversibly inhibit H+/K+-ATPase in gastric parietal cells, which inhibits secretion of gastric acid

Generic	Brand	Dose	Dosage Forms	Primary Side Effects	Key Monitoring	Pertinent Drug Interactions	Med Pearl	Top 200
Esomeprazole	Nexium	20–40 mg/day	Caps, granules for suspension, injection	• Diarrhea • Headache	S/S GERD/PUD	↓ absorption of ketoconazole and itraconazole (require acidic environment for absorption)	Zegerid is omeprazole + sodium bicarbonate (available as caps or suspension)	Yes
Lansoprazole	Prevacid	15–30 mg/day	Caps, orally disintegrating tabs, granules for suspension					Yes
Omeprazole	Prilosec	20 mg/day	Rx: Caps OTC: Tabs					Yes
Pantoprazole	Protonix	20–40 mg/day	Tabs, injection					Yes
Rabeprazole	Aciphex	20 mg/day	Tabs					Yes

Promotility Drug

Mechanism of action – dopamine antagonist; ↑ LES pressure and accelerates gastric emptying

Generic	Brand	Dose	Contra-indications	Primary Side Effects	Key Monitoring	Pertinent Drug Interactions	Med Pearl	Top 200
Metoclopramide	Reglan	40–60 mg/day	Seizures	• Dizziness • Fatigue • Drowsiness • Diarrhea • Extrapyramidal symptoms (EPS)	• S/S GERD • EPS	Use with antipsychotic agents may ↑ risk of EPS	Can also be used for diabetic gastroparesis; erythromycin is an alternative	Yes

Mucosal Protectant Drug

Mechanism of action – nonabsorbable aluminum salt that forms bonds with damaged and normal GI tissue; complex forms protective cover over ulcerated area

Generic	Brand	Dose	Contra-indications	Primary Side Effects	Key Monitoring	Pertinent Drug Interactions	Med Pearl	Top 200
Sucralfate	Carafate	4 g/day	None	Constipation	S/S PUD	May bind to numerous drugs (separate from other drugs by at least 2 hrs)	• Use cautiously in patients with chronic kidney disease (↑ risk of Al^{3+} toxicity) • Limited value in treatment of GERD; more useful in treatment of PUD	No

Prostaglandin Analog

Mechanism of action – prostaglandin E1 analog; replaces protective prostaglandins inhibited by NSAID therapy

Generic	Brand	Dose	Contraindications	Primary Side Effects	Key Monitoring	Pertinent Drug Interactions	Med Pearl	Top 200
Misoprostol	Cytotec	400–800 mcg/day	Pregnancy (abortifacient)	Diarrhea	S/S PUD	None	Women of childbearing age should have pregnancy test before initiating therapy; educate regarding appropriate use of contraception	No

Helicobacter pylori Treatment Regimens (for PUD)

Proton Pump Inhibitor	Drug #2	Drug #3	Drug #4	Comments
Three-Drug Regimen (PPI + two antibiotics; duration of therapy = 10–14 days; 14 days preferred)				
Esomeprazole 40 mg daily OR lansoprazole 30 mg 2x daily OR omeprazole 20 mg 2x daily OR pantoprazole 40 mg 2x daily OR rabeprazole 20 mg 2x daily	Amoxicillin 1,000 mg 2x daily	Clarithromycin 500 mg 2x daily		• Metronidazole can be used instead of amoxicillin or clarithromycin in patients with penicillin or macrolide allergy, respectively. • Rabeprazole regimen should be given for 7 days. • Prevpac is a compliance package that contains individual units of lansoprazole, amoxicillin, and clarithromycin.
Four-Drug Regimen (PPI + bismuth subsalicylate + metronidazole + tetracycline; duration of therapy = 14 days)				
Esomeprazole 40 mg daily OR lansoprazole 30 mg 2x daily OR omeprazole 20 mg 2x daily OR pantoprazole 40 mg 2x daily OR rabeprazole 20 mg daily	Bismuth subsalicylate 525 mg 4x daily	Metronidazole 500 mg 3x daily	Tetracycline 500 mg 4x daily	• Pylora contains bismuth, metronidazole, and tetracycline in each capsule. • Helidac is a compliance package that contains individual units of bismuth, metronidazole, and tetracycline. • It is fine alternatively use H$_2$ antagonist instead of PPI (would need to be used for 4–6 wks).

Storage and Administration Pearls

- Esomeprazole may be administered down a nasogastric (NG) or orogastric (OG) tube by opening the capsule, placing the granules in a syringe, and diluting with water; granules for oral suspension can also be placed in a syringe and diluted with water.

- Lansoprazole granules for oral suspension should *not* be administered via a NG/OG tube; to administer through these tubes, can open capsules and mix with apple juice, can dilute orally disintegrating tablets in water in a syringe, or a suspension can be made (will be compounded by pharmacy).

- Omeprazole suspension can be compounded by pharmacy for administration via NG/OG tube.

- Pantoprazole and rabeprazole tablets should *not* be crushed; cannot be given via NG/OG tube.

- Misoprostol should be administered with meals.

- Sucralfate should be administered 1 hour before meals.

Patient Education Pearls

- Lifestyle changes should be continued throughout the course of therapy.

- Patient should separate the administration of antacids from other medications by at least 2 hours.

- PPIs should be taken 15–30 minutes before breakfast; if patient is taking two daily doses, final dose should be taken before dinner (not at bedtime).

- A patient who is being treated for *H. pylori* should complete the entire course of therapy to facilitate eradication of the infection.

INFLAMMATORY BOWEL DISEASE

Definitions

Inflammatory bowel disease (IBD) is a broad-based term used to describe two conditions: ulcerative colitis (UC) and Crohn's disease (CD). Ulcerative colitis is a chronic inflammatory disease that consists of superficial mucosal lesions localized to the colon and rectum. CD is also a chronic inflammatory disease, but is characterized by transmural lesions that can occur anywhere along the GI tract. The etiology of both of these disorders is thought to be due to immunologic or infectious causes; however, environmental, psychological, or genetic factors may also contribute to the development of these diseases.

Diagnosis

Diagnosis is suspected on the basis of clinical presentation, but is confirmed through various studies, including sigmoidoscopy, colonoscopy, barium enema, and stool examination. A biopsy of the lesions is usually performed during the sigmoidoscopy or colonoscopy.

Signs and Symptoms

The following symptoms can occur with both UC and CD: fever, diarrhea, weight loss, rectal bleeding, and abdominal pain.

Clinical Findings Associated with Ulcerative Colitis or Crohn's Disease

Clinical Finding	Ulcerative Colitis	Crohn's Disease
Abdominal mass	No	Yes
Fistulas/strictures	No	Yes
Bowel involvement	Rectum/colon	Can affect anywhere from mouth to anus (often affects ileum)
Systemic complications (i.e., extraintestinal involvement)	Yes	Yes
Toxic megacolon	Yes	No
At risk for colorectal cancer	Yes	Rare
Pattern of inflammation	Continuous	Segmented ("cobblestone" appearance)

Guidelines

Guidelines for the treatment of ulcerative colitis (American College of Gastroenterology). *Am J Gastroenterol*, no. 99 (2004): 1371–85.

Guidelines for the treatment of Crohn's disease (American College of Gastroenterology). *Am J Gastroenterol*, no. 96 (2001): 635–43.

GUIDELINES SUMMARY

The goals of therapy are to induce and maintain remission, to prevent and resolve complications and systemic symptoms, and to maintain quality of life. There is no pharmacologic cure for these diseases; therefore, treatment focuses on management of symptoms.

- **Nonpharmacologic therapy**
  - Possible surgery when complications (e.g., fistulas, strictures, perforation) develop or to manage refractory disease
- **Pharmacologic therapy**
  - Adjunctive therapies: antidiarrheals (e.g., loperamide), antispasmodics (e.g., dicyclomine, propantheline, hyoscyamine)
  - Ulcerative colitis:
    - » Treatment based upon whether inflammation is distal (below the splenic flexure; topical therapy appropriate) or extensive (proximal to the splenic flexure; requires systemic therapy)
    - » Mild/moderate distal disease:
      - Active disease: Topical mesalamine (enema or suppository preferred), oral aminosalicylate, topical corticosteroid
      - Maintenance of remission: Topical mesalamine or oral aminosalicylate
    - » Mild/moderate extensive disease:
      - Active disease: oral aminosalicylate (1st-line), infliximab, oral corticosteroids, azathioprine, 6-mercaptopurine
      - Maintenance of remission: oral aminosalicylate (1st-line), infliximab, azathioprine, 6-mercaptopurine
    - » Severe disease:
      - Intravenous (IV) corticosteroids (1st-line), infliximab, IV cyclosporine
  - Crohn's disease:
    - » Mild/moderate active disease:
      - 1st-line: oral aminosalicylate
      - 2nd-line: metronidazole, ciprofloxacin, budesonide
    - » Moderate/severe disease:
      - 1st-line: prednisone or budesonide
      - 2nd-line: infliximab, methotrexate (intramuscularly or subcutaneously)
    - » Severe fulminant disease:
      - 1st-line: IV corticosteroids
      - 2nd-line: IV cyclosporine
    - » Maintenance therapy:
      - 1st-line: azathioprine, 6-mercaptopurine, or infliximab

Aminosalicylates

Mechanism of action – ↓ inflammation in GI tract by inhibiting prostaglandin synthesis and subsequent production of various immune mediators; sulfasalazine is cleaved in colon to mesalamine (responsible for therapeutic effect) + sulfapyridine (causes side effects); olsalazine and balsalazide also contain mesalamine

Generic	Brand	Dose	Dosage Forms	Contra-indications	Primary Side Effects	Key Monitoring	Med Pearl	Top 200
Sulfasalazine	• Azulfidine • Azulfidine EN • Sulfazine • Sulfazine EC	• Induction: 4–6 g/day • Maintenance: 2–4 g/day	Tabs, delayed-release (enteric-coated) tabs	• Aspirin allergy • Sulfa allergy • G6PD deficiency • Pregnancy (near term)	• Stevens-Johnson syndrome • Photosensitivity • Nausea/vomiting (N/V) • Headache • Folate deficiency • Hemolytic anemia • Agranulocytosis • Hepatitis	• S/S IBD • Liver function tests (LFTs) (with sulfasalazine) • Complete blood count (CBC) (with sulfasalazine)	• Mesalamine, olsalazine, and balsalazide are not sulfa derivatives; are poorly absorbed from GI tract (better tolerated than sulfasalazine) • Folic acid should be given to patients on sulfasalazine • Sulfasalazine may ↑ effects of warfarin and oral hypoglycemic • All may ↓ absorption of digoxin	No
Mesalamine	• Asacol • Canasa • Lialda • Pentasa • Rowasa	• Oral: Induction 2.4–4.8 g/day • Maintenance: 1.6–4.0 g/day • Rectal enema: 4 g at bedtime • Rectal suppository: 1 g at bedtime	Controlled-release caps, delayed-release tabs, rectal enema, rectal suppository	• Aspirin allergy • G6PD deficiency	• Nausea • Diarrhea • Headache • Malaise			Yes
Olsalazine	Dipentum	1–3 g/day	Caps					No
Balsalazide	Colazal	1.5–6.75 g/day	Caps					No

Corticosteroids

Generic	Brand	Dose	Dosage Forms	Contra-indications	Primary Side Effects	Key Monitoring	Med Pearl	Top 200
Mechanism of action – quickly ↓ inflammation during acute exacerbations of IBD								
Budesonide	Entocort EC	• Initial: 9 mg 1x daily for up to 2 mo • Maintenance: 6 mg 1x daily for up to 3 mo	Enteric-coated caps	None	• Hyperglycemia • ↑ appetite • Insomnia • Hypertension • Edema • Adrenal suppression • Osteoporosis • Cataracts • Delayed wound healing	• S/S IBD • Blood glucose • Blood pressure (BP) • Electrolytes	• Should only be used to treat acute exacerbation (4–8 wks) and then tapered • Budesonide has localized effect; has minimal systemic side effects	No
Methylprednisolone	Solu-Medrol	10–100 mg/day	Injection, tabs				• IV therapy given for severe exacerbations for 7–10 days, then switched to oral therapy	No
Prednisone	Sterapred	20–60 mg/day	Tabs					Yes

Immunosuppressants

Mechanism of action – ↓ production of inflammatory mediators (e.g., interleukins) through various mechanisms

Generic	Brand	Dose	Contra-indications	Primary Side Effects	Key Monitoring	Pertinent Drug Interactions	Med Pearl	Top 200
Azathioprine	Imuran	75–150 mg/day	• Pregnancy • Bone marrow suppression • Liver dysfunction	• Pancreatitis • Arthralgias • Nausea • Diarrhea • Rash • Bone marrow suppression • Hepatotoxicity	• Amylase/lipase (if symptoms) • CBC with differential • LFTs	• Allopurinol may ↑ risk of side effects (↓ azathioprine dose by 75%) • Aminosalicylates may ↑ risk of side effects • May ↓ effects of warfarin	• 6-mercaptopurine is active metabolite of azathioprine • Adjust dose in patients with renal dysfunction	No
6-Mercaptopurine	Purinethol	50–100 mg/day						No
Cyclosporine	Sandimmune	4–8 mg/kg/day IV	Renal failure	• Hypertension • Nephrotoxicity • Hypomagnesemia • Infection • Anaphylaxis	• BP • Blood urea nitrogen (BUN)/serum creatinine (SCr) • Electrolytes • S/S infection • Cyclosporine levels	• Cyclosporine is a CYP3A4 substrate and inhibitor • CYP3A4 inhibitors may ↑ levels/toxicity • CYP3A4 inducers may ↓ effects • May ↑ effects of other CYP3A4 substrates	• Used only for severe disease that has not responded to corticosteroids • Used only for 7–10 days (IV)	No
Methotrexate	Rheumatrex	IM or SC 15–25 mg/wk	• Pregnancy • Bone marrow suppression • Severe renal or hepatic dysfunction	• Hepatotoxicity • Bone marrow suppression • Pneumonitis • Rash • Nausea • Diarrhea	• LFTs • CBC with differential • Chest x-ray (if symptoms)	• NSAIDs and salicylates ↑ risk of toxicity • Penicillins, sulfonamides, and tetracyclines may ↑ risk of toxicity	• Only effective for CD • Adjust dose in patients with renal dysfunction	Yes

Biological Agents

Generic	Brand	Dose	Contra-indications	Primary Side Effects	Key Monitoring	Pertinent Drug Interactions	Med Pearl	Top 200
Mechanism of action – inhibits tumor necrosis factor							
Infliximab	Remicade	5 mg/kg IV at 0, 2, and 6 wks; then every 8 wks	• NYHA class III or IV heart failure • Active infection	• Infusion reactions (hypotension, fever, chills, urticaria, pruritus) • Delayed hypersensitivity (fever, rash, myalgia, headache, sore throat) • Infection (especially tuberculosis) • Heart failure exacerbation • Bone marrow suppression • Lymphoma • Hepatitis	• BP • LFTs • S/S infection • S/S heart failure • CBC with differential	Do not administer live vaccines	• Delayed hypersensitivity reaction may occur 3–10 days after administration • PPD should be done before initiating treatment	No

STORAGE AND ADMINISTRATION PEARLS

- Patients receiving infliximab should be pretreated with antihistamine, acetaminophen, and/or corticosteroid to prevent infusion-related reaction.
- Infliximab should be administered as an IV infusion over 2 hrs.
- If switching from prednisone to budesonide, prednisone should be tapered over a period of 2 wks.

PATIENT EDUCATION PEARLS

- Adherence to medication is very important as disease exacerbations can have a significant impact on quality of life.
- Mesalamine enemas and suppositories should be administered at bedtime to allow for direct contact of the drug with the rectal mucosa for at least 8 hours.
- Live vaccines should not be administered if a patient is receiving infliximab.
- Patients receiving azathioprine, 6-mercaptopurine, methotrexate, or infliximab are at increased risk for infection. They should wash their hands frequently and avoid crowds or other persons who are sick.
- Patients taking sulfasalazine should wear sunscreen and protective clothing. Sulfasalazine should be taken with meals to minimize GI effects. Patients taking sulfasalazine should take folic acid to prevent folate deficiency. Sulfasalazine may cause an orange discoloration of body fluids (urine, tears), which may stain clothing and contact lenses.
- Women receiving azathioprine, 6-mercaptopurine, or methotrexate should be counseled on using appropriate contraceptive methods.
- NSAIDs and high-dose salicylates (not the doses of aspirin used for prevention of cardiovascular diseases) should be avoided if the patient is receiving methotrexate.

LEARNING POINTS

- **GERD/PUD**
  - Antacids should be separated from other medications by at least 2 hours because of the risk for binding and ↓ the absorption of these drugs.
  - The majority of PUD cases are caused by either *H. pylori* infection or NSAIDs.
  - Three-drug regimen (PPI + two antibiotics [usually clarithromycin and amoxicillin]) is recommended for treatment of *H. pylori* infection.
  - The dosage of all H_2 antagonists needs to be adjusted in patients with renal insufficiency.

- Of all the H_2 antagonists, cimetidine is the most likely to be involved with drug interactions involving the CYP450 system.
- Of all the PPIs, only esomeprazole and pantoprazole are available as IV injection; also be familiar with the various dosage forms of the PPIs.

- **IBD**
  - Sulfasalazine should not be used in patients with sulfa allergies. The other aminosalicylates, mesalamine, olsalazine, and balsalazide can be used in these patients.
  - Folic acid should be administered to patients receiving sulfasalazine to prevent folate deficiency.
  - Know the various dosage forms of the aminosalicylates.
  - Be familiar with the side effects of systemic corticosteroids.
  - Methotrexate is only effective for CD.
  - PPD should be performed prior to starting infliximab therapy; drug should not be administered to patients with NYHA class III or IV heart failure.
  - Infliximab is associated with infusion reactions; patients need to be pretreated with antihistamine, acetaminophen, and/or corticosteroid.

PRACTICE QUESTIONS

1. Remicade is the brand name for which of the following drugs?

   (A) Azathioprine
   (B) Budesonide
   (C) Cyclosporine
   (D) Infliximab
   (E) Balsalazide

2. Which of the following is a contraindication for the use of metoclopramide?

   (A) Hyperkalemia
   (B) Myasthenia gravis
   (C) Porphyria
   (D) Seizure disorder
   (E) Sulfa allergy

ANSWERS

1. **D**

Remicade is the brand name for infliximab. Imuran is the brand name for azathioprine (A). Entocort EC is the brand name for oral budesonide (B). Sandimmune, Gengraf, and Neoral are brand names for cyclosporine (C). Colazal is the brand name for balsalazide (E).

2. **D**

Seizure disorder is a contraindication for the use of metoclopramide; therefore, choice (D) is correct.

Oncology

7

This chapter covers the following topics:

- **Hematologic malignancies (leukemia and lymphoma)**
- **Solid tumors (lung, colorectal, breast, prostate, and ovarian cancers)**
- **Supportive care**

 Suggested Study Time: **60 minutes**

Since many of the drugs used in chemotherapy are indicated for multiple types of cancer, the background information for all of the hematologic malignancies and solid tumors will be discussed first, with the drug therapies described in a chart at the end of the section. Because cancer therapy is generally protocol-driven, your focus should be mostly on toxicities and on certain cases where a specific drug is indicated on the basis of cell-surface markers such as CD20 or HER-2 overexpression. Supportive care (pain management, antinauseant and antiemetic agents, and colony-stimulating factors) are covered at the end of this chapter.

LYMPHOMA

Definitions

Lymphomas are tumors of the lymphoid cells. Hodgkin's lymphoma (or Hodgkin's disease, HD) is less common than other types of lymphoma and is marked by the presence of Reed-Steinberg cells. HD may have a genetic component; and while HD is not contagious, certain infections (particularly Epstein-Barr and HIV) may increase the risk of acquiring the disease. HD is more common in young adults (15–35 years) and those over 55.

Non-Hodgkin's lymphomas (NHLs) are a group of related cancers including follicular, diffuse large B-cell, and Burkitt's lymphoma. NHL is the fifth leading cause of cancer in the United States, and the incidence increases with age (median age of diagnosis is 50 years). Immunodeficiency and infections are risk factors for NHL, as is prior chemotherapy. The various types of NHL are typified by proliferation of malignant B or T lymphocytes. The cancer may be classified as either aggressive (fast-growing) or indolent (slow-growing).

Diagnosis

HD:

- Lymph node biopsy; presence of Reed-Sternberg cells
- CT scan, MRI, PET scan or bone marrow biopsy to determine staging

NHL:

- Lab values:
  - Elevated WBC
  - Lactate dehydrogenase levels may be high
- Lymph node or tissue biopsy
- Flow cytometry—cell surface marker analysis

Staging is the same for HD and NHL. Each stage is subdivided into A and B; B denotes the presence of systemic symptoms, specifically night sweats, weight loss, and fever:

- Stage 1: present in one lymph node or one part of tissue or organ
- Stage 2: present in at least two lymph nodes on the same side of the diaphragm
- Stage 3: present in lymph nodes above and below the diaphragm
- Stage 4: present in several parts of one or more tissues, or in an organ and distant lymph nodes
- Recurrent: disease returns after remission

Signs and Symptoms

HD:

- Painless enlargement of lymph nodes, especially in the neck
- Fever, night sweats, and/or weight loss in about 40% of cases
- Malaise
- Possible bone pain

NHL:

- Swollen lymph nodes on neck, underarms, and groin
- Fever, weight loss, and night sweats
- Fatigue
- Weakness

Guidelines

National Comprehensive Cancer Network, Clinical Practice Guidelines in Oncology, Version 1.2008: Hodgkin Disease/Lymphoma – Full Report, 2008. www.nccn.org/professionals/physician_gls/PDF/hodgkins.pdf.

National Comprehensive Cancer Network, Clinical Practice Guidelines in Oncology, Version 2.2008: Non-Hodgkin's Lymphoma – Full Report, 2008. www.nccn.org/professionals/physician_gls/PDF/nhl.pdf.

Guidelines Summary

HD:

- Gold standard: ABVD (Adriamycin [doxorubicin], bleomycin, vinblastine, dacarbazine)
- Also used:
  - Stanford V (mechlorethamine, doxorubicin, etoposide, vincristine, vinblastine, bleomycin, prednisone)
    - » Dose-intense, but cumulative doses are lower
    - » Reduces risks of infertility, secondary neoplasms, cardiac and pulmonary toxicity

NHL:

- Gold standard—combination chemotherapy:
  - CHOP (cyclophosphamide, doxorubicin [hydroxydaunorubicin], vincristine [Oncovin], prednisolone), or
  - CVP (no doxorubicin)
- Rituximab used if CD20 antigen is expressed (>90% of B-cell lymphomas)
  - Pretreat with diphenhydramine, steroids, H2 antagonist
  - May be added to CHOP or CVP
  - Ibritumomab yttrium 90 and tositumomab iodine 131 also target CD20
- Radiation therapy: Standard of care for early-stage follicular lymphoma, localized diffuse large B-cell lymphoma
- Relapsing cases: May require bone marrow transplantation

- Single-agent chemotherapy: May work for indolent cases (alkylating agents, purine nucleoside analogs).

Specific dosing depends on disease stage.

LEUKEMIA

Definitions

The leukemias are a group of blood malignancies characterized by unregulated growth of blood-forming cells in the bone marrow. These immature white cells crowd out normal cells in the bone marrow, leading to low red-cell, white-cell, and platelet counts. Four major types of leukemia exist: Acute lymphocytic (ALL), acute myeloid (AML), chronic lymphocytic (CLL), and chronic myeloid (CML) leukemias. Acute leukemias worsen rapidly; chronic leukemias worsen slowly. Exposure to radiation and chemicals (particularly benzene and formaldehyde) can increase leukemia risk.

Although the overall incidence of acute leukemias is low, they are the most common cancers in children, and ALL is the leading cause of cancer-related death in those under 35. AML occurs with increasing frequency in the elderly.

Diagnosis

- Bone marrow biopsy; send for morphologic examination
- AML diagnosis requires 20% blasts

Signs and Symptoms

- Weight loss, fatigue, malaise
- Palpitations and dyspnea on exertion
- Fever and chills; night sweats
- Bruising
- Bone pain

Guidelines

National Comprehensive Cancer Network, Clinical Practice Guidelines in Oncology, Version 1.2008: Acute Myeloid Leukemia – Full Report, 2008. www.nccn.org/professionals/physician_gls/PDF/aml.pdf.

National Comprehensive Cancer Network, Clinical Practice Guidelines in Oncology, Version 3.2008: Chronic Myelogenous Leukemia – Full Report, 2008. www.nccn.org/professionals/physician_gls/PDF/cml.pdf.

Guidelines Summary

AML:

- Anthracyclines and cytarabine are the most active agents for AML.
- Duration of remission is generally short; postremission therapy to prevent or delay relapse includes:
    - High-dose cytarabine
    - Allogenic or autologous hematopoietic stem cell transplantation (HSCT, bone marrow transplant)
- Gemtuzumab ozogamicin targets blasts expressing CD33.
    - Useful in older patients due to lower toxicity

CML:

- Philadelphia chromosome: abnormality characteristic of CML.
    - Results in bcr-abl fusion gene
    - Bone marrow makes tyrosine kinase enzyme; causes too many stem cells to form into white blood cells
- Tyrosine kinase inhibitors (primarily imatinib):
    - Target *bcr-abl* fusion gene
    - First-line treatment
- Interferon and conventional chemotherapy no longer considered first-line
- Allogenic hematopoietic stem cell transplant (alloHSCT): curative in many CML patients
    - Mortality is high
    - Busulfan and interferon-α increase post-transplant complications
    - Matched donor and younger age (below 50) required
    - No longer considered first-line

The National Comprehensive Cancer Network does not give guidelines for lymphocytic leukemia. Although protocols vary, methotrexate and cytarabine are commonly used in ALL. CLL is not currently considered curable; however, due to its often indolent time course, patients may live for years after diagnosis. Several biologic therapies targeting antigens expressed on B lymphocytes may be useful in appropriate cases of lymphocytic leukemia.

- Rituximab: Targets CD20
- Alemtuzumab: Targets CD52

LUNG CANCER

Definitions

Lung cancer is the leading cause of cancer death in men and women. Most lung cancers are non-small cell (NSCLC); while this type of cancer is slower-growing, it does not respond well to chemotherapy and only about 14% of patients can be cured. Small-cell lung cancer (SCLC) is very aggressive, and though it is chemotherapy-sensitive, most patients die within 2 years of diagnosis. Smoking is the primary risk factor for lung cancer; over 80% of patients have a history of smoking. Occupational exposure to asbestos, radon and other agents may also increase risk, as can certain genetic abnormalities and family history of the disease.

Diagnosis

- Chest x-ray, CT scans, and PET scan to detect lesions and determine extent of disease
- Pathological confirmation by sputum cytology or tumor biopsy

Signs and Symptoms

- Cough—most common
- Other lung-related symptoms (sputum production, dyspnea, wheezing); often misattributed to concomitant pulmonary conditions
- Weight loss, fever, bone pain
- Paraneoplastic syndromes:
    - Occur in 10% of cases; may be first sign or symptom:
    - Inappropriate secretion of antidiuretic hormone (SIADH)
    - Hypercalcemia
    - Eaton-Lambert myasthenic syndrome: muscle weakness and autonomic dysfunction

Guidelines

National Comprehensive Cancer Network, Clinical Practice Guidelines in Oncology, Version 2.2008: Non-Small Cell Lung Cancer–Full Report, 2008. www.nccn.org/professionals/physician_gls/PDF/nscl.pdf.

National Comprehensive Cancer Network, Clinical Practice Guidelines in Oncology, Version 1.2008: Small Cell Lung Cancer–Full Report, 2008. www.nccn.org/professionals/physician_gls/PDF/sclc.pdf.

Guidelines Summary

- Early-stage NSCLC: surgical resection is treatment of choice
- Radiation and chemotherapy: may also be used, and preferred with SCLC
- Advanced disease:
  - Cisplatin-based combination therapy
  - Bevacizumab is used in cases with vascular endothelial growth factor (VEGF) overexpression
- Recurrent disease:
  - Docetaxel or pemetrexed
  - Erlotinib in cases with EGFR overexpression; works only in small subset of patients

COLORECTAL CANCER

Definitions

Colorectal cancer is the third leading cause of cancer death in the United States. Incidence is highest in industrialized countries and may be linked to a higher-fat, lower-fiber diet in such locations. Genetic predisposition also plays a role in 5–10% of cases. Primary prevention strategies involve dietary change (increase calcium, fiber and antioxidants and decrease fat) and use of aspirin, NSAIDs, and COX-2 inhibitors. These drugs may inhibit free radical formation and the COX-2 overexpression that is seen in precancerous lesions in the colon. Regular use could decrease risk by up to 50%.

Diagnosis

- Fecal occult blood testing (FOBT) may decrease cancer mortality by one-third, but has a high false-negative rate as many early stage tumors do not bleed.
- FOBT plus immunochemical assays lead to improved specificity and sensitivity.
- Flexible sigmoidoscopy can detect lesions in distal and sigmoid colon; early detection and excision can decrease mortality by 60%.
- Colonoscopy is preferred screening method as it shows entire colon, but it requires more bowel preparation.
- Double-contrast barium enema plus flexible sigmoidoscopy may be used instead of colonoscopy.

Signs and Symptoms

- Change in bowel habits (diarrhea, constipation, stools narrower than usual)
- Rectal bleeding / blood in the stool

- Nausea, vomiting, and abdominal discomfort (gas pains or cramps, bloating)
- Fatigue (generally related to anemia)
- Weight loss
- Leg edema (result of lymph-node involvement)
- Hepatomegaly and jaundice

Guidelines

National Comprehensive Cancer Network, Clinical Practice Guidelines in Oncology, Version 1.2008: Colon Cancer – Full Report, 2008. www.nccn.org/professionals/physician_gls/PDF/colon.pdf.

Guideline Summary

- Surgical resection is treatment of choice (Stages I–III)
  - Complete resection of tumor and adjacent sections of tumor-free bowel; regional lymphadenectomy
- Adjuvant radiation therapy and chemotherapy: may be indicated for Stage II; standard therapy for Stage III
- Most common: 5-fluorouracil (5-FU) with leucovorin to enhance cytotoxicity
- Biologic therapies gaining popularity:
  - Bevacizumab: Targets VEGF
  - Cetuximab: Targets epidermal growth factor receptor (EGFR)

BREAST CANCER

Definitions

Breast cancer is the most common cancer in women and is second only to lung cancer as a cause of cancer death in women. Family history plays a large role in the development of breast cancer, with mutations in the BRCA1/BRCA2 tumor suppressor genes leading to high risk. Long-term progestin use and other endocrine factors (early menarche, late menopause, advanced age at first pregnancy) and lifestyle factors (high fat intake, alcohol consumption, obesity) also increase risk of developing breast cancer. Prognosis is poor in younger (under 35) and premenopausal patients, African Americans, and those with HER2/neu overexpression.

Diagnosis

- Palpable mass on physical examination
- Breast imaging techniques: mammography and/or ultrasound
- Biopsy if mass or cluster of calcifications is detected

Signs and Symptoms

- May be asymptomatic
- Painless lump: Initial sign in 90% of patients
- Stabbing or aching pain is initial sign in remaining 10%
- Nipple discharge, retraction, dimpling
- Scaly, red, or swollen skin of breast or nipple
- Advanced disease: bone pain, difficulty breathing, jaundice, abdominal enlargement, mental status changes

Guidelines

National Comprehensive Cancer Network, Clinical Practice Guidelines in Oncology, Version 2.2008: Breast Cancer–Full Report, 2008. www.nccn.org/professionals/physician _gls/PDF/breast.pdf.

Guideline Summary

- Early-stage treatment: Surgery and chemotherapy, with possible radiation therapy
- Adjuvant chemotherapy:
  - Anthracyclines: Most active against breast cancer
  - Taxanes
- Adjuvant endocrine therapy:
  - Antiestrogens: Tamoxifen gold standard in premenopausal women
  - Luteinizing hormone-releasing hormone (LH-RH) agonists: Useful in premenopausal women; may preserve fertility
  - Aromatase inhibitors: Anastrazole (more effective than tamoxifen in postmenopausal women)
- In metastatic cancer, endocrine therapy given first, then chemotherapy.
- Biologic therapy:
  - Trastuzumab: If tumor overexpresses HER2/neu; do not give with anthracyclines (additive cardiotoxicity)
  - Bevacizumab: Targets VEGF
  - Lapatinib: Targets HER2/neu and EGFR

PROSTATE CANCER

Definitions

Prostate cancer is the most common cancer in men, and the second most common cause of cancer death in men. One-third to one-half of men present with advanced disease, for which there is no cure. High-fat diet and hormonal factors are two of the primary risk factors; as prostate cancer is androgen-dependent, high levels of testosterone can fuel tumor growth. This may explain the increased incidence in African American men, who generally have testosterone levels 15% higher than Caucasian men.

Diagnosis

- Transrectal ultrasound or cystoscopy
- Biopsy: Only sure method of diagnosis

Signs and Symptoms

- Elevated prostate-specific antigen (PSA)
- Nodule on digital rectal exam of the prostate
- Localized disease: Generally asymptomatic; symptoms of prostatic enlargement may indicate cancer, benign prostatic hyperplasia, or infection; further investigation warranted
  - Urinary difficulty
  - Difficulty in having an erection
  - Blood in the urine or semen
- Advanced disease:
  - Bone pain
  - Anemia and fatigue, weight loss
  - Back pain
  - Edema of the legs

Guidelines

National Comprehensive Cancer Network, Clinical Practice Guidelines in Oncology, Version 1.2008: Prostate Cancer – Full Report, 2008. www.nccn.org/professionals/physician _gls/PDF/prostate.pdf.

Guideline Summary

- Prostatectomy performed
- Bilateral orchiectomy (removal of testes): reduces androgen levels but unacceptable to many patients
- Endocrine therapy: used to reduce androgen levels
- LH-RH agonists
  - Monotherapy is effective
  - Lower side-effect profile
- Antiandrogens
  - Monotherapy is less effective than LH-RH agonists
  - No sexual dysfunction; more accepted by younger patients
- Combined hormonal blockade; small survival advantage, but large financial cost and additional toxicities

OVARIAN CANCER

Definitions

Ovarian cancer typically occurs postmenopause. Risk factors include family history of ovarian or breast cancer, personal history of other types of cancer, nulliparity, and long-term estrogen therapy (without progesterone). Genetics also play a role; breast cancer and ovarian cancer are linked to mutation in BRCA1/BRCA2, along with other genetic alterations.

Diagnosis

- Ovarian size/contour on pelvic exam
- Elevation of CA-125 (antigen common to most ovarian cancers)
- Pelvic ultrasound
- Biopsy

Signs and Symptoms

Symptoms may be vague and nonspecific, but may include:

- Fatigue
- Back pain
- Bloating, constipation, abdominal pain
- Palpable abdominal mass, abdominal distention
- Hepatic and renal function abnormalities

Guidelines

National Comprehensive Cancer Network, Clinical Practice Guidelines in Oncology, Version 1.2008: Ovarian Cancer – Full Report, 2008. www.nccn.org/professionals/physician _gls/PDF/ovarian.pdf.

Guideline Summary

- Surgery and chemotherapy are used; radiation therapy is not often included unless the cancer is confined to one or both ovaries.
- Drug treatment generally involves taxane and/or platinum therapy.

Oncology Drugs

Note: None of the drugs contained in this table are in the Top 200 prescribed medications.

Mechanism of action – alkylating agents: alkylate DNA, making it more prone to breakage; most effective against rapidly dividing cells

Generic	Brand	Contraindications	Primary Side Effects	Key Monitoring	Pertinent Drug Interactions	Med Pearl
Cyclophosphamide	• Cytoxan (PO) • Neosar (IV)	None	• Alopecia • Hemorrhagic cystitis • Infertility • Nausea, vomiting, mucositis, stomatitis	• CBC with differential • Scr & BUN • UA	CYP3A4 inducers may increase levels of active metabolite, acrolein	• Maintain adequate hydration to avoid hemorrhagic cystitis • High emetogenic potential • Tablets should be taken with food • Injection can be taken by mouth
Chlorambucil	Leukeran (PO)	Hypersensitivity to any alkylating agent	• Bone marrow suppression • Infertility • Secondary leukemias • Seizures • Stevens-Johnson syndrome • Hepatotoxicity	• CBC wkly • WBC 2x wk for first 4–6 wks • LFTs	None	• Take on empty stomach • Avoid alcohol
Carmustine	BiCNU (IV) Gliadel (intracranial implant)	None	• Bone marrow suppression • Pulmonary fibrosis • Severe nausea, vomiting • Hypotension (IV) • Secondary leukemias (with long-term use) • Reversible elevation of LFTs	• CBC with differential • Pulmonary function tests • LFTS • BP during IV administration	• May decrease digoxin absorption • IV solution contains ethanol; do not give aldehyde-dehydrogenase inhibitors	Very high emetogenic potential

Oncology Drugs (cont'd)

Generic	Brand	Contraindications	Primary Side Effects	Key Monitoring	Pertinent Drug Interactions	Med Pearl
Mechanism of action – platinum-based agents: crosslink DNA, causing it to break						
Cisplatin	Generic (IV)	• Hypersensitivity to any platinum-containing compounds • Renal insufficiency • Pre-existing hearing impairment (cisplatin)	• Anaphylaxis • Dose-related myelosuppression, nausea and vomiting • Ototoxicity (cisplatin) • Renal toxicity with cumulative doses (esp. cisplatin)	• Serum creatinine and BUN • Electrolytes • Neurologic exam • CBC with differential • Urine output	• Administration with taxane derivatives may increase myelosuppression and decrease efficacy of platinum agents • May decrease digoxin levels (oxaliplatin)	• Do not administer doses exceeding 100 mg/m² 1x every 3 wks • High emetogenic potential
Carboplatin	Paraplatin (IV)					High emetogenic potential
Oxaliplatin	Eloxatin (IV)					• Moderate emetogenic potential • Warn patients to wear a scarf if being treated during cold weather to prevent laryngeal spasms
Mechanism of action – enzyme inhibitors: target enzymes responsible for DNA replication and repair						
Irinotecan	Camptosar (IV)	Concurrent therapy with ketoconazole or St. John's wort	• Bone marrow suppression, anemia • Severe, life-threatening diarrhea	• CBC with differential • Electrolytes (esp. if diarrhea)	• CYP3A4 substrate • Ketoconazole • St. John's wort	• Diarrhea may be early or late onset • High emetogenic potential
Etoposide	VePesid (PO)	None	• Bone marrow suppression • Hepatotoxicity	• CBC with differential • LFTs	CYP3A4 substrate	• Do not give IV push (may cause hypotension) • Do not give IM (necrosis)
Mechanism of action – antimitotics (spindle poisons): interfere with mitotic spindle; prevent chromosome segregation and lead to cell death						
Vincristine	Oncovin (IV)	None	• Peripheral neuropathy (dose-limiting) • Paralytic ileus (secondary to neurologic toxicity) • Photosensitivity • Hepatotoxicity	• Neurological examination • LFTs • Change in frequency of bowel movements	CYP3A4 substrate	• *Do not* give intrathecally (fatal) • All patients should be on a prophylactic bowel management regimen • Avoid extravasation (vesicant)

Oncology Drugs *(cont'd)*

Generic	Brand	Contraindications	Primary Side Effects	Key Monitoring	Pertinent Drug Interactions	Med Pearl
Vinblastine	Generic (IV)	None	• Neurotoxicity • Bone marrow suppression (dose-limiting)	CBC with differential	CYP3A4 substrate	• *Do not* give intrathecally (fatal) • Avoid extravasation (vesicant) • May cause metallic taste
Paclitaxel	Taxol (IV)	Hypersensitivity to Cremophor	• Bone marrow suppression (dose-limiting) • Peripheral neuropathy • Cardiac rhythm abnormalities • Hepatotoxicity • Mucositis, stomatitis (severe)	• CBC with differential • Monitor for cardiac abnormalities • LFTs	• CYP3A4 substrate • Administer prior to platinum derivatives to limit myelosuppression and enhance efficacy • May decrease digoxin absorption	Pretreat with dexamethasone, diphenhydramine, and H2RA
Paclitaxel nanoparticles bound to albumin	Abraxane (IV)	Baseline neutrophils <1,500/mm^3	• Bone marrow suppression • Cardiac disturbances (abnormal ECG 60%) • Dose-related sensory neuropathy • Hepatotoxicity • Visual disturbances	• CBC • BP (during infusion) • Baseline ECG	• Substrate of CYP2C9 and CYP3A4 • Administer prior to platinum derivatives to limit myelosuppression and enhance efficacy • May decrease digoxin absorption	No need for pretreatment with steroids
Docetaxel	Taxotere (IV)	• Hypersensitivity to polysorbate 80 • Baseline neutrophils <1,500/mm^3	• Significant, dose-dependent fluid retention • Hepatotoxicity • Bone marrow suppression • Decrease in LVEF • Infusion-related reactions	• CBC with differential • LFTs • Weight, signs of edema	• CYP3A4 substrate • Administer prior to platinum derivatives to limit myelosuppression and enhance efficacy	• Avoid doses >100 mg/m^2 • Pretreat with corticosteroids for 1–5 days to prevent fluid retention and hypersensitivity reactions

Oncology Drugs *(cont'd)*

Mechanism of action – antimetabolite nucleoside analogs

Generic	Brand	Contraindications	Primary Side Effects	Key Monitoring	Pertinent Drug Interactions	Med Pearl
Cytarabine	Cytosar (IV)	None	• Potent bone marrow suppression • Cytarabine syndrome: myalgia, bone pain, rash, conjunctivitis, and fever	CBC with differential and platelets	May decrease levels of digoxin	• Pretreat with corticosteroid; may prevent cytarabine syndrome • May be administered IM, IT, or SQ at concentrations <100 mg/mL
	DepoCyt (IT)	Active meningeal infection	• Chemical arachnoiditis (nausea, vomiting, headache, & fever) • Neurotoxicity	Monitor closely for signs of immediate reactions and neurotoxicity	None reported; limited systemic exposure	• Co-administer dexamethasone to lessen chemical arachnoiditis • Moderate emetogenic potential
5-Fluorouracil	Adrucil (IV)	• Dihydropyrimidine dehydrogenase (DPD) deficiency • Hypersensitivity • Pregnancy	• Hand-and-foot syndrome • Vomiting, diarrhea, mucositis, stomatitis • Bone marrow suppression	CBC with differential and platelets	Warfarin: may increase aPTT and bleeding time; monitor	• Leucovorin increases effectiveness and toxicity; dose of fluorouracil may need to be decreased

Mechanism of action – antimetabolite folic acid antagonist

Generic	Brand	Contraindications	Primary Side Effects	Key Monitoring	Pertinent Drug Interactions	Med Pearl
Methotrexate	Trexall (PO) Generic (IV, IM)	• Severe renal or hepatic impairment • AIDS • Pre-existing blood dyscrasias	• Renal damage • Bone marrow suppression • Stevens-Johnson syndrome • Severe diarrhea and ulcerative stomatitis • Neurotoxicity	• CBC • Serum creatinine • LFTs	NSAIDs: may cause severe bone marrow suppression, aplastic anemia, or GI toxicity	• Give leucovorin rescue 24 hrs after dosing to limit toxicity; do not administer concurrently

Oncology Drugs *(cont'd)*

Generic	Brand	Contraindications	Primary Side Effects	Key Monitoring	Pertinent Drug Interactions	Med Pearl
Mechanism of action – hormonal agents: treat cancers in which growth is accelerated by hormones						
Leuprolide	Lupron (SQ)	• Spinal cord compression • Undiagnosed abnormal vaginal bleeding	• Abnormal menses • Exacerbation of endometriosis • Hot flashes/sweats • Decrease in bone mineral density (is used >6 mos) • Spinal cord compression and urinary tract obstruction in prostate cancer • Tumor flare • Depression, mood disturbances	• LH and FSH levels • Serum testosterone (males), estradiol (females) • Bone mineral density	None	• Administered daily • Rotate injection sites
	Lupron depot (IM)					• Administered every 1–6 mos, depending on dosage • Rotate injection sites
	Eligard (SQ depot formulation)					
Tamoxifen	Nolvadex (PO)	• Concurrent warfarin therapy • History of DVT or pulmonary embolism	• Serious, life-threatening thromboembolic events • Increased risk of endometrial cancer • Ocular effects • Hot flashes • Altered menses • Mood disturbances, depression	Annual gynecologic exams	• CYP3A4 substrate • Warfarin: significant enhancement of anticoagulant effects	• Bone pain may indicate a good therapeutic response; manage with mild analgesic • Used in premenopausal women
Anastrozole	Arimidex (PO)	None	• Decrease in bone mineral density • Hyperlipidemia • Mood disturbances	• Bone mineral density • LDL and total cholesterol	Estrogen derivatives diminish therapeutic effects	Used in postmenopausal women
Mechanism of action – anthracyclines: intercalate DNA and generate reactive oxygen species						
Daunorubicin	Cerubidine (IV)	Pre-existing severe myocardial insufficiency or arrhythmia	• Dose-related cardiotoxicity • Severe bone marrow suppression • Skin necrosis (if extravasation occurs) • Red coloration of body fluids	CBC with differential ECG, LVEF	• CYP2D6 substrate • Trastuzumab, bevacizumab, and taxane derivatives (increased cardiotoxicity)	• Greatest risk of irreversible myocardial damage at cumulative dose >500 mg/m² • Never administer IM or SQ (skin necrosis and ulceration)
Doxorubicin	Adriamycin (IV)		• Dose-related cardiotoxicity • Severe bone marrow suppression • Secondary leukemias			

Storage and Administration Pearls

- 5-FU IV solution may be mixed with water, grape juice, or soda and given by mouth.
- Do not administer live vaccines during chemotherapy cycles.

Patient Education Pearls

- Patient should not breastfeed or attempt to become pregnant while taking chemotherapy.
- Because Bexxar and Zevalin contain radioactive isotopes, patients should be instructed on proper handwashing, special disposal of bodily waste, and other ways to limit exposure to family members postdischarge.

SUPPORTIVE CARE

About 55% of cancer patients experience nausea and vomiting during the first week of chemotherapy. 5HT3 antagonists are useful in most cases, but should be used only for prevention of nausea and vomiting. Corticosteroids should be given unless contraindicated, as they are synergistic with the 5HT3 antagonists; other drug therapies depend on the type of nausea and vomiting experienced.

- Benzodiazepines: Treatment of choice for anticipatory nausea and vomiting (caused by the sights and smells of the chemotherapy environment)
- Aprepitant: Useful for delayed nausea and vomiting caused by drugs with high emetic potential (cisplatin, cyclophosphamide, doxorubicin)
- Prochlorperazine or metoclopramide: May be used in less severe cases

Pain is one of the most common symptoms associated with cancer and occurs in up to 75% of advanced cases, greatly affecting quality of life. Cancer pain frequently requires much higher analgesic doses than pain from other causes. As a result, cancer pain is often undertreated.

For uncontrolled pain, drug choice depends on prior opioid use and severity of pain. If opioids have not been used:

- Severe pain: Rapid titration with short-acting opioids
- Moderate pain: Slower titration with short-acting opioids
- Mild pain: NSAID, acetaminophen, or slow titration with short-acting opioids

Morphine, codeine, oxycodone, oxymorphone, hydromorphone, and fentanyl are the most commonly used opioids for cancer pain; all are short-acting agents unless given in a controlled-release dosage form. These formulations are recommended only for non–opioid naïve patients, as they cannot be easily titrated. Methadone is occasionally used in cancer pain, and has a longer half-life and duration of action. Patients taking controlled-release formulations should also receive a prescription for a short-acting, fast-onset analgesic for breakthrough pain. Likewise, patient-controlled analgesia devices should have on-demand bolus doses available for acute pain, with a lockout setting to reduce the risk of overdose.

Neutropenia and its major complication, neutropenic fever, are major concerns in many types of cancer. The nadir, or lowest, concentration of WBCs in the peripheral blood usually occurs 1–2 weeks following the administration of chemotherapy, and is typically proportional to the dose. Subsequent chemotherapy is delayed until the absolute neutrophil count (ANC) recovers, which explains the 3-to-4-week cycle length of most chemotherapy regimens. Classification of ANC is:

- Normal: 3,000–7,000 neutrophils/mm^3
- Mild neutropenia: 500–1,000/mm^3
- Moderate neutropenia: 100–500/mm^3
- Severe neutropenia: <100/mm^3

Colony-stimulating factors (CSF) such as filgrastim have been shown to shorten the duration of neutropenia, but they have little effect on mortality and are very expensive. CSFs do decrease hospitalizations, however, and clinical judgment should be used to determine which patients are most likely to benefit. Because infection leads to death in a large percentage of neutropenic patients (possibly up to 30%), anti-infective therapy is frequently needed. Broad-spectrum bactericidal antibiotics are generally used (third- and fourth-generation cephalosporins, carbapenems, or quinolones with or without aminoglycosides or β-lactams), with antipseudomonal activity being particularly important. If antifungal therapy is needed, amphotericin B is the drug of choice.

Anemia is also common in cancer patients. Treatment of anemia is currently the subject of much controversy; use of erythropoiesis-stimulating agents (ESA), including erythropoietin and darbepoetin, is no longer supported in myeloid malignancies due to a 2008 meta-analysis showing a 10% increase in mortality compared to patients not receiving erythropoietin. The hypothesis is that the drug may be stimulating cancer growth. This finding may not apply to solid tumors; more information is needed.

Antiemesis Drugs

Generic	Brand	Dose	Contraindications	Primary Side Effects	Key Monitoring	Pertinent Drug Interactions	Med Pearl	Top 200
Mechanism of action – 5HT3 antagonists; prevent release of serotonin in GI mucosa								
Ondansetron	Zofran	16–24 mg PO or 8–12 mg IV	Current nausea and vomiting (useful only for prevention)	• Headache • Constipation or diarrhea	None	CYP3A4 substrate	• Single dose prior to chemotherapy; repeat doses do not increase effect	No
Granisetron	Kytril	2 mg PO or 1 mg IV		• Fatigue • Dry mouth			• Can give IV ondansetron and dolasetron by mouth	No
Dolasetron	Anzemet	100 mg IV/PO		• Transient elevations in liver function tests			• Aloxi effective in preventing delayed nausea and vomiting	No
Palonosetron	Aloxi	0.25 mg IV						No
Mechanism of action – neurokinin-1 (NK-1) antagonist; blocks substance P from NK-1 receptor								
Aprepitant	Emend	Day 1: 125 mg Days 2–3: 80 mg	None	• Asthenia • Fatigue • Diarrhea • Hiccups • Dizziness • Dehydration	Monitor levels of chemotherapy agents metabolized by CYP3A4	• Inhibits CYP3A4 • Induces CYP2C9	• Use in combination with 5HT3 and steroid • Prevents delayed nausea and vomiting	No
Mechanism of action – corticosteroids; potentiate antiemetic properties of 5HT3 antagonists								
Dexamethasone	Decadron	8–40 mg daily	Systemic fungal infections	• Hyperglycemia • Immunosuppression • Adrenal suppression • Insomnia • Mood changes, anxiety • GI irritation • Weight gain	• Hgb • Fecal occult blood • Serum potassium • Glucose	• CYP3A4 substrate • Ethanol • Echinacea	• Synergistic with 5HT3 antagonists • Use as single agents for mild chemo-induced nausea and vomiting	Yes
Methylprednisolone	Solu-Medrol	40–125 mg daily			• Glucose			Yes
Mechanism of action – dopamine-2 antagonists								
Metoclopramide	Reglan	10–20 mg PO q2 hrs	With drugs causing dystonic reactions GI obstruction, perforation, or hemorrhage	• Dystonic reactions • Sedation, fatigue	• Dystonic reactions • Glucose	• Ethanol • Antipsychotic agents	Should not drive or operate heavy machinery while taking this drug	No

Cancer Pain Drugs

Mechanism of action: narcotic opioid analgesics; stimulate the μ opioid receptor, inhibiting pain pathways

Generic	Brand	Dose	Contraindications	Primary Side Effects	Key Monitoring	Pertinent Drug Interactions	Med Pearl	Top 200
Codeine	Various	15–60 mg q4–6 hrs	• Increased intracranial pressure • Severe respiratory depression • Severe or acute asthma • Paralytic ileus	• Drowsiness • Dizziness • Palpitations, hypotension • Nausea • Constipation • Xerostomia	• Pain release • Respiratory status • Mental status • Blood pressure	CNS depressants	• Usually in combination with aspirin, acetaminophen, or NSAIDs • Poor metabolizers of CYP2D6 cannot convert to morphine and receive no pain relief; start immediately on another drug	Yes (combination products)
Morphine	Injectable: generic	0.8–80 mg/hr				• Alcohol, CNS depressants • Mixed agonist/antagonist analgesics (could precipitate withdrawal) • Skeletal muscle relaxants • Cimetidine • Neuroleptics • MAOIs • Fentanyl is a CYP3A4 substrate	• Drug of choice for severe pain • Use immediate-release products to titrate and to control breakthrough pain • Do not crush controlled-release products; Kadian and Evinsa may be opened • Do not give Kadian through NG tube	Yes
	Immediate release: generic (tablet, liquid suppository) Roxanol (liquid)	• 5–30 mg q4h PO • 10–20 mg q4h rectally						

Cancer Pain Drugs *(cont'd)*

Generic	Brand	Dose	Contraindications	Primary Side Effects	Key Monitoring	Pertinent Drug Interactions	Med Pearl	Top 200
	Extended release: • MS Contin • Evinsa • Kadian • Oramorph	Varies widely in opioid-tolerant patients; no max dose in chronic pain	• Increased intracranial pressure • Severe respiratory depression • Severe or acute asthma • Paralytic ileus	• Drowsiness • Dizziness • Palpitations, hypotension • Nausea • Constipation • Xerostomia	• Pain release • Respiratory status • Mental status • Blood pressure	• Alcohol, CNS depressants • Mixed agonist/antagonist analgesics (could precipitate withdrawal) • Skeletal muscle relaxants • Cimetidine • Neuroleptics • MAOIs • Fentanyl is a CYP3A4 substrate		
Hydromorphone	Dilaudid (tablets, liquid, injection, suppository)	2.5–10 mg q3–6 hrs PO 1–2 mg q4–6 hrs SQ or IM					• More potent than morphine • Short half-life; requires frequent dosing	No
Oxycodone	• OxyContin • Percocet (with acetaminophen)	10–30 mg q4h (IR) 10 mg q12h (CR); titrate dosage upward as needed					Do not crush CR tabs	Yes
Fentanyl	Actiq, Fentora (transmucosal)	100–200 mcg per episode					• Actiq and Fentora should be used for breakthrough pain only; they are not interchangeable • Duragesic should be used only for chronic pain in patients who are opioid-tolerant	No
	Duragesic (transdermal)	25–100 mcg/hr						Yes
Hydrocodone (available only in combination products)	With acetaminophen: • Vicodin • Lortab • Lorcet • Anexsia With ibuprofen: • Vicoprofen	1 tablet (5–10 mg) q4–6 hrs Maximum of 5 tabs/24 hrs					Other drugs limit ability to titrate upward	Yes

Colony-Stimulating Factors

Generic	Brand	Dose	Contra-indications	Primary Side Effects	Key Monitoring	Pertinent Drug Interactions	Med Pearl	Top 200
Mechanism of action – stimulate production of white blood cells								
Filgrastim	Neupogen	300–480 mcg SQ daily	Hypersensitivity to *E. coli*	• Bone pain • Hypertension	CBC with differential	Use lithium with caution, as it can potentiate neutrophil release	• Requires daily administration • Neutrophil-specific	No
PEG-Filgrastim	Neulasta	6 mg SQ with each chemotherapy cycle		• Swelling • Redness • Hypersensitivity reactions • Can act as tumor growth factor			• PEG unit increases half-life; can give 1x per chemotherapy cycle • Neutrophil-specific	No
Sargramostim	Leukine	250–500 mcg SQ daily	• Hypersensitivity to yeast • Excessive leukemic myeloid blasts in bone marrow	• Fever, chills • Bone pain • Myalgia • Hypertension • Hypersensitivity reactions			• Requires daily administration • Stimulates formation of all WBCs except lymphocytes	No

Storage and Administration Pearls

- Dolasetron injection may be diluted in apple or apple-grape juice and taken orally; stable for 2 hours.
- Zofran ODT contains phenylalanine; sensitive patients may take IV solution orally.

Patient Education Pearls

- Kadian and Evinsa may be opened and sprinkled on applesauce; do not chew, crush, or let dissolve, or too much drug will be absorbed too quickly.
- Patient should take morphine with food if it causes stomach upset.
- Patient should not take echinacea if she is taking corticosteroids.

LEARNING POINTS

- Chemotherapy protocols vary tremendously; you should focus more on the toxicity profile of the most commonly used drugs and less on dosing and specific drug combinations.
- Because of the increasing importance of pharmacogenomics, you should know what drugs target specific receptors (Herceptin – HER2 receptor, Erbitux – EGFR, Rituxan – CD20 cell surface protein, etc.).
- Leucovorin is used as a rescue agent in patients receiving methotrexate but enhances the effect of 5-FU.
- To treat nausea and vomiting, most patients should receive a corticosteroid, a 5HT3 antagonist, and possibly a benzodiazepine. For severe cases, aprepitant should be added.
- Short-acting opioids are the pain management drugs of choice for cancer pain. As severity increases, titration should be performed more quickly.

PRACTICE QUESTIONS

1. Effective anti-androgen therapy in prostate cancer consists of which of the following?

       I. An LH-RH agonist
      II. A testosterone antagonist
    III. Bilateral orchiectomy

  (A) I only
  (B) II only
  (C) I and II
  (D) I or III
  (E) I, II, and III

2. Which of the following chemotherapeutic agents is associated with profound acute- and late-onset diarrhea?

  (A) Irinotecan
  (B) Doxorubicin
  (C) Daunorubicin
  (D) Trastuzumab
  (E) Methotrexate

3. The mechanism of action of Emend is

  (A) 5HT3 receptor antagonist.
  (B) neurokinin-1 receptor antagonist.
  (C) D2 receptor antagonist.
  (D) benzodiazepine receptor agonist.
  (E) histamine receptor antagonist.

ANSWERS

1. **D**

Either an LH-RH agonist (I) or a bilateral orchiectomy (III) is considered adequate anti-androgen therapy in prostate cancer. Therefore, (D) is correct. Testosterone antagonists (II) are not generally considered as solo agents, and in most studies have been shown to provide limited (if any) survival benefit when added to LH-RH agonist therapy. The major use for testosterone blockers is to prevent adverse effects from the initial testosterone surge that accompanies the initiation of LH-RH agonist therapy.

2. **A**

Of the drugs listed, only irinotecan exhibits major GI adverse effects. The other drugs are more likely to lead to cardiomyopathy (trastuzumab, doxorubicin, and daunorubicin) or neuro-, nephro-, and hepatotoxicity (methotrexate).

3. **B**

Emend (aprepitant) is a highly selective emetogenic agent that works against the neurokinin-1 receptor. It has little to no affinity for the other receptor targets of chemotherapy-induced or postoperative nausea and vomiting.

Psychiatric Disorders

8

This chapter covers the following disease states:

- **Depression**
- **Anxiety**
- **Bipolar disorder**
- **Schizophrenia**

 Suggested Study Time: **45 minutes**

DEPRESSION

Definition

Depression, or major depressive disorder, is a complex mood disorder that has many subtypes and is due to multiple etiologies. Depression can be classified as single-episode, recurrent, or chronic, and as depression with or without psychotic features, with typical or atypical symptoms, etc.

Diagnosis

The diagnosis of depression is based on the Diagnostic and Statistical Manual of Mental Disorders, 4th Edition (DSM IV). Criteria for diagnosis are based primarily on symptoms. Five or more of the following symptoms must have been present during the same 2-week period and must represent a change from previous functioning; at least one of the symptoms is either (*1*) depressed mood or (*2*) loss of interest or pleasure.

- Depressed mood most of the day, nearly every day
- Markedly diminished interest or pleasure in all, or almost all, activities

- Significant weight loss when not dieting, or weight gain
- Insomnia or hypersomnia nearly every day
- Psychomotor agitation or retardation nearly every day
- Fatigue or loss of energy nearly every day
- Feelings of worthlessness or of excessive or inappropriate guilt
- Diminished ability to think or concentrate, or indecisiveness
- Recurrent thoughts of death (not just fear of dying), recurrent suicidal ideation without a specific plan, or a suicide attempt or a specific plan for committing suicide

Signs and Symptoms

Signs and symptoms are detailed in the diagnostic criteria.

GUIDELINES

American Psychiatric Association practice guidelines for the treatment of patients with major depressive disorder. American Journal of Psychiatry, no. 157 (4 Suppl) (2000): pp 1–45.

GUIDELINES SUMMARY

- The primary goal of therapy is remission of symptoms.
- There are various antidepressant medications available. Clinical evidence indicates that, in general, efficacy is similar between classes.
- Initial choice of pharmacotherapy agent is based on anticipated side effects, tolerability of these side effects for an individual patient, patient preference, quantity and quality of clinical evidence, and cost.
- First-line options for most patients include selective serotonin reuptake inhibitors (SSRIs), desipramine, nortriptyline, bupropion, and venlafaxine. Because of the potential for serious side effects and drug interactions, monoamine oxidase inhibitors (MAOIs) should be reserved for patients who do not respond to other therapies.
- An adequate therapy trial requires at least 6–8 weeks. Dose adjustments or treatment changes are made at 6-to-8-week intervals at the earliest.

Antidepressants

Mechanism of action – selective serotonin reuptake inhibitors (SSRIs): inhibit reuptake of serotonin, allowing more serotonin availability in synapses

Generic	Brand	Dose & Max Mg (frequency)	Contra-indications	Primary Side Effects	Key Monitoring Parameters	Pertinent Drug Interactions	Med Pearls	Top 200
Citalopram	Celexa	10–60 mg daily (q day)	MAOI; Pimozide; Hypersensitivity	• Lightheadedness • Syncope • Sweating • Diarrhea • Nausea • Xerostomia • Confusion • Dizziness • Somnolence • Tremor • Hallucinations • Disorder of ejaculation • Impotence • Rhinitis • Fatigue	• Reduction or resolution of symptoms • Withdrawal symptoms from abrupt discontinuation • Abnormal bleeding • Worsening of depression, suicidality, or unusual behavior at initiation of therapy or when changing dose	• Other serotonergic medications, such as MAOI, SSRI, triptans, linezolid, St. John's wort, tramadol	Racemic mixture R and S isomer	Yes
Escitalopram	Lexapro	10–20 mg daily (q day)					Only contains the S isomer of citalopram	Yes
Fluoxetine	• Prozac • Prozac Wkly • Sarafem • Rapiflux	20–60 mg daily (q day) or 80 mg wkly (q week)				• Other serotonergic medications such as MAOI, SSRI, triptans, linezolid, St. John's wort, tramadol, phenytoin • Drugs metabolized by cytochrome P450	Allow 5 wks washout prior to MAOI due to long half-life	Yes
Fluvoxamine	Luvox	50–300 mg daily (q day)	MAOI; Pimozide; Thioridazine; Alosetron; Astemizole; terfenadine; Tizanidine; hypersensitivity					No
Paroxetine	Paxil	20–60 mg daily (q day)	MAOI; Pimozide; Thioridazine; hypersensitivity			Other serotonergic medications such as MAOI, SSRI, triptans, linezolid, St. John's wort, tramadol		Yes
Sertraline	Zoloft	50–200 mg daily (q day)	MAOI; Pimozide; disulfiram-like compounds (oral concentrate); Linezolid; hypersensitivity				Oral concentrate contains alcohol	Yes

Antidepressants (cont'd)

Mechanism of action – tricyclic antidepressants (TCAs): increased synaptic concentration of norepinephrine and serotonin

Generic	Brand	Dose & Max Mg (frequency)	Contra-indications	Primary Side Effects	Key Monitoring Parameters	Pertinent Drug Interactions	Med Pearls	Top 200
Amitriptyline	• Elavil • Vanatrip	50–300 mg daily (q day–TID)	• MAOI • Post-MI acute recovery • Hypersensitivity	• Anticholinergic symptoms • Weight gain • Bloating • Blurred vision • Xerostomia • Constipation • Asthenia • Dizziness • Somnolence • Headache • Fatigue	• Reduction or resolution of symptoms • Withdrawal symptoms from abrupt discontinuation • Worsening of depression, suicidality, or unusual behavior at initiation of therapy or when changing dose • Blood pressure • ECG in patients with cardiac disease or hyperthyroidism	Other serotonergic medications such as MAOI, SSRI, triptans, linezolid, St. John's wort, tramadol	• Dangerous in overdose situations • Avoid in patients with high suicidality • Avoid dispensing large quantities • Also used for sleep disorders	Yes
Amoxapine	Ascendin	50–600 mg daily (BID–TID)						No
Clomipramine	Anafranil	75–250 mg daily (divided TID)						No
Desipramine	Norpramin	100–300 mg daily (q day or divided doses)						No
Doxepin	• Sinequan • Prudoxin • Zonalon	25–300 mg daily (q day–TID)						No
Imipramine	Tofranil	100–300 mg daily (q day–divided)						No
Nortriptyline	• Pamelor • Aventyl	25 mg TID–QID; max: 150 mg daily						Yes
Protriptyline	Vivactil	15–60 mg daily (TID–QID)						No
Trimipramine	Surmontil	75–300 mg daily (q day–TID)						No

Antidepressants *(cont'd)*

Mechanism of action – selective serotonin and norepinephrine reuptake inhibitors: inhibit the reuptake of serotonin and norepinephrine to allow higher available synaptic concentrations

Generic	Brand	Dose & Max Mg (frequency)	Contra-indications	Primary Side Effects	Key Monitoring Parameters	Pertinent Drug Interactions	Med Pearls	Top 200
Duloxetine	Cymbalta	30–120 mg daily (q day)	• MAOI • Hypersensitivity • Uncontrolled narrow-angle glaucoma	• Palpitations • Diaphoresis • Constipation • Decreased appetite • Diarrhea • Nausea • Xerostomia • Asthenia • Dizziness • Insomnia • Somnolence • Vertigo • Blurred vision • Polyuria • Reduced libido • Cough • Nasopharyngitis • Fatigue	• Reduction or resolution of symptoms • Withdrawal symptoms from abrupt discontinuation • Worsening of depression	Other serotonergic medications such as MAOI, SSRI, Triptans, Linezolid, St. John's wart, Tramadol;	Doses greater than 60 mg did not provide additional benefit in generalized anxiety disorder	Yes
Venlafaxine	• Effexor • Effexor XR	37.5–375 mg daily (q day–TID)	• MAOI • Hypersensitivity	• Hypertension • Sweating • Weight loss • Constipation • Loss of appetite • Nausea • Xerostomia • Insomnia or somnolence • Erectile dysfunction	• Reduction or resolution of symptoms • Withdrawal symptoms from abrupt discontinuation • Worsening of depression • Blood pressure • Heart rate • Lipid panel • Cough • Progressive dyspnea • Chest discomfort • Ocular pressure			Yes

Antidepressants *(cont'd)*

Generic	Brand	Dose & Max Mg (frequency)	Contra-indications	Primary Side Effects	Key Monitoring Parameters	Pertinent Drug Interactions	Med Pearls	Top 200
Nefazodone	Serzone	200–600 mg daily (BID)	• Previous nefazodone-induced hepatic damage • Hypersensitivity • Astemizole • Carbamazepine • Cisapride • Triazolam • Terfenadine • Pimozide	• Lightheadedness • Constipation • Indigestion • Nausea • Xerostomia • Asthenia • Confusion • Dizziness • Headache • Insomnia • Memory impairment • Somnolence	• Reduction or resolution of symptoms • Withdrawal symptoms from abrupt discontinuation • Worsening of depression			No

Antidepressants *(cont'd)*

Mechanism of action – monoamine oxidase inhibitors (MAOIs): increase epinephrine, norepinephrine, dopamine, and serotonin

Generic	Brand	Dose & Max Mg (frequency)	Contra-indications	Primary Side Effects	Key Monitoring Parameters	Pertinent Drug Interactions	Med Pearls	Top 200
Isocarboxazid	Marplan	20–60 mg daily (BID–QID)	• Cardiovascular disorder • Hypertension • Cerebrovascular disorder • Concurrent administration of interacting medications • General anesthesia • History of headache • Hypersensitivity • Pheochromocytoma • Severe renal function impairment	• Weight gain • Constipation • Xerostomia • Dizziness • Headache • Insomnia • Somnolence • Blurred vision • Anxiety • Mania	• Reduced depression and associated symptoms • Blood pressure • Liver function • Worsening of depression, suicidality, or unusual changes in behavior	• Other serotonergic medications such as SSRI, triptans, linezolid, St. John's wort, tramadol • Concurrent administration of antihistaminic, sedative, or anesthetic substances • Bupropion • Buspirone • Narcotics • Barbiturates • ethanol	Used very infrequently due to poor side-effect profile and frequency of drug interactions	No
Phenelzine	Nardil	45–90 mg daily (TID–QID)	• Cardiovascular disorder • Hypertension • Cerebrovascular disorder • Concurrent administration of interacting medications • General anesthesia • History of headache • Hypersensitivity • Pheochromocytoma • Severe renal function impairment			• Dextromethorphan • Excessive caffeine • Foods containing high concentrations of tyramine • Meperidine • SSRI • Sympathomimetic drugs • MAOI • TCA • Maprotiline • Carbamazepine • Cyclobenzaprine		No
Tranylcypromine	Parnate	30–60 mg daily (divided doses)						

Antidepressants *(cont'd)*

Generic	Brand	Dose & Max Mg (frequency)	Contra-indications	Primary Side Effects	Key Monitoring Parameters	Pertinent Drug Interactions	Med Pearls	Top 200
Selegiline	Emsam	6 mg daily transdermal patch (q day)	• Cardiovascular disorder • Hypertension • Cerebrovascular disorder • Concurrent administration of interacting medications • General anesthesia • History of headache • Hypersensitivity • Pheochromocytoma • Severe renal function impairment			• Other serotonergic medications such as SSRI, triptans, linezolid, St. John's wort, tramadol • Concurrent administration of antihistaminic, sedative, or anesthetic substances • Bupropion • Buspirone • Narcotics • Barbiturates • Ethanol • Dextromethorphan • Excessive caffeine • Foods containing high concentrations of tyramine • Meperidine • SSRI • Sympathomimetic drugs • MAOI • TCA • Maprotiline • Carbamazepine • Cyclobenzaprine	Used primarily for Parkinson's disease and less frequently for depression	No

Antidepressants *(cont'd)*

Mechanism of action — selective serotonin norepinephrine and dopamine reuptake inhibitor (SSNDRI); inhibits the reuptake of both serotonin and norepinephrine, increasing available concentrations in the synapse

Generic	Brand	Dose & Max Mg (frequency)	Contra-indications	Primary Side Effects	Key Monitoring Parameters	Pertinent Drug Interactions	Med Pearls	Top 200
Bupropion	• Wellbutrin • Wellbutrin SR • Wellbutrin XL • Zyban	100–450 mg daily (q day–QID)	• MAOI • Bulimia or anorexia • Patients in withdrawal from alcohol • Seizure disorders	• Taste disturbance • Agitation • Increased seizure activity	• Reduction or resolution of symptoms • Withdrawal symptoms from abrupt discontinuation • Worsening of depression • Seizure activity	MAOI	• Also used for smoking cessation • Mostly dopamine reuptake activity	Yes

Mechanism of action — tetracyclic antidepressants: increase available synaptic concentrations of norepinephrine, serotonin, or both

Generic	Brand	Dose & Max Mg (frequency)	Contra-indications	Primary Side Effects	Key Monitoring Parameters	Pertinent Drug Interactions	Med Pearls	Top 200
Maprotiline	Ludiomil	75–225 mg daily (BID–TID)	• MAOI • Hypersensitivity • Seizure disorder • Post-MI acute recovery period	• Hypotension • Tachyarrhythmia • Rash • Weight gain • Constipation • Nausea • Pancreatitis • Reduced salivation • Vomiting • Xerostomia	• Reduction or resolution of symptoms • Withdrawal symptoms from abrupt discontinuation • Worsening of depression	MAOI		No
Mirtazapine	• Remeron • Remeron Solutab	15–45 mg daily (q HS)		• Increased appetite • Hyperlipidemia • Weight gain • Constipation • Elevated transaminases		• MAOI • Clonidine • Tramadol • Fluoxetine • Fluvoxamine • Linezolid • Olanzapine • Venlafaxine	Dosed at bedtime due to somnolence	Yes

Storage and Administration Pearls

- Store at room temperature in a dry place that is protected from light.

PATIENT EDUCATION PEARLS

- It may take several weeks for medication to demonstrate maximal efficacy. Allow adequate trial before determining if medication is ineffective.
- Patients should not abruptly discontinue their medication. They should consult with a healthcare professional to determine appropriate tapering procedures.
- Patients on MAO inhibitors should avoid excessive caffeine intake, chocolate, and foods containing high levels of tyramine, including red wine, aged cheeses, avocado, eggplant, figs, and soy-based foods.

ANXIETY

Definition

Anxiety disorders consist of a number of disorders, including generalized anxiety disorder (GAD) and panic disorder. This chapter focuses on these two most common subtypes of anxiety disorders. The pathophysiology of anxiety is poorly understood but is theoretically linked to abnormal function of several neurotransmitters, including GABA, serotonin, and norepinephrine.

Diagnosis

GAD diagnosis is based on the presence of anxiety or excessive worry (1) that has been present on most days over at least 6 months, and (2) over which the patient feels a lack of control. Three or more subjective symptoms must be present in order to make the diagnosis.

Panic disorder is a complex disorder characterized by panic attacks. During a panic attack, at least four psychic and somatic symptoms will be present. In order to be diagnosed with panic disorder, a patient must have a history of recurrent panic attacks

Signs and Symptoms

- Subjective symptoms of GAD include restlessness, feeling easily fatigued, difficulty concentrating, irritability, muscle tension, and sleep difficulties.

- Psychic symptoms of panic disorder include depersonalization, fear of dying, derealization, fear of losing control, and fear of going "crazy."

- Somatic symptoms of panic disorder include sweating, trembling, shaking, choking, chest pain, nausea, abdominal pain, palpitations, tachycardia, shortness of breath, dizziness, light-headedness, chills, and hot flashes.

Summary of Treatment Recommendations

- Goals of therapy include improvement in overall functionality and quality of life through reduction of symptom frequency and intensity. Complete remission of illness is the long-term treatment goal.

- Treatment options are detailed in the medication charts and no consensus exists as to the preferred initial therapy or order of options thereafter.

- Many clinicians prefer the SSRIs as initial therapy due to their favorable side-effect profile as compared to other therapies. Subsequently, other antidepressants such as venlafaxine or tricyclics can be utilized. Benzodiazepines are commonly used, especially in acute situations. Although efficacious, these agents lend themselves to issues related to dependence, increased fall risk in the elderly, and potential for negative cognitive effects in general. Buspirone is a unique treatment option that is effective but requires 2 to 3 weeks to reach efficacy; thus, it is not useful in acute situations.

Anxiolytics

Mechanism of action – benzodiazepines bind to GABA receptors, causing an influx of chloride which results in hyperpolarization and a less excitable state; metabolized by CYP450, benzodiazepines have a potential interaction with all CYP450 inhibitors and inducers

Generic	Brand	Dose & Max Mg (frequency)	Contra-indications	Primary Side Effects	Key Monitoring Parameters	Pertinent Drug Interactions	Med Pearls	Top 200
Alprazolam	• Xanax • Xanax XR • Nirazax ODT • Alprazolam • Intensol	• IR: 0.25–2 mg (q day–TID) • XR: 0.5–3 mg (q day) • Max: 4 mg/day	• Hypersensitive • Narrow-angle glaucoma	• Somnolence • Ataxia • Dizziness • Changes in appetite • Decreased libido • Confusion • Constipation • Blurred vision	• Orthostasis • Excessive sedation • Signs of withdrawal • Periodic BMPs • LFTs and CBCs in chronic therapy	• Ketoconazole • Itraconazole • Alcohol • CNS depressants • Digoxin • Fluoxetine • Propoxyphene • Nefazodone	• Schedule C-IV • Pregnancy category D • Smoking decreases concentration up to 50% • Pediatric dosing	Yes
Chlordiazepoxide	Librium	5–25 mg (TID–QID)				• Alcohol • CNS depressants • Ketoconazole	• CrCl <10% give 50% of recommended dose • IV injection available • Avoid in elderly • Schedule C-IV • Pregnancy category D	No
Clonazepam	• Klonopin, • Klonopin Wafers	• 0.5–2 mg (BID) • ODT: 0.125–2 mg (BID)					• Decrease dose by 50% in elderly and hepatic disease • Pregnancy category D • Schedule C-IV	Yes
Clorazepate	• Gen-XENE • Tranxene T-Tab • Tranxene-SD • Tranxene	• IR: 3.75–15 mg (BID–QID) • ER: 11.25–22.5 mg (q day)					• Avoid in elderly • Schedule C-IV • Pregnancy category D	No
Diazepam	• Valium • Diazepam Intensol	2–10 mg (BID–QID)					• IV and liquid dosage forms available • Schedule C-IV • Pregnancy category D	Yes

Anxiolytics *(cont'd)*

Generic	Brand	Dose & Max Mg (frequency)	Contra-indications	Primary Side Effects	Key Monitoring Parameters	Pertinent Drug Interactions	Med Pearls	Top 200
Lorazepam	• Ativan • Lorazepam • Intensol	• 0.5–2 mg (BID–TID) • Max: 10 mg/day					• Available in IV and liquid form • Schedule C-IV • Pregnancy category D	Yes
Oxazepam		10–30 mg (TID–QID)					• Schedule C-IV • Pregnancy category D	No
Mechanism of action – selective serotonin reuptake inhibitors (SSRIs): selectively inhibit the reuptake of serotonin by presynaptic neuronal membranes with little to no effect on norepinephrine or dopamine reuptake								
Citalopram	Celexa	Details above in antidepressants table			Unlabeled use for panic disorder (PD), generalized anxiety disorder (GAD), post-traumatic stress disorder (PTSD), and obsessive–compulsive disorder (OCD)			Yes
Escitalopram	Lexapro				Indicated for GAD			Yes
Fluoxetine	• Prozac • Sarafem				Indicated for OCD, PD			Yes
Paroxetine	Paxil, Paxil CR				Indicated for PD, PTSD, GAD, OCD, social anxiety disorder (SAD)			
Sertraline	Zoloft				Indicated for OCD, PD, SAD, PTSD			
Fluvoxamine	Luvox				Indicated for OCD			No
Mechanism of action – nonselective beta-adrenergic blocker which competitively blocks response to beta1- and beta2-adrenergic stimulation in the heart muscle, vascular smooth muscle, and bronchial muscles								
Propranolol (nonselective BB)	• Inderal, Inderal LA • InnoPran XL • Propranolol • Intensol	10–80 mg 1 hr prior to anxiogenic event	• Hypersensitivity • Severe bradycardia • Heart block • Uncompensated CHF • Severe COPD or asthma	• Dizziness • Fatigue • GI upset • Hypotension	• Heart rate • Blood pressure	Inhibitors/inducers of CYP450 (major CYP1A2), non-dihydropyridine CCBs	Unlabeled for situational anxiety, acute panic	No

Anxiolytics *(cont'd)*

Generic	Brand	Dose & Max Mg (frequency)	Contra-indications	Primary Side Effects	Key Monitoring Parameters	Pertinent Drug Interactions	Med Pearls	Top 200
Mechanism of action – exact mechanism is unknown; high affinity for 5-HT$_{1A}$ and 5-HT$_2$ receptors, mild affinity for dopamine D$_2$ receptors								
Buspirone	BuSpar	• 5–30 mg (BID–TID) • Max 60 mg/day		• Headache • Dizziness • Nausea • Hostility • Confusion • Drowsiness	• Mental status • Symptoms of anxiety • Pseudo-parkinsonism	• MAOIs • Nondihydropyridine CCBs • Inhibitors/inducers of CYP450 • Macrolides • SSRIs	• Pregnancy category B • Avoid use in renal and hepatic impairment • Pediatric dosing for 6 yrs and older • Takes 2–3 wks to reach efficacy	Yes
Mechanism of action – selective norepinephrine reuptake inhibitor (SNRI): inhibits reuptake of neuronal serotonin and norepinephrine; may have weak inhibitory effect on reuptake of dopamine								
Venlafaxine	• Effexor • Effexor XR	• 25–100 mg (q day) • ER: 37.5–150 mg (q day) • Max: 225 mg/day	• Hypersensitivity • Concurrent use of MAOI	• Drowsiness • Dizziness • Insomnia • Xerostomia • Weakness (generalized) • Changes in appetite	• Blood pressure • Cholesterol • Mental status • Symptoms/signs of serotonin syndrome	• Alcohol • CNS depressants–SSRIs • TCAs • MAOIs • Buspirone • Tramadol • Lithium • Haloperidol • Clozapine • Nefazodone • Trazodone	• Labeled for GAD, PD, SAD • Pregnancy category C • **Black box warning** for suicidal ideation • Use with caution in renal impairment	Yes

Anxiolytics *(cont'd)*

Mechanism of action – inhibits neuronal reuptake of serotonin and norepinephrine; also blocks 5-HT$_2$ and alpha1 receptors

Generic	Brand	Dose & Max Mg (frequency)	Contra-indications	Primary Side Effects	Key Monitoring Parameters	Pertinent Drug Interactions	Med Pearls	Top 200
Nefazodone	Serzone	• 50–250 mg (q day–BID) • Max: 600 mg/day	• Hypersensitivity • Acute liver disease • Elevated LFTs • Concurrent use of carbamazepine • Cisapride • Pimozide	• Headache • Drowsiness • Insomnia • Dizziness • Xerostomia • Nausea • Constipation • Hypotension • Edema	LFTS: D/C at 3x ULN and do not reintroduce, mental status	• Triazolam • Alprazolam • Lovastatin • Simvastatin • Other statins to lesser extent • Digoxin • Alcohol • CNS depressants • Inhibitors/ inducers of CYP3A4	• Does not inhibit REM sleep • Unlabeled use in GAD, PD, PTSD, SAD • **Black box warning** for suicidal ideation • Pregnancy category C	No

Mechanism of action – competes with histamine for H$_1$-receptor sites on effector cells in GI, blood vessels, and respiratory tract

Generic	Brand	Dose & Max Mg (frequency)	Contra-indications	Primary Side Effects	Key Monitoring Parameters	Pertinent Drug Interactions	Med Pearls	Top 200
Hydroxyzine	Vistaril	10–100 mg (QID)	• Hypersensitivity • Early pregnancy	• Dizziness • Drowsiness • fatigue • Xerostomia • Blurry vision • Urinary retention	• Blood pressure • Mental status • Serum creatinine/ BUN with chronic use	• Antihistamines • MAOIs • CNS depressants	• Use with caution in BPH, respiratory disease, glaucoma • Pregnancy category C • Avoid in elderly • Avoid in renal impairment	Yes

Mechanism of action – appears to affect the thalamus and limbic system; also appears to inhibit multineuronal spinal reflexes

Generic	Brand	Dose & Max Mg (frequency)	Contra-indications	Primary Side Effects	Key Monitoring Parameters	Pertinent Drug Interactions	Med Pearls	Top 200
Meprobamate	Miltown	• 200–400 mg (TID–QID) • Max: 2,400 mg/day	• Hypersensitivity to carbamates • Porphyria	• Drowsiness • Ataxia • Nausea, vomiting, diarrhea • Anorexia • Hypotension	• Signs/ symptoms of withdrawal • Mental status • LFTs with chronic use	• Alcohol • CNS depressants	• Schedule C-IV • Pregnancy category D • Dose adjustment in hepatic and renal insufficiency	No

STORAGE AND ADMINISTRATION PEARLS

- Tablets and capsules should all be stored at room temperature, in dry area out of direct sunlight.
- Keep liquid preparations from freezing or overheating. Do not expose to temperatures >77ºF (25° C).

PATIENT EDUCATION PEARLS

- Take as directed by physician.
- Patients should *not* abruptly discontinue any anxiety medication.
- SSRIs, SNRIs, MAOIs may take up to several weeks (2–4 weeks) to see effect
- Patients should avoid alcohol when taking any of these medications.
- Patients should avoid driving or operating heavy machinery while taking benzodiazepines until they know how they respond to the medication.

BIPOLAR DISORDER

Definition

Bipolar disorder is an episodic, lifelong illness with symptoms of depression alternating with symptoms of mania or hypomania. Bipolar disorder is classified on the basis of the frequency of alternating symptoms and the subtype of manic symptoms demonstrated. Bipolar I disorder is defined as one or more manic episodes plus one or more major depressive episodes. Bipolar II disorder is defined as one or more episodes of major depression and one or more hypomanic episodes with no history of a full manic or mixed episode.

Diagnosis

The diagnosis of bipolar disorder is based on the DSM IV criteria for each of the subtype mood disorders (mania, hypomania, depression, mixed episode). Bipolar disorder diagnosis requires that a patient exhibits diagnosed episodes of both major depression plus manic, hypomanic or mixed episodes. Acute manic symptoms are hallmarks of the disorder and consist of elevated, expansive, or irritable mood lasting for at least 1 week or requiring hospitalization. Hypomania is defined as symptoms of mania that do not meet the criteria for manic episode and last for at least 4 days. Mixed episode is one that meets criteria for major depression and a manic episode for at least 1 week.

Signs and Symptoms

Acute mania requires that three of the following symptoms must be present: flight of ideas or racing thoughts, decreased need for sleep, inflated self-esteem or grandiosity, more talkative than usual or pressured speech, distractibility, psychomotor agitation, and excessive involvement in pleasurable activities with high potential for negative consequences.

Major depressive symptoms are detailed in the depression section of this chapter.

GUIDELINES

Texas Implementation of Medication Algorithms: update to the algorithms for the treatment of bipolar disorder. *Journal of Clinical Psychiatry*, no. 66 (2005): 870–86.

GUIDELINES SUMMARY

- First-line treatment options for patient with acute manic episodes include lithium, valproate, aripiprazole, quetiapine, risperidone, ziprasidone, olanzapine, or carbamazepine. Antipsychotic medications are detailed in medication charts later in this chapter.
- First-line treatment options for acute depressive episodes include lamotrigine monotherapy or lamotrigine in combination with antimania therapy.
- Maintenance therapy generally consists of continuation of therapy used in acute phases. Lithium and valproate have long history of clinical success in maintenance therapy.

Mood Stabilizers

Generic	Brand	Dose & Max mg (frequency)	Contra-indications	Primary Side Effects	Key Monitoring Parameters	Med Pearls	Top 200
Mechanism of action — lithium: altered sodium transport leads to a shift toward intraneuronal metabolism of catecholamines; the specific mechanism in mania is not fully understood							
Lithium	• Tablets • Lithobid extended-release tablets	• 300–1,200 mg daily (TID) • 300–1,200 mg daily (BID)	• Significant renal or cardiovascular disease • Dehydration	• Diarrhea • Vomiting • Drowsiness • Muscle weakness • Lack of coordination • Ataxia • Blurred vision • Tinnitus	Serum drug concentration 0.6–1.5 mEq/L	Significant drug interactions with ACE inhibitors and diuretics which decrease lithium clearance and increase toxicity	Yes
Mechanism of action — valproic acid: not fully understood; thought to increase gamma amino butyric acid (GABA) concentrations in the brain							
Valproic acid (divalproex sodium)	• Depakote • Depakote ER • Depakene • Depacon	10–60 mg/kg/day	• Hepatic dysfunction • Hypersensitivity • Urea cycle disorders	• Hepatic impairment • Thrombocytopenia • Hyperammonemia • Weight gain • Pancreatitis	• Serum drug concentrations (50–100 mcg/mL) • Liver function tests at baseline and periodically • Periodic CBC and serum ammonia levels	• Highly teratogenic • Available in oral capsules, tablets, extended-release tablets, sprinkle caps, oral syrup, and IV solution • Drug interactions detailed in neurological disorders chapter	Yes
Mechanism of action — oxcarbazepine: blocks voltage-sensitive sodium channels, resulting in stabilization of hyperexcitable neuronal membranes							
Oxcarbazepine	Trileptal tablets and oral suspension	600–2,400 mg daily (BID)	Hypersensitivity	• Sedation • Dizziness • Ataxia • Nausea • Rash (Stevens-Johnson possible) • Hyponatremia	Periodic Na, renal function; serum concentrations 12–30 mcg/mL	• CrCl <30 mL/min requires half of initial dose • Drug interactions detailed in neurological disorders chapter	Yes
Mechanism of action — lamotrigine: affects sodium channels stabilizing neuronal membranes; the exact mechanism in bipolar disorder is unknown							
Lamotrigine	• Lamictal • Oral tablets, chewable tablets	25–700 mg daily (once to BID)	• Hypersensitivity • History of Stevens-Johnson rash	• Stevens-Johnson rash • Other rash • Diplopia • Dizziness • Headache	• Response to therapy • Presence of side effects	• Risk of rash increased when combined with VPA • Slow dose titration necessary • Drug interactions detailed in neurological disorders chapter	Yes

Storage and Administration Pearls

- All medications should be stored at room temperature in a dry area away from direct sunlight.
- Patient may take medications with food if GI upset occurs.

Patient Education Pearls

- It is important that medications be continued once the symptoms have resolved.
- Patients should discuss any new medications with a healthcare professional prior to use due to risk of drug interactions.

SCHIZOPHRENIA

Definition

Schizophrenia is a psychiatric disorder that manifests as symptoms including hallucinations or delusions, and has a dramatic impact on the affected individual's functionality and quality of life. The pathophysiology is not fully understood, but theories suggest an excessive firing of dopamine and potential activity of additional neurotransmitters such as norepinephrine, serotonin, and glutamate.

Diagnosis

Persistent disturbances in social, occupational, and self-care functioning must be present for at least 6 months, with 1 month of symptoms including at least two of the following: hallucinations, delusions, disorganized speech, behavior or negative symptoms.

SIGNS AND SYMPTOMS

There are multiple subtypes of schizophrenia and symptoms vary widely between them, ranging from catalepsy or stupor to disorganized speech. Potential symptoms include auditory or visual hallucinations, delusions, disorganized speech or behavior, flat or inappropriate affect, and catatonic behavior.

GUIDELINES

American Psychiatric Association. Practice guideline for the treatment of patients with schizophrenia. 2nd Ed. Arlington, VA. American Psychiatric Association, no. 114 (2004): p. 1–114.

GUIDELINES SUMMARY

For many years, atypical antipsychotics were considered the obvious first-line choice because of significantly reduced incidence of extrapyramidal side effects. Recently, considerable controversy has surfaced, because of the ability of these medications to increase the risk of the metabolic syndrome. At this time, choice of either class is appropriate as first-line therapy. It should be considered, however, that atypical agents have better efficacy in treating negative symptoms.

- Goals of therapy include: Reduce or eliminate symptoms, minimize adverse effects of pharmacological treatment, and prevent relapse.
- Atypical and typical antipsychotics have similar efficacy profiles. Decision on first-line therapy is based on consideration of side-effect profiles, adherence issues, history of response, and cost.

Typical Antipsychotics

Mechanism of action – phenothiazines: block postsynaptic mesolimbic dopaminergic receptors in the brain

Generic	Brand	Dose & Max Mg (frequency)	Contra-indications	Primary Side Effects	Key Monitoring Parameters	Pertinent Drug Interactions	Med Pearls	Top 200
Chlorpromazine	Thorazine	• 10–200 mg (BID–QID) • Max: 2,000 mg/day	• Hypersensitivity • Severe CNS depression • Coma	• Orthostatic hypotension • Drowsiness • Xerostomia • Constipation	• Vital signs • Mental status • Lipid profile • Fasting blood glucose • Severity of EPS • LFTs • Involuntary movement • Neuroleptic malignant syndrome (NMS) • CBCs	• Alcohol • CNS depressants • Lithium • Warfarin • Other phenothiazine • Propranolol • Pindolol • Valproic acid • Phenytoin • Atropine	• Available in IV • May produce false-positive PKU test results and pregnancy • Pregnancy category C	No
Fluphenazine	Prolixin	• 1–10 mg (TID–QID) • Max: 40 mg/day	• Hypersensitivity • Severe CNS depression • Coma	• Nausea • Urinary retention • Blurred vision • Photosensitivity			• Available as elixir and injection • Pregnancy category C	No
Perphenazine	Trilafon (only generic available)	• 2–16 mg (BID–QID) • Max: 64 mg/day	• Subcortical brain damage • Blood dyscrasias • Hepatic disease	• Extrapyramidal symptoms (EPS)			Pregnancy category C	No
Trifluoperazine	Stelazine (only generic available)	• 1–10 mg (q day–BID) • Max: 40 mg/day					• Pregnancy category C • False-positives on PKU and pregnancy tests	No
Prochlorperazine	• Compazine • Compro (suppository)	• 5–15 mg (TID–QID) • 2.5–25 mg (BID) • Max: 150 mg/day					False-positives on PKU and pregnancy tests	No
Thioridazine	Mellaril (only generic available)	• 10–200 mg (BID–QID) • Max: 800 mg/day				• Alcohol • CNS depressants • Propranolol • Pindolol • Drugs that prolong Q-T interval	• Pregnancy category C • **Black box warning** for altered cardiac conduction • Use with caution in respiratory disease and hepatic disease	No

Typical Antipsychotics *(cont'd)*

Mechanism of action – haloperidol: not well established; thought to block postsynaptic mesolimbic dopaminergic D_2 receptors in the brain

Generic	Brand	Dose & Max Mg (frequency)	Contra-indications	Primary Side Effects	Key Monitoring Parameters	Pertinent Drug Interactions	Med Pearls	Top 200
Haloperidol	• Haldol • Haldol Deconade (Injection)	• 0.5–20 mg (BID-TID) • 50–100 mg/ml (q day) • Max: 100 mg/day	• Hypersensitivity • Parkinson's disease • Severe CNS depression • Bone marrow suppression • Severe cardiac or hepatic disease • Coma	• Xerostomia • Drowsiness • Constipation • Nausea • Urinary retention • Blurred vision • EPS • Dyspepsia • Priapism	• Vital signs • CBCs • Mental status • EKG at baseline • EPS • Involuntary movement	• Alcohol • CNS depressants • Antiparkinson medication • Lithium • Inhibitors/ inducers of CYP450	• Available in IV and liquid dosage form • Pregnancy category C • IV form uses sesame oil	No

Mechanism of action – Pimozide: a potent, centrally acting dopamine-receptor antagonist

Generic	Brand	Dose & Max Mg (frequency)	Contra-indications	Primary Side Effects	Key Monitoring Parameters	Pertinent Drug Interactions	Med Pearls	Top 200
Pimozide	Orap	• 1–2 mg (q day) • Max: 0.2 mg/kg or 10 mg, whichever is less	• Severe CNS depression • Coma • History of dysrhythmia • Prolonged QT syndrome • Hypokalemia, hypomagnesemia • Drugs that are inhibitors of CYP3A4 (azole antifungals, fluvoxamine, macrolide antibiotics)	• Somnolence • Drowsiness • Rash • Xerostomia • Constipation • Diarrhea • Increased appetite • Taste disturbance • Impotence • Weakness • Visual disturbance • Speech disorder • Hypotension	• Vital signs • CBCs • Mental status • EKG at baseline • EPS • Involuntary movement	• Alcohol • CNS depressants • Anticonvulsants • Propranolol • macrolide antibiotics • Lithium • Sertraline • TCAs • CYP3A4 inhibitors	• FDA-labeled for Tourette's disorder • Pregnancy category C	No

Typical Antipsychotics *(cont'd)*

Generic	Brand	Dose & Max Mg (frequency)	Contra-indications	Primary Side Effects	Key Monitoring Parameters	Pertinent Drug Interactions	Med Pearls	Top 200
Mechanism of action – loxapine: blocks postsynaptic mesolimbic D_1 and D_2 receptors in the brain, and also possesses serotonin $5\text{-}HT_2$ blocking activity								
Loxapine	Loxitane	• 5–50 mg (BID–QID) • Max: 250 mg/day	• Hypersensitivity • Severe CNS depression • Coma	• Hypotension • Nausea • Constipation • Vomiting • Xerostomia • Weakness • Sexual disturbance • Dizziness	• Vital signs • Mental status • EPS • CBCs • Thyroid function tests • Involuntary movement	• Lorazepam • Alcohol • CNS depressants • TCAs • Anticonvulsants • Lithium	• Use with extreme caution in patients with thyroid disease • False-positive PKU test • Pregnancy category C	No
Mechanism of action – Molindone: exerts effect on the ascending reticular activating system								
Molindone	Moban	• 5–50 mg (TID–QID) • Max: 225 mg/day	• Severe cardiovascular disorders • Hypersensitivity	• Drowsiness • Xerostomia • constipation • Hypotension • Tachycardia	• Vital signs • Mental status • EPS • CBCs	• Phenytoin • Tetracycline • Alcohol • CNS depressants	Pregnancy category C	No
Mechanism of action – thiothixene: blocks postsynaptic dopamine receptors, resulting in inhibition of dopamine-mediated effects; also has alpha-adrenergic blocking activity.								
Thiothixene	Navane	• 1–20 mg (TID) • Max: 60 mg/day	• Hypersensitivity • Severe CNS depression • Circulatory collapse • Blood dyscrasias • Coma	• Hypotension • Dizziness • GI upset • Constipation • Libido changes • Tachycardia • Insomnia	• Vital signs • CBCs • Thyroid function tests • EPS	• Alcohol • CNS depressants	May cause false-positive pregnancy tests,	No

Atypical Antipsychotics

Generic	Brand	Dose & Max Mg (frequency)	Contra-indications	Primary Side Effects	Key Monitoring Parameters	Pertinent Drug Interactions	Med Pearls	Top 200
Aripiprazole	• Abilify • Abilify Discmelt • Oral tablet, disintegrating tablet, solution, immediate IM injection	• 10–30 mg PO daily (q day) • 9.75 IM (q 2 hours up to 30 mg/day)	Hypersensitivity	• Weight gain • Constipation • Nausea • Vomiting • Akathisia • Dizziness • Hyperglycemia • Hyperlipidemia • Anxiety • Restlessness • Sedation • Prolonged QT interval • Hyperprolactinemia (rare) • EPS (rare) • Tardive dyskinesia (rare)	• Blood sugar • Fasting lipid panel, BP, and heart rate • Weight/BMI • Symptoms of psychosis or EPS • ECG	• Ranolazine • Carbamazepine • Quinidine • Ketoconazole • Medications that prolong QT interval	Among the lowest risk of metabolic syndrome	Yes
Olanzapine	• Zyprexa • Oral tablets; oral disintegrating tablets; immediate IM injection	• 10–20 mg IM daily (q day) • 10–30 mg IM daily					Higher degree of weight gain than some other atypicals	Yes
Paliperidone	Invega	• 6–12 mg daily (q day)					• Major active metabolite of risperidone • Newest med in this class, least clinical evidence	No
Quetiapine	• Seroquel • Oral tablets, extended-release tablets	• IR: 50–750 mg daily (BID–TID) • ER: 300–800 mg daily (q day)					Dosed HS due to somnolence	Yes
Risperidone	• Risperdal • Risperdal Consta • Risperdal M–Tab • Tablet, liquid, disintegrating tablet, long-acting injection	• 2–16 mg PO daily (q day–BID) • 25–50 mg IM Q 2 wks					Sedation often leads to HS dosing	

Atypical Antipsychotics *(cont'd)*

Generic	Brand	Dose & Max Mg (frequency)	Contra-indications	Primary Side Effects	Key Monitoring Parameters	Pertinent Drug Interactions	Med Pearls	Top 200
Ziprasidone	Geodon	40–160 mg daily (BID)	• Hx of cardiac arrhythmias • Uncompensated heart failure • Hypersensitivity • Acute or recent MI • QT prolongation history • Drugs that cause QT prolongation				Lower risk of metabolic syndrome when compared to other atypicals	Yes
Clozapine	Clozaril FazaClo	12.5–900 mg daily (q day–TID)	• Hx of clozapine-induced agranulocytosis or severe granulocytopenia • Myeloproliferative disorder • Paralytic ileus • CNS depression or comatose states • Other agents that cause agranulocytosis	• Hypotension • Tachyarrhythmia • Rash • Weight gain • Agranulocytosis • Neuroleptic malignant syndrome (rare)	• WBC and ANC wkly for 6 mos, q 2 wks for 6 mos and then q 4 wks • S/S of psychotic behavior • Blood sugar, fasting lipid panel • Symptoms of neuroleptic malignant syndrome • BP and heart rate • Orthostatic hypotension • ECG	• Droperidol • Buspirone • Carbamazepine • Lithium • Tramadol • Zotepine	• Used less frequently than other atypicals due to requirement for frequent monitoring • Effective in treatment of refractory cases and in patients at high risk for suicide	No

Storage and Administration Pearls

- All medications should be stored at room temperature in a dry area away from direct sunlight.
- Patient may take medications with food if GI upset occurs.

Patient Education Pearls

- Grapefruit juice should be avoided when taking these medications.
- Alcohol should be avoided due to excessive CNS depression.
- Driving or operating heavy machinery should be avoided until patients know how they respond to medication.
- All medications can take up to several weeks (2–4 weeks) to see full effect.
- Medications should *not* be abruptly discontinued.
- Patients should not self-adjust dose.
- Patients should report to a physician any side effects that disrupt their daily life (i.e., EPS).

LEARNING POINTS

- The most commonly used antidepressants are the SSRIs. These agents may take several weeks to reach maximal efficacy.
- Bupropion is the antidepressant of choice in patients with sexual side effects resulting from other classes of antidepressants.
- The treatment of anxiety and panic disorder may include acute therapies such as benzodiazepines but may also include chronic prophylactic therapies with antidepressants.
- Mood stabilizer therapy is the mainstay of treatment for bipolar disorder. Lithium has a narrow therapeutic window and requires therapeutic serum monitoring.
- While atypical antipsychotic medications exhibit fewer extrapyramidal side effects than typical agents, they do carry a greater risk of metabolic side effects such as weight gain, hyperglycemia, and hyperlipidemia. Atypical antipsychotics are more effective in treating the negative symptoms of schizophrenia.

PRACTICE QUESTIONS

1. Which of the following is first-line in the treatment of acute depressive episode in a patient with bipolar disorder?

   (A) Lithium
   (B) Valproic acid
   (C) Oxcarbazepine
   (D) Lamictal
   (E) Carbamazepine

2. Which of the following medications can be used in the treatment of anxiety?

   I.   Clonazepam
   II. Venlafaxine
   III. Hydroxyzine

   (A) I only
   (B) III only
   (C) I and II only
   (D) II and III only
   (E) I, II, III

ANSWERS

1. **D**

According to the guidelines, first-line treatment options for acute depression episodes include lamotrigine as monotherapy or in combination with antimania agents. Lithium and valproic acid (B) are used as first-line treatment options for acute manic episodes. Oxcarbazepine (C) and carbamazepine (E) would also be used as first-line treatment options of acute manic episodes. Maintenance therapy may consist of a combination of medications for both depression and manic episodes.

2. **E**

All of the named medications can be used in the treatment of anxiety. Clonazepam (I) is a benzodiazepine, which is commonly used for the acute treatment of anxiety. Venlafaxine (II) is generic Effexor, which is labeled for GAD, PD, and SAD. Hydroxyzine (III) competes with histamine and can also be used in the treatment of anxiety.

Bone and Joint Disorders

9

This chapter covers the following disease states:

- **Osteoarthritis**
- **Rheumatoid arthritis**
- **Osteoporosis**
- **Gout**

 Suggested Study Time: **40 minutes**

OSTEOARTHRITIS

Definition

Osteoarthritis (OA) is a disease of the cartilage resulting from an imbalance between cartilage destruction and formation with subsequent bony proliferation within the joint, which results in pain, potentially decreased range of motion, and local inflammation.

Diagnosis

The diagnosis of OA is based on history, physical exam, and radiographs. History and physical exam will reveal symptoms and signs consistent with OA (detailed below) and should be used to rule out other potential conditions such as rheumatoid arthritis. Radiologic changes may include joint space narrowing, osteophytes, or subchondral bone sclerosis.

Signs and Symptoms

Osteoarthritis signs: Physical exam may reveal tenderness, crepitus, and/or enlargement of the affected joints. Radiologic evaluation is necessary to identify presence of OA and disease progression. Radiographic changes may not be easily identifiable in early, mild disease but with disease progression may include narrowing of the joint spaces, presence of osteophytes, subchondral bony sclerosis, and eventual subluxation and deformity.

Osteoarthritis symptoms: Patients with OA present with pain, stiffness, and instability of joints that can be unilateral or bilateral. The pain is often worsened with weight-bearing activity and is described as deep and aching. Stiffness may resolve with motion but may limit physical activity. Commonly affected joints include the hands, knees, and hips.

Guidelines

American College of Rheumatology Subcommittee on Osteoarthritis Guidelines: Recommendations for medical management of osteoarthritis of the hip and knee. Arthritis & Rheumatism, no. 43(9): 1905–15. www.rheumatology.org/publications/guidelines/oa-mgmt/oa-mgmt.asp.

Guidelines Summary

The goals of therapy are to decrease pain and stiffness, maintain/improve joint mobility and limit functional impairment, and increase the quality of life.

- Nonpharmacological therapy: Rest, physical therapy, and weight loss
- Pharmacological therapy:
  - First-line: Scheduled acetaminophen up to a maximum daily dose of 4 g
  - Second-line: Nonsteroidal anti-inflammatory drugs (NSAIDs); specific agent chosen based on cost, prior response, and gastrointestinal risk factors
  - Third-line: Narcotic analgesics or hyaluronate injections
  - Adjunctive therapy: Topical capsaicin cream, glucosamine sulfate

Drugs for Osteoarthritis

Generic	Brand	Dose & Max Mg (frequency)	Contraindications	Primary Side Effects	Key Monitoring Parameters	Pertinent Drug Interactions	Med Pearls	Top 200
Mechanism of action – decreases pain through inhibition of central cyclo-oxygenase, which in turn inhibits prostaglandin synthesis								
Acetaminophen	Tylenol	• 325–1,000 • TID–QID	• Hepatic disease • Alcoholism	Very few	Pain relief	Alcohol	OTC Best if taken on scheduled basis vs. PRN	No
Tramadol	• Ultram • Ultram ER	• IR 25–400 daily (q 4–6 hrs) • ER 100–300 daily	Hypersensitivity	Confusion, sedation, rash, stomach upset, orthostatic hypotension	Pain relief, renal and hepatic function periodically	• Alcohol • Opioids • SSRIs • MAOIs • Warfarin	Renal dose adjustment for CrCl <30 mL/min	Yes
Mechanism of action – induces the release of substance P, the principle chemomediator of pain impulses from the periphery								
Capsaicin Cream	Various	0.025–0.1% applied 3–4x daily	Do not apply to wounds or damaged skin	Localized stinging	Pain relief	None	• OTC • Must be used regularly for 2 wks or more for maximal efficacy	No
Mechanism of action – nonsteroidal anti-inflammatory drugs (NSAIDs): decrease pain and inflammation by inhibition of prostaglandin synthesis through inhibition of cyclooxygenase enzymes.								
Aspirin	Various	• IR 325–3,600 daily (q 4–6 hrs) • XR product 650–1,300 TID	• Allergy • Fever in children • Active bleeding	• GI (upset stomach, bleeding) • Rash	Pain relief, GI symptoms	• Warfarin • Other NSAIDs • ACE inhibitors	• OTC • Anti-inflammatory only at high doses (>3 g/day)	No
Nonacetylated salicylates								
Salsalate	Various	500–3,000 daily (BID–TID)	Hypersensitivity	• GI (upset stomach, bleeding) • Rash • Diminished renal function	Pain relief, GI symptoms	• Other salicylates • Warfarin • ACE inhibitors	• Monitor serum salicylate levels with chronic use or very high doses • Desired range 10–30 mg/100 ml	No
Diflunisal	None	500–1,500 daily (BID)		• Edema			Administer with food	No

Drugs for Osteoarthritis *(cont'd)*

Generic	Brand	Dose & Max Mg (frequency)	Contraindications	Primary Side Effects	Key Monitoring Parameters	Pertinent Drug Interactions	Med Pearls	Top 200
Acetic acids								
Etodolac	None	200–1,200 daily (Q 6–8 hrs)	Hypersensitivity	• GI (upset stomach, bleeding) • Rash • Diminished renal function • á blood pressure • Edema	• Pain relief • GI symptoms • Renal function • Blood pressure	• Other salicylates • Warfarin • Lithium • ACE inhibitors	Administer with food	Yes
Diclofenac	• Cataflam • Voltaren	50–150 daily (BID–TID)						Yes
Indomethacin	• Indocin • Indocin SR	• IR 25–200 daily (BID–TID) • SR 75–150 1x daily		• GI (upset stomach, bleeding) • Rash • Diminished renal function • á blood pressure • Edema • CNS disturbances			• Most commonly used for treatment of gout • Fat-soluble, crosses blood brain barrier • Administer with food	Yes
Ketorolac	Toradol	• 30 mg IM or 15 mg IV initial; 10 mg PO q 4–6 hrs up to 40 mg daily	• Active PUD or bleeding • History of GI bleeding • Severe renal impairment • Labor and delivery	• GI (upset stomach, bleeding) • Rash • Diminished renal function • á blood pressure • Edema			• Only approved for moderate-severe pain for ≤5 days duration • Available IM and IV as well	No
Nabumetone	Relafen	500–2,000 daily (q day–BID)	Hypersensitivity				Administer with food	No

Drugs for Osteoarthritis *(cont'd)*

Generic	Brand	Dose & Max Mg (frequency)	Contraindications	Primary Side Effects	Key Monitoring Parameters	Pertinent Drug Interactions	Med Pearls	Top 200
Propionic acids								
Fenoprofen	Nalfon	200–3,200 daily (TID–QID)	Hypersensitivity	• GI (upset stomach, bleeding) • Rash • Diminished renal function • High blood pressure • Edema	• Pain relief • GI symptoms • Renal function • Blood pressure	• Other salicylates • Warfarin • ACE inhibitors • Lithium	Administer with food	No
Flurbiprofen	Ansaid	50–300 daily (BID–QID)						No
Ibuprofen	• Motrin • Advil	200–3,200 daily (TID–QID)					• Available OTC and Rx (400–800 mg tabs) • Administer with food • Available in pediatric preparations	Yes
Ketoprofen	• Orudis • Oruvail • Rhodis • Apo-Keto-E	• IR: 50–300 daily (TID–QID) • SR: 75–200 daily						No
Naproxen	• Naprosyn • EC • Naprosyn • Naprelan	• IR: 250–1,500 daily (BID) • EC: 375–1,500 daily (BID) • CR: 375–1,500 daily (BID)					• Available OTC and Rx • Administer with food	Yes
Naproxen sodium	Anaprox	275–1,650 daily (BID)						Yes
Oxaprozin	Daypro	600–1800 daily (1x daily)					Administer with food	No

Drugs for Osteoarthritis *(cont'd)*

Generic	Brand	Dose & Max Mg (frequency)	Contraindications	Primary Side Effects	Key Monitoring Parameters	Pertinent Drug Interactions	Med Pearls	Top 200
Fenamates								
Meclofenamate	None available	50–400 daily (q 4–6 hrs)	Hypersensitivity	GI (upset stomach, bleeding); rash; diminished renal function; á blood pressure; edema	Pain relief, GI symptoms, renal function, blood pressure	Other salicylates, warfarin, ACE inhibitors, lithium	Administer with food	No
Oxicams								
Piroxicam	Feldene	10–20 daily (1x daily)	Hypersensitivity	GI (upset stomach, bleeding); rash; diminished renal function; á blood pressure; edema	Pain relief, GI symptoms, renal function, blood pressure	Other salicylates, warfarin, ACE inhibitors, lithium	More COX-2 selectivity than traditional NSAIDs; slightly less GI symptoms	Yes
Meloxicam	Mobic	7.5–15 daily (1x daily)						Yes
Selective COX-2 Inhibitors								
Celecoxib	Celebrex	50–200 daily (q day–BID)	Hypersensitivity	GI (upset stomach, bleeding— less than other NSAIDs); rash; diminished renal function; á blood pressure; edema	Pain relief, GI symptoms, renal function, blood pressure	Other salicylates (including aspirin), warfarin, ACE inhibitors, lithium	• Lower incidence of GI toxicity than with nonselective NSAIDs • Concern about cardiovascular adverse effects prompted withdrawal of similar drug from market (rofecoxib)	Yes

Drugs for Osteoarthritis *(cont'd)*

Narcotic Analgesics – Stimulate opioid receptors in the brain

Generic	Brand	Dose & Max Mg (frequency)	Contraindications	Primary Side Effects	Key Monitoring Parameters	Pertinent Drug Interactions	Med Pearls	Top 200
Hydrocodone/ APAP	• Various • Lortab • Vicodin	• 5–60 mg hydrocodone daily (q4–6 hrs)	• Hypersensitivity • Severe hepatic impairment • Alcoholism	• Constipation • CNS depression • Confusion • Sedation • Respiratory depression • Hypotension • Bradycardia	• Presence of side effects (constipation, confusion) • Pain relief • Respiratory rate • Blood pressure • Heart rate	• Alcohol • Other CNS depressants	• Take with food • Often need laxative in addition • High abuse potential	Yes
Propoxyphene/ APAP	• Various • Darvocet	65–600 mg propoxyphene (q 4–6 hrs)						Yes
APAP/Codeine	• Various • Tylenol #3	7.5–360 mg codeine daily (q4–6 hrs)						Yes
Morphine	Various	See chapter on pain management						No
Oxycodone/ APAP	• Various • Percocet • Roxicet	5–40 mg daily oxycodone (q6 hrs PRN)						Yes

Adjunctive Therapies/Nuatritional Supplements

Generic	Brand	Dose & Max Mg (frequency)	Contraindications	Primary Side Effects	Key Monitoring Parameters	Pertinent Drug Interactions	Med Pearls	Top 200
Glucosamine Sulfate	Various	500–1,500 daily (q day–BID)	Unknown	• Itching • GI upset	• Pain relief • Presence of side effects	Unknown	• Nutritional supplement • Available OTC • Conflicting clinical trial data	No

Storage and Administration Pearls

- NSAIDs should be administered with food to decrease the risk of gastrointestinal side effects.
- Capsaicin cream may take several weeks for maximal efficacy to be demonstrated. Regular daily use, 2–4 times daily for 4 weeks, is considered an adequate trial.

Patient Education Pearls

- Take NSAIDs with food to avoid stomach upset.
- Avoid alcohol when taking acetaminophen or narcotic analgesics due to the risk of liver damage.
- Avoid driving or operating heavy machinery while taking narcotics.
- Capsaicin cream may take 2–4 weeks to become effective. Allow an adequate trial before determining efficacy.
- Wash your hands very thoroughly after capsaicin application.

RHEUMATOID ARTHRITIS

Definition

Rheumatoid arthritis (RA) is an autoimmune disease characterized by chronic inflammation of the synovial tissue lining the joint capsule. The erosive synovitis is generally symmetrical and extra-articular involvement may also occur, including rheumatoid nodules, cardiopulmonary disease, lymphadenopathy, splenomegaly, and neurological dysfunction.

Diagnosis

RA diagnosis is based on history and physical, laboratory evidence, and radiographic evaluation. History and physical will reveal consistent signs and symptoms of RA. Laboratory evidence will demonstrate rheumatoid factor presence in 60–70% of affected patients, elevated erythrocyte sedimentation rate and c-reactive protein, and radiographic evidence of joint space narrowing or erosions.

Signs and Symptoms

- Symmetrical symptoms of joint pain and stiffness (especially in the morning) for more than 6 weeks' duration
- Joint tenderness, erythema, swelling, and, potentially, rheumatoid nodules

Guidelines

American College of Rheumatology Guidelines for the Management of Rheumatoid Arthritis. Arthritis and Rheumatism, no. 46(2) (2002): 328–46.

Guidelines Summary

- Disease-modifying antirheumatic drug (DMARD) should be initiated within 3 months of diagnosis to retard disease progression.
- Methotrexate is first-line DMARD in absence of contraindication.
- NSAIDs are useful for symptomatic relief during onset of DMARD and PRN otherwise. NSAIDs do not alter disease progression in RA.
- Corticosteroids are used as adjunctive therapy in patient with refractory symptoms.
- Biologic agents are used when methotrexate has been demonstrated to be ineffective as monotherapy. Additional DMARDs may be tried prior to use of biologics.
- Biologic therapies increase the risk of serious infections and should not be initiated in a patient with an active infection.

Drugs for Rheumatoid Arthritis

Generic	Brand	Dose & Max mg (frequency)	Contra-indications	Primary Side Effects	Key Monitoring Parameters	Pertinent Drug Interactions	Med Pearls	Top 200
Mechanism of action — corticosteroids: exert anti-inflammatory and immunosuppressive effects by inhibiting prostaglandins and leukotrienes, which results in decreased inflammation, decreased pain, and a potential decrease in joint destruction								
Prednisone	Various	5–60 daily initially; individualized	• Systemic fungal infection • Hypersensitivity	• High blood sugar • High blood pressure • Reduced bone mineral density • Fluid retention • Impaired wound healing	Blood sugar, blood pressure, bone mineral density, presence of edema/weight	Warfarin	Side effects generally present with chronic and/or long-term use	Yes
Disease-modifying antirheumatic drugs (DMARDs)								
Mechanism of action — inhibits cytokine production, inhibits purine biosynthesis, thereby decreasing inflammation in affected joints								
Methotrexate	• Rheumatrex • Trexall	7.5 mg 1x wkly	• Hypersensitivity • Alcoholism • Severe hepatic impairment • Immunodeficiency • Significant blood dyscrasias/anemias • Pregnancy • CrCl <40 mL/min	• GI upset (nausea, diarrhea, abdominal pain) • Stomatitis • Thrombo-cytopenia • Leukopenia • ↑ liver enzymes • Malaise • Fatigue • Fever/chills • Infections	• Pain relief • Liver function tests • Periodic CBC • Folate	Salicylates, sulfonamides, phenytoin	• May supplement folic acid to decrease adverse effects and prevent folate deficiency • Myelosuppression is biggest concern • Should be taken with food	No
Mechanism of action — not fully understood; thought to be related to immunosuppressant properties								
Hydroxychloroquine	Plaquenil	200–600 daily (1x daily)	• Hypersensitivity • Retinal changes with agent in past	Macular damage, corneal deposits, retinopathy; rash; nausea, diarrhea	Ocular exams q 3 mos	Cyclosporine, digoxin	Older drug without risk of myelosuppression but ocular risk	Yes

Drugs for Rheumatoid Arthritis *(cont'd)*

Generic	Brand	Dose & Max mg (frequency)	Contra-indications	Primary Side Effects	Key Monitoring Parameters	Pertinent Drug Interactions	Med Pearls	Top 200
Mechanism of action – leflunomide: inhibits pyrimidine synthesis, thereby decreasing lymphocyte proliferation and inflammation								
Leflunomide	Arava	Load 100 mg daily for 3 days; 20 mg daily maintenance	• Hepatic disease • Pregnancy • Immunodeficiency	• Diarrhea • Elevated liver enzymes • Alopecia • Rash	ALT monthly x 6 mos, then periodically	Cholestyramine, rifampin	• Oral DMARD with low risk of bone marrow toxicity • Appropriate contraception should be used • Highly teratogenic	No
Mechanism of action – not fully understood; related to anti-inflammatory properties								
Sulfasalazine	Azulfidine	250–2,000 daily (BID)	Hypersensitivity to any sulfa-containing drug	• Frequent diarrhea, nausea, vomiting • Rash • Urticaria • Photosensitivity • Leukopenia • Alopecia • Stomatitis • Elevated liver enzymes	• Response to therapy • Presence of adverse effects • CBC • Liver enzymes	Warfarin, methotrexate, cyclosporine, digoxin, thiopurines	• Warfarin interaction very clinically significant • Monitor INR closely	No
Biologics								
Mechanism of action – binds to and inhibits the cytokine tumor necrosis factor (TNF), thereby inhibiting the subsequent inflammatory cascade								
Etanercept	Enbrel	50 mg subcutaneously 1x wk	• Sepsis • Active infection • Hypersensitivity	• Local injection site reactions • Infections	Response to therapy	Anakinra; cyclophosphamide	• Refrigerate prior to use • Discontinue temporarily if infection occurs • Can be self-administered • Can be used alone or in combination with MTX	

Drugs for Rheumatoid Arthritis *(cont'd)*

Generic	Brand	Dose & Max mg (frequency)	Contra-indications	Primary Side Effects	Key Monitoring Parameters	Pertinent Drug Interactions	Med Pearls	Top 200
Mechanism of action – monoclonal antibody that binds to TNF and prevents interaction with TNF receptors on inflammatory cells								
Infliximab	Remicade	3–10 mg/kg IV infusion at initiation; wks 2 and 6 and q8 wks thereafter	• Active infection • Hypersensitivity	• Infections (upper respiratory common) • Acute infusion reactions (fever, chills, rash)	Response to therapy	Anakinra	• *Always* used in combination with MTX • Dose limited to ≤5 mg/kg in patients with heart failure	
Mechanism of action – monoclonal antibody that binds to TNF, blocking its interaction with cell surface receptors and decreasing inflammation								
Adalimumab	Humira	40 mg sub-cutaneously q other wk to wkly	• Active infection • Untreated latent tuberculosis	Injection-site reactions; infections	• Tuberculin skin test (PPD) prior to initiation • Ongoing monitoring for response to therapy and presence of infection • Response to therapy	Anakinra	• Caution use in patients with heart failure • Discontinue during serious infections • Used as monotherapy or in combination with MTX or other DMARDs	
Mechanism of action – Binds to interleukin-1 receptors on target cells, thereby preventing release of chemotactic factors and adhesion molecules and subsequently decreasing inflammation and connective tissue damage								
Anakinra	Kineret	100 mg subcutaneously daily	• Hypersensitivity • Active infections	Injection-site reactions (inflammation, ecchymosis); infections; neutropenia	• CBC periodically • Response to therapy • Presence of adverse effects	Etanercept, infliximab, adalimumab	Used alone or in combination with DMARDs (other than TNF blockers)	

Storage and Administration Pearls

- NSAIDs should be administered with food to decrease risk of gastrointestinal side effects.

- Oral methotrexate should be administered with food to avoid stomach upset.

- The following medications should be refrigerated to 2–8°C (36–46°F): methotrexate injectable, etanercept, infliximab, adalimumab, anakinra. These medications should *not* be frozen and should be protected from light.

- The following medications are administered through subcutaneous injection: etanercept, adalimumab, anakinra.

- Methotrexate is administered orally or through intramuscular injection.

- Infliximab cannot be self-administered and is delivered through intravenous infusion.

- The following medications are available in prefilled syringes and/or pen devices: etanercept, adalimumab, anakinra.

Patient Education Pearls

- Promptly report any signs of infection to your physician. A temporary withdrawal of medication may be necessary during this time.

- Do not receive live vaccines while you are on biologic therapies.

- Appropriate administration of injectable therapies is as follows:

  - Visually inspect the products for particulate matter or discoloration. Do not use if either is present.

  - Methotrexate is injected intramuscularly.

  - All other injectables are subcutaneous administration.

  - Rotate injection site.

  - Do not inject into tender, bruised, hard, or ulcerated skin.

  - Do not reuse needles or syringes.

  - Properly dispose of needles in a puncture-proof container.

OSTEOPOROSIS

Definition

Osteoporosis is a condition of low bone mass, which results in increased fragility of bone and subsequent increased risk of fracture. Potential etiologies of the characteristic decreased bone mass include age-related physiologic changes, disorders of estrogen or testosterone levels, or use of medications associated with drug-induced osteoporosis. Although more common in women, osteoporosis also occurs in men.

Normal bone physiology includes constant bone remodeling, which consists of bone formation via osteoblasts and bone resorption via osteoclasts. Bone mineral density (BMD) reflects the balance between resorption and formation. Osteoporosis occurs when there is an imbalance between formation and resorption resulting in a decreased BMD.

Diagnosis

The diagnosis of osteoporosis is most commonly based on the results of BMD measurement with dual energy x-ray absorptiometry (DXA) at the hip and spine. Results of the DXA are reported as the T score. The T score represents the number of standard deviations away from the mean BMD for a young, healthy individual. Normal BMD would be considered any T score greater than –1, while osteopenia would be a T score –1 to –2.5; a T score of less than –2.5 would be diagnostic for osteoporosis. Osteoporosis can also be diagnosed based on the occurrence of a nontraumatic fracture.

Signs and Symptoms

Typical signs of osteoporosis include kyphosis; shortened stature, and nontraumatic fractures of the vertebrae, hip, or forearm. Some patients may have symptoms of bone pain, and often vertebral fractures go undiagnosed as patients complain of chronic back pain. In a patient with risk factors for osteoporosis, radiographic investigation of back pain is warranted. Pain and physical changes associated with osteoporosis may lead to depression and lowered self-esteem.

Guidelines

American Association of Clinical Endocrinologists medical guidelines for clinical practice for the prevention and treatment of osteoporosis: 2001 Edition, with selected updates for 2003. *Endocr Pract*, no. 9(6) (2003): 544–64. www.aace.com/pub/pdf/guidelines/osteoporosis2001Revised.pdf.

Guidelines Summary

- Oral calcium and vitamin D supplementation is an important prerequisite to pharmacological therapy. Without adequate calcium and vitamin D available, other therapies will be limited in their ability to improve bone architecture.

- Bisphosphonates are the first-line therapy for the prevention and treatment of osteoporosis in patients without contraindications.

- Oral bisphosphonates are approved for prevention and treatment of osteoporosis (including glucocorticoid-induced osteoporosis) in men and women.

- Raloxifene is recommended as an alternative choice for the treatment of osteoporosis in patients with contraindications to bisphosphonates or in patients who are unable to comply with the appropriate bisphosphonate administration instructions.

- Calcitonin is reserved for third-line therapy because of a lack of compelling evidence indicating fracture reductions and lack of long-term data. Calcitonin is approved for the treatment of acute pain secondary to vertebral fractures and is well tolerated, so may have specific role in certain situations.

- Teriparatide is approved for treatment of osteoporosis and is indicated in patients with a history of fracture secondary to osteoporosis and in those with multiple risk factors for fracture who have not responded or are intolerant to bisphosphonate therapy.

Drugs for Osteoporosis

Generic	Brand	Dose & Max	Contra-indications	Primary Side Effects	Key Monitoring Parameters	Pertinent Drug Interactions	Med Pearls	Top 200
Mechanism of action — bisphosphonates: adsorb to bone apatite and inhibit osteoclast activity								
Alendronate	Fosamax	• 10 mg daily or 70 mg 1x wk (treatment) • 5 mg daily or 35 mg 1x wk (prevention)	Esophageal stricture; hypersensitivity; inability to sit upright or stand for 30 minutes; CrCl <35 mL/min; hypocalcemia	Nausea, dyspepsia, esophageal irritation, ulceration, muscle pain	Bone mineral density (BMD)	NSAIDs/ASA increase risk of GI symptoms	• Must be taken with at least 8 oz of water ≥30 minutes prior to other medications/food • Patient should remain upright for 30 min or more	Yes
Risedronate	Actonel	5 mg daily or 35 mg 1x wk						Yes
Ibandronate	Boniva	(PO) 2.5 mg daily or 150 mg 1x month						Yes
Zoledronic acid	Reclast	5 mg IV infusion 1x year	Hypersensitivity; CrCl <35 mL/min	Hypotension, agitation, confusion, fever, nausea, constipation, hypocalcemia, muscle pain	BMD	Aminoglycosides	Annual IV infusion	No
Mechanism of action — selective estrogen receptor modulators: through selective binding to estrogen receptors, decreases bone resorption and reduces biochemical markers of bone turnover								
Raloxifene	Evista	60 mg 1x daily	• Hypersensitivity • History of pulmonary embolism or deep vein thrombosis • Pregnancy/lactation	Hot flushes, leg cramps, thrombo-embolism	BMD; presence of adverse effects	Cholestyramine, warfarin	• Monitor INR closely for patients on warfarin (expect INR increase) • Lipid effects include decreased LDL with no effect on HDL/triglycerides	Yes

Drugs for Osteoporosis *(cont'd)*

Generic	Brand	Dose & Max	Contra-indications	Primary Side Effects	Key Monitoring Parameters	Pertinent Drug Interactions	Med Pearls	Top 200
Miscellaneous Agents								
Mechanism of action – inhibits bone resorption through inhibition of osteoclast activity, to a small decrease stimulates bone formation through stimulation of osteoblast activity								
Calcitonin	• Miacalcin Nasal Spray • Injection	• 200 units (1 spray) daily intranasally • 100 units q other day (SQ or IM)	Hypersensitivity	Nasal irritation and dryness, rhinitis	BMD	None	• Refrigerate • Keep nasal spray at room temp while in use (<86°F/30°C) • Discard unused nasal spray after 30 days	No
Mechanism of action – acts as a parathyroid hormone (PTH) agonist; thereby increases bone formation by the stimulation of osteoblast activity and increases renal reabsorption of calcium								
Teriparatide (Parathyroid hormone)	Forteo	20 mcg 1x daily SQ	• Hypersensitivity • Primary hyperparathyroidism • Hypercalcemia • Paget's disease	Orthostatic hypotension, dizziness, nausea, hypercalcemia	BMD	Digoxin (may predispose to digoxin toxicity)	Reduces risk of vertebral and nonvertebral fractures	No

Storage and Administration Pearls

- Oral bisphosphonates should be taken on an empty stomach first thing in the morning with at least 8 oz of water. At least 30 to 60 minutes should pass prior to ingestion of any medication or food. Patient should remain upright for 30 to 60 minutes after taking dosage.

- Zoledronic acid solution for injection should be refrigerated prior to use. Intravenous infusion administered only by healthcare professional.

- Calcitonin injection and nasal spray should be refrigerated at 2–8°C (36–46°F). Nasal spray can be kept at room temperature up to 86°F (30°C) during use.

- Nasal spray should be primed prior to use. Discard unused portion after 30 days.

- Calcitonin injection can be administered subcutaneously or intramuscularly.

- Teriparatide injection is available in a prefilled pen device and should be refrigerated at 2–8°C (36–46°F). The product should not be frozen, and any unused portion should be discarded after 28 days of use.

Patient Education Pearls

- Take oral bisphosphonates on an empty stomach first thing in the morning with at least 8 oz of plain water. You should then remain upright for 30–60 minutes and avoid lying down. Avoid ingestion of food, beverages (other than water), and other medications for 30–60 minutes after taking this medication.

- Calcitonin nasal spray should be primed prior to use and any unused portion should be discarded after 30 days.

- Teriparatide injection should be refrigerated at all times and should be discarded after 28 days of use.

GOUT

Definition

Gout is a syndrome of acute or chronic recurrent arthritis characterized by deposits of monosodium urate crystals in synovial fluid and/or tissues and is most often associated with hyperuricemia. Hyperuricemia can result from either an overproduction or underexcretion of uric acid. Overproduction of uric acid is most common in myeloproliferative and lymphoproliferative disorders. A decrease in the renal excretion of uric acid can be the result of renal dysfunction, certain drugs, or a number of predisposing conditions, including obesity and hypothyroidism. Acute gouty attacks may be precipitated by a number of conditions including stress, trauma, and alcohol ingestion.

Diagnosis

The diagnosis of gout is based on clinical presentation along with the presence of uric acid crystals detected on joint aspiration of the synovial fluid of affected joints. Evaluation of a 24-hour urinary uric acid will allow classification of the patient as a uric acid overproducer (urinary uric acid excretion ≥600 mg) or a uric acid underexcretor (urinary uric acid >600 mg), which will assist in pharmacotherapeutic decisions.

Signs and Symptoms

Patients presenting with acute gouty arthritis complain of a quick onset of excruciating pain, inflammation, and swelling that most commonly affects the first metatarsophalangeal (MTP) joint and can also affect the feet, ankles, heels, knees, wrists, fingers, and elbows. Severe cases of gout can result in uric acid nephrolithiasis, nephropathy, or urate deposits (tophi) in affected joints.

Summary of Treatment Recommendations

Treatment of Acute Gouty Arthropathy

- Asymptomatic hyperuricemia does not require therapy.
- First-line treatment for gout includes the use of a nonsteroidal anti-inflammatory drug (NSAID). The majority of acute gout attacks will respond to an NSAID within 72 hours of therapy. Indomethacin is the most common NSAID used in the treatment of gout, but other NSAIDs are also appropriate. Please see the medication chart in the osteoarthritis section of this chapter for more specific NSAID information.
- If patients have a contraindication to the use of an NSAID, evaluation of the time course of symptoms is necessary.
  - If gout symptoms have been present for less than 48 hours, colchicine is recommended for acute treatment.
  - If gout symptoms have been present for more than 48 hours, use of a corticosteroid is recommended.
- If the patient demonstrates an inadequate response to either NSAIDs or colchicine, corticosteroids should be considered.
- The use of oral (preferred) or parenteral corticosteroids is recommended for multijoint involvement, while an intraarticular corticosteroid can be used to target one specific symptomatic joint.
- Allopurinol should never be used in the treatment of acute gout. This agent is reserved for chronic prophylactic therapy in patients with multiple gout exacerbations each year.
  - If allopurinol is used in the treatment of an acute gout exacerbation, the symptoms may be worsened due to the mobilization of uric acid stores.

Prophylaxis of Gout

- Colchicine maintenance therapy is indicated for prophylaxis in patients with only slightly elevated serum uric acid levels.

- Allopurinol is indicated for prophylaxis of gout exacerbations in patients with a moderately elevated serum uric acid level and a history of nephrolithiasis, tophi, serum creatinine >2.0 g/dL, or urinary uric acid excretion indicative of overproduction.

- Uricosuric drugs are indicated for prophylaxis of gout exacerbations in patients who are not candidates for allopurinol therapy and have a urinary uric acid excretion indicative of underexcretion.

- When initiating prophylactic therapy in a patient with gout, colchicine should be initiated with either allopurinol or a uricosuric and continued for the first 3–6 months of therapy to avoid causing an exacerbation.

Drugs for Gout

Generic	Brand	Dose & Max	Contra-indications	Primary Side Effects	Key Monitoring Parameters	Pertinent Drug Interactions	Med Pearls	Top 200
Mechanism of action – colchicine: inhibits lactic acid production, decreases uric acid deposition, reduces phagocytosis, and decreases inflammation							
Colchicine	None	1 mg followed by 0.5 mg q2 hrs until symptoms resolve, diarrhea occurs, or 8 mg taken	Hypersensitivity; serious GI, renal, hepatic or cardiac disorders	• Diarrhea, nausea, vomiting • Rare: bone marrow suppression, aplastic anemia, thrombocytopenia	• Response to therapy • Serum uric acid • GI symptoms • Periodic CBC	None significant	• Patients may be provided with a prescription to be filled on a PRN basis and used during an exacerbation • Used for treatment and prophylaxis	Yes
Mechanism of action – xanthine oxidase inhibitor: by inhibition of xanthine oxidase, impairs the conversion of xanthine to uric acid, thereby decreasing the production of uric acid							
Allopurinol	Zyloprim	100–800 mg daily (renal dose adjustment necessary)	Hypersensitivity	Skin rash, leukopenia, GI upset	Response to therapy, serum uric acid, renal function	Mercaptopurine, azathioprine	Renal dose adjustment	Yes
Mechanism of action – uricosuric agents: increase the renal clearance of uric acid by inhibiting tubular reabsorption							
Sulfinpyrazone	Anturane	50–800 mg daily (BID)	• Hypersensitivity • CrCl <50 mL/min • History of renal calculi • Overproducers of uric acid • Peptic ulcer disease (PUD)	GI upset, rash, stone formation	• Response to treatment • Serum uric acid • Renal function	Warfarin (á INR), salicylates	May precipitate acute gouty attacks; avoid use during acute gouty arthritis	No
Probenecid	None	250–2,000 mg daily (BID)	• Hypersensitivity • CrCl <50 mL/min • History of renal calculi • Overproducers of uric acid • PUD	GI upset, rash, stone formation	• Response to treatment • Serum uric acid • Renal function	Methotrexate (á MTX levels), salicylates	May precipitate acute gouty attacks; avoid use during acute gouty arthritis	No

Storage and Administration Pearls

- Medications should be stored in a dry place and protected from light.

Patient Education Pearls

- Patient should drink plenty of water (6–8 eight-oz glasses) while taking sulfinpyrazone or probenecid to avoid formation of kidney stones.

LEARNING POINTS

- First-line therapy for mild to moderate osteoarthritis is acetaminophen.
- NSAIDs and other pain medication should be administered with food to minimize stomach upset.
- Biologic therapies for rheumatoid arthritis suppress immunity and therefore cannot be initiated during infection and may be temporarily withdrawn during active infection.
- Biologic therapy for rheumatoid arthritis requires parenteral administration.
- First-line therapy for osteoporosis is the bisphosphonate class. Frequency of administration varies greatly from once daily to once annually. Oral formulations require very specific adherence to administration instructions to avoid esophageal side effects.
- Allopurinol is used for gout prophylaxis only and should be avoided during acute attacks because of its ability to exacerbate acute gout arthropathy by mobilizing uric acid stores.

PRACTICE QUESTIONS

1. Pharmacists dispensing narcotic analgesics to patients with severe osteoarthritis should inform the patients that

    (A) medication will work better on an empty stomach.
    (B) if taken as directed, there is little potential for addiction.
    (C) it is okay to consume small amounts of alcohol with the medication.
    (D) they may need to take a stool softener or laxative with the medication.
    (E) they may need to take acetaminophen between doses.

2. Which of the following is NOT correctly matched with its trade name?

    (A) Methotrexate – Rheumatrex
    (B) Hydroxychloroquine – Azulfidine
    (C) Leflunomide – Arava
    (D) Etanercept – Enbrel
    (E) Infliximab – Remicade

ANSWERS

1. **D**

Narcotic analgesics may cause constipation and often require the need for a laxative or stool softener. Narcotics may cause stomach upset and should be taken with food (A). Narcotics are controlled substances and have the potential for addiction and abuse even if taken correctly (B). Narcotics may cause CNS depression and should not be used with any amount of alcohol (C). Many narcotics are formulated in combination with acetaminophen, so recommending extra acetaminophen between dosing intervals may provide over the daily recommendation of acetaminophen (E) and should not be advised.

2. **B**

Hydroxychloroquine is generic for Plaquenil. Azulfidine is the brand name for sulfasalazine. The other answer choices are correctly matched with their trade names. Methotrexate (A) is generic for Rheumatrex or Trexall.

Pain Management

10

This chapter covers the following drug classes:

- **Nonsteroidal anti-inflammatory drugs (NSAIDs)**
- **Non-opioid pain management**
- **Opioid pain management**

The text also provides an overview of basic treatment and management of pain.

 Suggested Study Time: **30 minutes**

PAIN MANAGEMENT

Definitions

Pain management can be a very complicated and a very involved condition because pain is subjective and therapy must be individualized. Such objective measures as tachycardia are not reliable. There are five main types of pain: Acute, chronic, chronic cancer, breakthrough, and neuropathic pain. Acute pain usually requires only temporary therapy for less than 30 days. Chronic pain is persistent and adversely affects the function or well-being of the patient for longer than 6 months. Non-narcotic preparations should be used when possible; however, patients are at greater risk for potential addiction and dependences. Often, chronic pain will intensify, requiring more complex regimens and combination therapy with narcotics and non-narcotics. Chronic cancer pain occurs in 60–90% of patients with cancer. It is similar to chronic nonmalignant pain. Breakthrough pain is intermittent and occurs at a greater intensity over baseline chronic pain. Neuropathic pain is characterized by a burning or tingling feeling, and can often be treated using anticonvulsants and antidepressants (also known as co-analgesics) with great success.

Diagnosis

Because pain is identified principally through self-reports and is very much subjective, it is challenging for a clinician to accurately assess and is virtually impossible to diagnose.

- Pain is always subjective.
- No neurophysiological or laboratory test can measure pain.
- The clinician must accept the patient's report of pain.

Signs and Symptoms

- Objective observations such as grimacing, limping, or tachycardia may be helpful in assessing patients, but theses signs are often absent in patients with chronic pain caused by structural lesions.
- Pain intensity scales help patients communicate the signs and symptoms and pain intensity. This assessment can help guide treatments.
- Most adults and children above the age of 7 can score their pain intensity on a verbal numerical rating scale: 0 = no pain; 10 = the worst pain imaginable.

Guidelines

Institute for Clinical Systems Improvement, March 2007. Assessment and Management of Chronic Pain. www.icsi.org/pain_chronic_assessment_and_management_of_14399/pain_chronic_assessment_and_management_of_guideline_.html.

Guidelines Summary

- Drug therapy is the mainstay of management for acute pain and cancer pain in all age groups, including neonates, infants, children, and adults. The drugs discussed in this review are classified into three categories: Nonopioid analgesics, including acetaminophen and nonsteroidal anti-inflammatory drugs (NSAIDs); opioid pain management; and co-analgesics. The drug classes can be used in monotherapy and combination for pain.
- As the pain increases, so does the dose of medications, the migration to stronger medications, and the use of combinations of medications with different mechanisms of actions.
- Acetaminophen and NSAIDs are useful for acute and chronic pain arising from a variety of causes, including surgery, trauma, arthritis, and cancer.
- NSAIDs are indicated for pain involving inflammation because acetaminophen lacks clinically effective anti-inflammatory agents.

- NSAIDs differ from opioid analgesic by the following mechanisms:
  - NSAIDs are both analgesics and inflammatory in nature.
  - There is a dose ceiling of affect in relationship with adverse affects.
  - NSAIDs do not produce physical or psychological dependence.
  - NSAIDs are antipyretic.
- Initiation of opioid analgesics should be based on a pain-directed history and physical that includes repeated pain assessment.
  - Opioid analgesics should be added to nonopioids to manage acute pain and cancer-related pain that does not respond to nonopioids alone.
  - There is enormous variability in doses of opioids required to provide pain relief, even among opioid-naïve patients.
  - It is important to give each analgesic an adequate trial. As a result, a clinician will increase the opioid dose until unacceptable side effects appear before changing to another opioid.
  - It is recommended to administer analgesics on a regular schedule if pain is present most of the day. This allows the patient to stay ahead of the pain.
    - » For chronic pain, consider having a scheduled long-acting agent on board and a short-acting agent for times of breakthrough pain.
- Patient-controlled intravenous opioid administration (PCA) for acute pain is a commonly used technique for pain control.
  - PCA is used with a microprocessor-controlled infusion pump.
  - PCA is most often used for the IV administration of opioids for acute pain.
  - PCA allows patients considerable control over the experience of pain.
  - PCA is not recommended in situations in which oral opioids could readily manage pain.

Nonnarcotic Oral and Nonsteroidal Anti-inflammatory Drugs (NSAIDs)

Mechanism of action – decreases pain through inhibition of central cyclo-oxygenase, which in turn inhibits prostaglandin synthesis

Mechanism of action – NSAIDs: decrease pain and inflammation by inhibition of prostaglandin synthesis through inhibition of cyclooxygenase enzymes

Generic	Brand	Dose & Max Mg (frequency)	Contra-indications	Primary Side Effects	Key Monitoring Parameters	Pertinent Drug Interactions	Med Pearls	Top 200
Acetaminophen	Tylenol	• 325–1,000 TID–QID • Max: 4,000 mg	• Hepatic disease • Alcoholism	Very few	Pain relief	Alcohol	• OTC • Best if taken on scheduled basis vs. PRN	Yes
Aspirin	Various	• IR: 325–3,600 daily (q4–6 hrs) • XR product 650–1,300 TID • Max: 5.4 g/day	• Allergy • Fever in children • Active bleeding	GI (upset stomach, bleeding); rash	Pain relief, GI symptoms	• Warfarin • Other NSAIDs • ACE inhibitors	• OTC • Anti-inflammatory only at high doses (>3 g/day)	Yes
Nonacetylated salicylates								
Salsalate	Various	• 500–3,000 daily (BID–TID) • Max: 3 g/day	Hypersensitivity	• GI (upset stomach, bleeding) • Rash • Diminished renal function • Edema	Pain relief, GI symptoms	• Other salicylates • Warfarin • ACE inhibitors	• Monitor serum salicylate levels with chronic use or very high doses • Desired range 10–30 mg/100 ml	No
Diflunisal	None	500–1,500 daily (BID)	Hypersensitivity				Administer with food	No

Nonnarcotic Oral and Nonsteroidal Anti-inflammatory Drugs (NSAIDs) *(cont'd)*

Generic	Brand	Dose & Max Mg (frequency)	Contra-indications	Primary Side Effects	Key Monitoring Parameters	Pertinent Drug Interactions	Med Pearls	Top 200
Acetic acids								
Etodolac	None	200–1,200 daily (q 6–8 hrs)	Hypersensitivity	• GI (upset stomach, bleeding) • Rash • Diminished renal function • ã blood pressure • Edema	• Pain relief • GI symptoms • Renal function • Blood pressure	• Other salicylates • Warfarin • Lithium • ACE inhibitors	Administer with food	No
Diclofenac	Cataflam Voltaren	50–150 daily (BID–TID)	Hypersensitivity	• GI (upset stomach, bleeding) • Rash • Diminished renal function • ã blood pressure • Edema	• Pain relief • GI symptoms • Renal function • Blood pressure	• Other salicylates • Warfarin • Lithium • ACE inhibitors	Administer with food	Yes
Indomethacin	Indocin Indocin SR	• IR: 25–200 daily (BID–TID) • SR: 75–150 1x daily • Max: 200 mg/day	Hypersensitivity	• GI (upset stomach, bleeding) • Rash • Diminished renal function • ã blood pressure • Edema • CNS disturbances	• Pain relief • GI symptoms • Renal function • Blood pressure	• Other salicylates • Warfarin • Lithium • ACE inhibitors	• Most commonly used for treatment of gout • Fat-soluble, crosses blood-brain barrier • Administer with food	Yes
Ketorolac	Toradol	30 mg IM or 15 mg IV initial; 10 mg PO q 4–6 hrs up to 40 mg daily	• Active PUD or bleeding • History of GI bleeding • Severe renal impairment • Labor and delivery	• GI (upset stomach, bleeding) • Rash • Diminished renal function • ã blood pressure	• Pain relief • GI symptoms • Renal function • Blood pressure	• Other salicylates • Warfarin • Lithium • ACE inhibitors	Only approved for moderate–severe pain for ≤5 days' duration, due to risk of renal and GI dysfunction	No
Nabumetone	Relafen	500–2,000 daily (Q day–BID)	Hypersensitivity				Administer with food	Yes

Nonnarcotic Oral and Nonsteroidal Anti-inflammatory Drugs (NSAIDs) *(cont'd)*

Generic	Brand	Dose & Max Mg (frequency)	Contra-indications	Primary Side Effects	Key Monitoring Parameters	Pertinent Drug Interactions	Med Pearls	Top 200
Propionic acids								
Fenoprofen	Nalfon	200–3,200 daily (TID–QID)	Hypersensitivity	• GI (upset stomach, bleeding)	• Pain relief	• Other salicylates	Administer with food	No
Flurbiprofen	Ansaid	50–300 daily (BID–QID)	Hypersensitivity	• Rash	• GI symptoms	• Warfarin	Administer with food	No
Ibuprofen	Motrin Advil	• 200–3,200 daily (TID–QID) • Max: 3.2 g/day	Hypersensitivity	• Diminished renal function • á blood pressure	• Renal function • Blood pressure	• Lithium • ACE inhibitors	• Available OTC and Rx (400–800 mg tabs) • Administer with food • Available in pediatric preparations	Yes
Ketoprofen	Orudis Oruvail Rhodis	• IR: 50–300 daily (TID–QID) • SR: 75–200 daily	Hypersensitivity				• Available OTC and Rx • Administer with food	No
Naproxen	Naprosyn EC Naprosyn Naprelan	• IR: 250–1,500 daily (BID) • EC: 375–1,500 daily (BID) • CR: 375–1,500 daily (BID)	Hypersensitivity				• Available OTC and Rx • Administer with food	Yes
Naproxen sodium	Anaprox	275–1,650 daily (BID)	Hypersensitivity				• Available OTC and Rx • Administer with food	Yes
Oxaprozin	Daypro	600–1,800 daily (1x daily)	Hypersensitivity				Administer with food	No

Nonnarcotic Oral and Nonsteroidal Anti-inflammatory Drugs (NSAIDs) *(cont'd)*

Generic	Brand	Dose & Max Mg (frequency)	Contra-indications	Primary Side Effects	Key Monitoring Parameters	Pertinent Drug Interactions	Med Pearls	Top 200
Fenamates								
Meclofenamate	Meclomen	50–400 daily (q 4–6 hrs)	Hypersensitivity	• GI (upset stomach, bleeding) • Rash • Diminished renal function • á blood pressure	• Pain relief • GI symptoms • Renal function • Blood pressure	• Other salicylates • Warfarin • Lithium • ACE inhibitors	Administer with food	No
Oxicams								
Piroxicam	Feldene	10–20 daily (1x daily)	Hypersensitivity	• GI (upset stomach, bleeding) • Rash • Diminished renal function • á blood pressure	• Pain relief • GI symptoms • Renal function • Blood pressure	• Other salicylates • Warfarin • Lithium • ACE inhibitors	• More COX -2 selectivity than traditional NSAIDs • Slightly less GI symptoms	Yes
Meloxicam	Mobic	7.5–15 daily (1x daily)	Hypersensitivity					Yes
Selective COX -2 Inhibitors								
Celecoxib	Celebrex	50–200 daily (q day–BID)	Hypersensitivity	• GI (upset stomach, bleeding—less than other NSAIDs) • Rash • Diminished renal function • á blood pressure; edema	• Pain relief • GI symptoms • Renal function • Blood pressure	• Other salicylates (including aspirin) • Warfarin • Lithium • ACE inhibitors	• Lower incidence of GI toxicity than with NSAIDs • Concern about cardiovascular adverse effects prompted withdrawal of similar drug from market (rofecoxib)	Yes

Narcotic Analgesics

Narcotic analgesics: stimulate opioid receptors in the brain

Generic	Brand	Dose & Max Mg (frequency)	Contra-indications	Primary Side Effects	Key Monitoring Parameters	Pertinent Drug Interactions	Med Pearls	Top 200
Hydrocodone/APAP	• Various • Lortab • Vicodin	5–60 mg hydrocodone daily (q4–6 hrs)	Hypersensitivity, severe hepatic impairment, alcoholism	• Constipation • CNS depression • Confusion • Sedation • Respiratory depression • Hypotension • Bradycardia	• Presence of side effects (constipation, confusion) • Pain relief • Respiratory rate • Blood pressure • Heart rate	• Alcohol • Other CNS depressants	• Take with food • Often need laxative in addition • High abuse potential	Yes
Propoxyphene/APAP	• Various • Darvocet	65–600 mg propoxyphene (q4–6 hrs)		• Constipation • CNS depression • Confusion • Sedation • Elevated liver transaminases	• Presence of side effects • Pain relief • Liver transaminases periodically		• Take with food • Often need laxative in addition • High abuse potential	Yes
APAP/Codeine	• Various • Tylenol #3	7.5–360 mg codeine daily (q4–6 hrs)		• Constipation • CNS depression • Confusion • Sedation • Respiratory depression • Hypotension • Bradycardia	• Presence of side effects (constipation, confusion) • Pain relief • Respiratory rate • Blood pressure • Heart rate			Yes
Morphine	Various	No max					• Take with food • Often need laxative in addition • High abuse potential • Initiate IR and switch to CR/ER	Yes

Narcotic Analgesics *(cont'd)*

Generic	Brand	Dose & Max Mg (frequency)	Contra-indications	Primary Side Effects	Key Monitoring Parameters	Pertinent Drug Interactions	Med Pearls	Top 200
Oxycodone/APAP	• Various • Percocet • Roxicet	5–40 mg daily oxycodone (q 6 hrs PRN)		• Constipation • CNS depression • Confusion • Sedation	• Presence of side effects (constipation, confusion) • Pain relief	• Alcohol • Other CNS depressants	• Take with food • Often need laxative in addition • High abuse potential	Yes
Fentanyl	• Duragesic • Actiq • Fentora	• Infusion, injection, lozenge, tab, transdermal patch • No max • Dosages different for each delivery system		• Respiratory depression • Hypotension • Bradycardia	• Respiratory rate • Blood pressure • Heart rate	CYP 450 3A4	• Patch takes 24 hrs to begin working • Fentanyl remains in patch at 72 hrs; fold in half to avoid diversion	Yes
Hydromorphone	• Dilaudid • Dilaudid – HP	• 3, 6, 12, 18, 24, 30 mg • No max	Hypersensitivity, asthma, respiratory depression, CNS depression			None	• Tolerance can develop • High potential for abuse • Dilaudid-HP is highly concentrated	Yes
Meperidine	Demerol	Injection, PCA pump, tablet 25–100 mg	• Avoid in renal failure • Avoid hepatic disease		• Same as above; add seizure due to potential metabolite-normeperidine	• CYP 450 – 2B6, 2C19, 3A4	• Not recommended as an analgesic • Use less than 48 hrs and in doses less than 600 mg/day	No
Methadone	Dolophine	• Initial opioid naive: 2.5–10 mg q 8–12 hrs • No max	Same as above but add concurrent use of selegiline		• Pain relief, mental status, blood pressure	• CYP 450 • Inhibits: 2D6, 3A4	Long half-life and difficult to titrate	Yes

Analgesic Adjuncts

Mechanism of action – increases synaptic concentration of norepinephrine, desensitization of adenyl cyclase, downregulation of serotonin receptors

Generic	Brand	Dose & Max Mg (frequency)	Contraindications	Primary Side Effects	Key Monitoring Parameters	Pertinent Drug Interactions	Med Pearls	Top 200
Desipramine	Norpramin	• Initial: 75–150 mg • Max: 300 mg	Use of MAOI past 14 days; acute recovery phase following a myocardial infarction	• Orthostatic hypotension • Tachycardia • Anticholinergic	• Blood pressure • Suicidal ideation	CYP 450 inhibits 1A2, 2C9, 2D6, 2E1	• Increased suicidal behavior in young adults age 18–24 yrs • Chronic pain is an unlabeled indication	No
Amitriptyline	Elavil	• Initial: 50–150 mg/day • Max: 400 mg						Yes

Mechanism of action – induces the release of substance P, the principle chemomediator of pain impulses from the periphery

Generic	Brand	Dose & Max Mg (frequency)	Contraindications	Primary Side Effects	Key Monitoring Parameters	Pertinent Drug Interactions	Med Pearls	Top 200
Gabapentin	Neurontin	• Initial 300 mg TID • Max: 3,600	None	• Somnolence • Dizziness • Peripheral edema	Pain scale	Sedative effects: CNS depressants, alcohol, opiates	Chronic pain is not an official indication	Yes
Pregabalin	Lyrica	• Initial: 75 mg BID • Max: 450 mg/day					• Controlled substance (C5) • Has official FDA indication for neuropathic pain associated with diabetes	Yes

Mechanism of action – binds to μ-opiate receptors in the CNS, causing inhibition of ascending pain pathways

Generic	Brand	Dose & Max Mg (frequency)	Contraindications	Primary Side Effects	Key Monitoring Parameters	Pertinent Drug Interactions	Med Pearls	Top 200
Tramadol	• Ultram • Ultram ER	• IR: 25–400 daily (q 4–6 hrs) • ER: 100–300 daily	Hypersensitivity	• Confusion • Sedation • Rash • Stomach upset • Orthostatic hypotension	• Pain relief • Renal and hepatic function periodically	• Alcohol • Opioids • SSRIs • MAOIs • Warfarin	• Renal dose adjustment for CrCl <30 mL/min • Not a controlled substance	Yes

Mechanism of action – induces the release of substance P, the principal chemomediator of pain impulses from the periphery

Generic	Brand	Dose & Max Mg (frequency)	Contraindications	Primary Side Effects	Key Monitoring Parameters	Pertinent Drug Interactions	Med Pearls	Top 200
Capsaicin Cream	Various	0.025–0.1% applied 3–4x daily	Do not apply to wounds or damaged skin	Localized stinging	Pain relief	None	• OTC • Must be used regularly for 2 wks or more for maximal efficacy	No

STORAGE AND ADMINISTRATION PEARLS

- Do not freeze acetaminophen suppositories.
- Hydrolysis of aspirin occurs upon exposure to water or moist air, resulting in salicylate and acetate, which possess a vinegar-like odor. Do not use if a strong odor is present.
- Ibuprofen, indomethacin, ketoprofen, and ketoralac must be protected from light.
- With codeine, protect injection from light.
- Amitriptyline, oxycodone, fentanyl, hydromorphone, meperidine, methadone all need to be protected from light.

PATIENT EDUCATION PEARLS

- The patient should always take exactly what is prescribed. Never increase the dose without discussing with the prescriber
- The narcotic medications may cause physical and psychological dependence.
- While using pain medications, it is recommended not to use alcohol or other prescription or OTC medications.

LEARNING POINTS

- NSAIDs are both analgesics and inflammatory in nature.
- No NSAID is any more effective than any other in the general population.
- Symptoms of overdose for narcotic medications include: CNS depression, bradycardia, hypotension, respiratory depression, miosis, apnea, pulmonary edema, and convulsions.
- Onset of action of most pain medication occurs within 45 minutes, with peak drug effect in 1 to 2 hours after oral administration for most immediate-release medications.
- PCA provides the important advantage of medication that is rapidly administered when needed, delaying pain exacerbation.
- In chronic pain, continuous opioid administration is recommended with controlled release medication, transdermal patch, or infusion. Short-acting medications should be available for breakthrough pain.

PRACTICE QUESTIONS

1. Which of the following is NOT a muscle relaxer?

   (A) Baclofen
   (B) Relafen
   (C) Robaxin
   (D) Parafon Forte
   (E) Zanaflex

2. Which of the following drugs is/are contraindicated for a patient with a history of a GI bleed?

       I. Aspirin
      II. Warfarin
     III. Toradol

   (A) I only
   (B) III only
   (C) I and II only
   (D) II and III only
   (E) I, II, and III

ANSWERS

1. **B**

Relafen (nabumetone) is an NSAID, so (B) is correct. The other choices are all muscle relaxer: Baclofen (Lioresal), Robaxin (methocarbamol), Parafon Forte (chlorzoxazone), and Zanaflex (tizanidine).

2. **E**

Aspirin, warfarin, and Toradol are all contraindicated for someone who has had a GI bleed, so (E) is correct. Aspirin and Toradol inhibit prostaglandins, which protect the lining of the stomach. Warfarin and aspirin both increase the bleeding time.

Ophthalmologic Disorders

11

This chapter covers the following disorder:

- **Glaucoma**

 Suggested Study Time: **10 minutes**

GLAUCOMA

Definitions

Glaucoma is a group of eye disorders caused by damage to an area of the optic nerve (optic disk), which results in loss of visual sensitivity and field. The two types of glaucoma include open-angle and closed-angle glaucoma. Open-angle glaucoma is the most common form of this disorder and can be due to either genetic causes (most prevalent is primary open-angle glaucoma [POAG]) or other factors such as trauma, surgery, or medications (secondary open-angle glaucoma). Although it was previously believed that an increased intraocular pressure (IOP) was solely responsible for the damage to the optic disk, it appears that factors such as ischemia, changes in blood flow, and auto-immune factors may also play a role.

Given that up to 70% of all cases of glaucoma in the United States are characterized as POAG, the discussion in this chapter focuses only on this form of the ocular disorder.

Diagnosis

The diagnosis of POAG is based on the presence of characteristic changes to the optic disk and visual field loss with or without an increased IOP. An increased IOP does not need to be present to confirm the diagnosis of POAG. In general, an IOP greater than 21 mmHg is considered to be elevated.

Signs and Symptoms

Symptoms for glaucoma usually do not develop until significant damage to the optic disk and significant visual field loss has already occurred. Patients may complain of blind spots, reduced peripheral vision, and changes in color perception.

Guidelines

American Academy of Ophthalmology. http://one.aao.org/CE/PracticeGuidelines/default.aspx.

Overview of Treatment

Because the above guidelines do not specify which drugs should be used as 1st-line or 2nd-line therapy, this section should not be considered as a "Guidelines Summary" but rather as a general overview of the pharmacologic treatment of glaucoma.

The initial goal is to achieve at least a 20% reduction in the IOP. Additional lowering may be necessary based upon the baseline IOP, the extent of damage to the optic disk, and the extent of visual field loss.

- β-blockers, prostaglandin analogs, or α$_2$ agonists (brimonidine) are considered 1st-line therapy for POAG. These agents can be used as monotherapy or in combination with each other.
  - If a patient does not tolerate or does not respond at all (no reduction in IOP) to an agent, an alternative drug should be used.
  - If a patient partially responds to an agent (some reduction in IOP, but not at goal), addition of another drug should be considered.
- Topical carbonic anhydrase inhibitors can be considered if the patient does not respond to or tolerate one of the above 1st-line agents.
- Cholinergic agonists and dipivefrin are usually considered as last-line drug therapies because of their increased risk of side effects.
- Laser or surgical procedures may also be considered during the course of therapy.

β-Blockers

Mechanism of action — ↓ IOP by ↓ production of aqueous humor

Generic	Brand	Dose	Contra-indications	Primary Side Effects	Key Monitoring	Pertinent Drug Interactions	Med Pearl	Top 200
Betaxolol (β₁- selective)	• Betoptic • Betoptic-S	• Solution: 1–2 drops 2x daily • Suspension: 1 drop 2x daily	• Sinus bradycardia • ≥2nd-degree heart block (in absence of pacemaker) • Decompensated heart failure • Severe chronic obstructive pulmonary disease/ asthma	Local: Burning, stinging, tearing, blurred vision, dry eyes • Systemic: • Bradycardia • Heart block • Hypotension • Heart failure exacerbation • Bronchospasm • Fatigue	IOP every 2–4 wks until target achieved, then every 6 mo	• ↑ risk of systemic side effects with oral β-blockers • ↑ risk of bradycardia or heart block with digoxin, verapamil, diltiazem, or clonidine	• All have similar efficacy in ↓ IOP • Tachyphylaxis may occur with long-term use • Effect on IOP may be lessened in patients receiving oral β-blockers	No
Carteolol (nonselective, ISA properties)	Only available generically	1 drop 2x daily						No
Levobunolol (nonselective)	• AKBeta • Betagan	1 drop 1–2x daily						No
Metipranolol (nonselective)	OptiPranolol	1 drop 2x daily						No
Timolol (nonselective)	• Solution: Timoptic, Betimol, Istalol • Gel-forming solution: Timoptic-XE	• Solution: 1 drop 1–2x daily • Gel-forming solution: 1 drop 1x daily						No

Prostaglandin Analogs

Mechanism of action – ↓ IOP by ↑ outflow of aqueous humor

Generic	Brand	Dose	Contra-indications	Primary Side Effects	Key Monitoring	Pertinent Drug Interactions	Med Pearl	Top 200
Bimatoprost	Lumigan	1 drop 1x daily in evening	Hypersensitivity	Change in iris, eyelash, and eyelid pigmentation (become darker) • Growth of eyelashes • Eyelid edema • Itching, redness, blurred vision, dry eyes	IOP every 2–4 wks until target achieved, then every 6 mo	No significant interactions	• Do not exceed 1x daily dosing (may worsen IOP) • Iris discoloration is not reversible (highest incidence with latanoprost) • Eyelid discoloration and eyelash changes may be reversible • Travatan Z does not contain benzalkonium chloride	Yes
Latanoprost	Xalatan	1 drop 1x daily in evening						Yes
Travoprost	• Travatan • Travatan Z	1 drop 1x daily in evening						Yes

α$_2$-Agonists

Mechanism of action – ↓ IOP by ↓ production of aqueous humor (brimonidine may also ↑ outflow of aqueous humor)

Generic	Brand	Dose	Contra-indications	Primary Side Effects	Key Monitoring	Pertinent Drug Interactions	Med Pearl	Top 200
Apraclonidine	Iopidine	1 drop 3x daily	Concurrent or recent use (within 14 days) of monoamine oxidase inhibitors	Local effects: • Eyelid edema • Itching, redness, burning Systemic effects: • Dizziness • Fatigue • Dry mouth • Headache • Hypotension • Bradycardia	IOP every 2–4 wks until target achieved, then every 6 mo	↑ risk of systemic side effects with CNS depressants (e.g., alcohol, opiates, sedatives, barbiturates)	• Structurally similar to clonidine • Apraclonidine primarily used to control postoperative ↑ IOP	No
Brimonidine	Alphagan P	1 drop 3x daily						Yes

Carbonic Anhydrase Inhibitors

Mechanism of action — ↓ IOP by ↓ production of aqueous humor

Generic	Brand	Dose	Contra-indications	Primary Side Effects	Key Monitoring	Pertinent Drug Interactions	Med Pearl	Top 200
Brinzolamide	Azopt	1 drop 3x daily	Sulfa allergy (risk of cross-sensitivity)	• Eyelid reactions • Burning, stinging, tearing, blurred vision • Bitter taste in mouth	IOP every 2–4 wks until target achieved, then every 6 mo	No significant interactions	• Topical therapy rarely associated with systemic side effects	No
Dorzolamide	Trusopt	1 drop 3x daily					• Oral carbonic anhydrase inhibitor therapy (e.g., acetazolamide) may be used in patients refractory to maximal doses of topical therapy; associated with higher risk of side effects	No

Cholinergic Agonists (Direct-Acting)

Mechanism of action — ↓ IOP by ↑ outflow of aqueous humor

Generic	Brand	Dose	Contra-indications	Primary Side Effects	Key Monitoring	Pertinent Drug Interactions	Med Pearl	Top 200
Carbachol	Isopto Carbachol	1–2 drops 2–3x daily	Ocular inflammatory condition (may worsen condition)	• Impaired night vision • Headache • Eyelid twitching • Stinging, burning, tearing	IOP every 2–4 wks until target achieved, then every 6 mo	No significant interactions	• Patients with darker eyes may require higher concentrations of pilocarpine to ↓ IOP	No
Pilocarpine	• Solution: Isopto Carpine • Gel: Pilopine HS	1–2 drops 3–4x daily At bedtime					• Pilocarpine concentrations >4% may be associated with ↑ risk of systemic side effects (e.g., ↑ urinary frequency, sweating, vomiting, salivation, bronchospasm, bradycardia)	No

Nonspecific Adrenergic Agonists

Mechanism of action — ↓ IOP by ↑ outflow of aqueous humor

Generic	Brand	Dose	Contraindications	Primary Side Effects	Key Monitoring	Pertinent Drug Interactions	Med Pearl	Top 200
Dipivefrin	• AKPro • Propine	1 drop 2x daily	Closed-angle glaucoma	Tearing, burning, stinging, blurred vision	IOP every 2–4 wks until target achieved, then every 6 mo	No significant interactions	• Prodrug of epinephrine • Least effective in ↓ IOP	No

Combination Drugs

Generic	Brand
Timolol/brimonidine	Combigan
Timolol/dorzolamide	Cosopt

STORAGE AND ADMINISTRATION PEARLS

- Most ophthalmic preparations (gels, solutions, suspensions) should be stored at room temperature.
  - Latanoprost should be refrigerated until opened; once opened, the bottle can be stored at room temperature.
- Ophthalmic suspensions should be shaken well prior to using.

PATIENT EDUCATION PEARLS

- Patient should be educated on the appropriate administration of ophthalmic preparations:
  - Wash and dry hands.
  - If suspension is being used, shake the bottle well.
  - Contact lenses should be removed prior to administration.
  - Tilt head back and look at the ceiling.
  - Pull down the lower eyelid to form a pocket into which the medication will be instilled.
  - Place the dropper over the eye, look up, and then place a single drop in the eye.
  - To avoid contamination, the tip of the dropper should not touch any part of the eye.
  - Close the eyes for several minutes. Do not rub the eyes.
- If the patient is using more than one ophthalmic drug, administration of these drugs should be separated by at least 10 minutes to prevent loss of the initially administered drug.
- Patient should be educated on use of nasolacrimal occlusion when administering eyedrops to minimize the development of systemic side effects and to enhance drug efficacy.
  - Once the eyedrop is instilled, instruct patient to close eye and place index finger over nasolacrimal drainage system in the inner corner of the eye for 1–3 minutes.

LEARNING POINTS

- Know examples of ophthalmic β-blockers, prostaglandin analogs, and α2 agonists.
- β-blocker eyedrops can cause systemic adverse effects. Use caution in patients also receiving oral β-blocker therapy.
- Prostaglandin analogs can cause pigmentation changes in the iris, eyelid, and eyelashes.
- Carbonic anhydrase inhibitors should not be used in patients with sulfa allergies.
- Know combination drug products.

PRACTICE QUESTIONS

1. Which of the following medications is likely to cause a darkening of the iris of the eye?

    (A) Apraclonidine
    (B) Carbachol
    (C) Dorzolamide
    (D) Latanoprost
    (E) Timolol

2. Lumigan belongs to which of the following classes of drugs?

    (A) Alpha-2-agonist
    (B) Antihistamine
    (C) Beta-blocker
    (D) Cholinergic agonist
    (E) Prostaglandin analog

ANSWERS

1. **D**

Latanoprost, an ophthalmic prostaglandin analog, is likely to cause darkening of the iris, so choice (D) is correct. This class of drugs may also cause increased pigmentation of the eyelid and eyelashes.

2. **E**

Lumigan, the brand name for bimatoprost, is a prostaglandin analog, so choice (E) is correct.

Hematologic Disorders

12

This chapter covers the following diseases:

- **Iron deficiency anemia**
- **Anemia of chronic kidney disease and dialysis**
- **Pernicious anemia**

 Suggested Study Time: **45 minutes**

IRON DEFICIENCY ANEMIA

Definitions

Iron deficiency anemia (IDA) is a common disorder worldwide. In the United States, most cases are caused by menstrual blood loss, GI blood loss, and increased iron requirements of pregnancy. Decreased iron absorption or increased iron requirements may also lead to iron deficiency.

Diagnosis

- Evidence of a source of blood loss should be sought.
- Iron deficiency anemia is classically described as a microcytic anemia.
- The differential diagnosis includes thalassemia, sideroblastic anemias, some types of anemia of chronic disease, and lead poisoning.
- Serum ferritin is the preferred initial diagnostic test. Total iron-binding capacity, transferrin saturation, serum iron, and serum transferrin receptor levels may be helpful if the ferritin level is between 46 and 99 ng/mL (46 and 99 mcg/L); bone marrow biopsy may be necessary in these patients for a definitive diagnosis.
- Laboratory tests include:

- MCV: Normal in early iron deficiency; eventual decreases
- HCT: Falls below 30%
- Platelet count: May increase
- Serum ferritin: Less than 10 ng/mL in women and 20 ng/mL in men
- Total iron-binding capacity (TIBC): Increased >420 ug/dL

Signs and Symptoms

There are many symptoms of IDA. Different patients will experience different combinations of symptoms; and if the anemia is mild, the symptoms may not be noticeable. Some of the symptoms are: Pale skin color, fatigue, irritability, dizziness, weakness, shortness of breath, sore tongue, brittle nails, decreased appetite (especially in children), and frontal headaches.

Guidelines

American Family Physicians, Citation: American Family Physician, no. 75 (2007): 671–8. www.aafp.org/afp/20070301/671.pdf.

Guidelines Summary

Routine iron supplementation is recommended for high-risk infants 6 to 12 months of age. In children, adolescents, and women of reproductive age, a trial of iron is a reasonable approach if the review of symptoms, history, and physical examination are negative; however, the hemoglobin should be checked at 1 month. If there is not a 1–2 g/dL increase in the hemoglobin level in that time, possibilities include malabsorption of oral iron, lack of compliance, continued bleeding, or presence of an unknown lesion.

Transfusion should be considered for patients of any age with IDA who are complaining of symptoms such as fatigue or dyspnea on exertion. Transfusion should also be considered for asymptomatic cardiac patients with hemoglobin less than 10 g/dL (100 g/L). However, oral iron therapy is usually the first-line therapy for patients with IDA. As noted in the etiology section, iron absorption varies widely based on type of diet and other factors.

- Bone marrow response to iron is limited to 20 mg/day of elemental iron.
- An increase in the hemoglobin level of 1 g/dL (10 g/L) should occur every 2 to 4 weeks on iron therapy.
- It may take up to 4 months for the iron stores to return to normal after the hemoglobin has corrected. Iron sulfate in a dose of 300 mg provides 60 mg of elemental iron, whereas 325 mg of iron gluconate provides 36 mg of elemental iron.

- Sustained-release formulations of iron are not recommended as initial therapy because they reduce the amount of iron that is presented for absorption to the duodenal villi.

- Gastrointestinal absorption of elemental iron is enhanced in the presence of an acidic gastric environment.

- This can be accomplished through simultaneous intake of ascorbic acid (i.e., vitamin C).

- Although iron absorption occurs more readily when taken on an empty stomach, this increases the likelihood of stomach upset because of iron therapy. Increased patient adherence should be weighed against the inferior absorption.

- Laxatives, stool softeners, and adequate intake of liquids can alleviate the constipating effects of oral iron therapy.

- Indications for the use of intravenous iron include:
  - Chronic uncorrectable bleeding
  - Intestinal malabsorption
  - Intolerance to oral iron: Often results in nonadherence by the patient
  - Hemoglobin levels less than 6 g/dL (60 g/L) with signs of poor perfusion in patients who would otherwise receive transfusion (e.g., those who have religious objections).

Drugs for Iron Deficiency Anemia

Generic	Brand	Dose	Contraindications	Primary Side Effects	Key Monitoring	Pertinent Drug Interactions	Med Pearl	Top 200
Mechanism of action – replaces iron found in hemoglobin, myoglobin; allows the transportation of oxygen via hemoglobin								
Ferrous sulfate, gluconate, fumarate	• Sulfate: Feosol, Fer-In-Sol, Fer-Iron, Slow-FE • Gluconate	• Sulfate: Treatment: 300 mg BID • Gluconate/ Fumarate: 60 mg BID Prophylaxis 1x daily	Hypersensitivity to iron salts, hemochromatosis (GI absorbs excess iron), hemolytic anemia	• GI irritation • Epigastric pain • Nausea • Dark stools • Vomiting • Stomach cramping • Constipation	• Serum iron • Total iron-binding capacity • Reticulocyte count • Hemoglobin	• Absorption: tetracyclines, fluoroquinolones, levodopa, methyldopa, penicillamine • PPIs and H$_2$ blockers can affect iron absorption	• The advantage of iron dextran is the ability to administer large doses (200 to 500 mg) at one time • One major drawback of iron dextran is the risk of anaphylactic reactions that can be fatal	Yes
Mechanism of action – release iron from the plasma; eventually replenishes the depleted iron stores in the bone marrow								
Dextran 40, 70	Dexferrum	IV: 500–1,000 mL at 20–40 mL/min for 5 days	• Hypersensitivity to dextran • Thrombocytopenia • Hypofibrinogenemia	• Mild hypotension • Tightness in the chest • Wheezing	• Circulatory overload • Anaphylactoid reaction • Hemoglobin	Enhance the anticoagulant effect of abciximab	• Rifabutin often will be used with drug interaction to prevent the use of rifampin • Test dose is required	No
Sodium ferric gluconate	Ferrlecit	IV: 125 mg/10 mL infused approximately 8x	Use in any anemia not caused by iron deficiency	• Angina, bradycardia • Hypotension • Agitation • Chills, dizziness, fatigue	• Hematocrit • Electrolytes • Vital signs	Decrease the absorption of oral iron	• A safer form of parenteral iron compared to dextran • No test dose is required	No
Mechanism of action – iron sucrose is dissociated by the reticuloendothelial system into iron and sucrose; increases serum iron levels								
Iron sucrose	Venofer	IV: 100 mg administered 1–3x/wk during dialysis	• Evidence of iron overload • Anemia not caused by iron deficiency	• Hypotension • Peripheral edema • Headache and nausea	• Circulatory overload • Anaphylactoid reaction • Hemoglobin • Hematocrit • Electrolytes • Vital signs	Decrease the absorption of oral iron	Safety profiles are similar to sodium ferric gluconate	No

Storage and Administration Pearls

- Sodium ferric gluconate and iron sucrose should not be frozen.
- Iron is a leading cause of fatal poisoning in children. Store out of children's reach and in child-resistant containers.

Patient Education Pearls

- If taking rifampin, report any tingling or numbness in hands of feet.
- If taking streptomycin, maintain adequate hydration.

ANEMIA OF CHRONIC KIDNEY DISEASE AND DIALYSIS

Definitions

Anemia of kidney disease and dialysis is attributed primarily to decrease endogenous EPO production and may occur as the creatinine clearance declines below approximately 50 mL/min. Eventually, the patient may require dialysis to filtrate metabolic waste. There are several types of dialysis, including:

- Hemodialysis, which diffuses small molecular-weight solutes across a semipermeable membrane
- Peritoneal dialysis, which uses the peritoneum as a dialysis membrane
- Ultrafiltration and hemofiltration, which removes large volumes of fluid with minimal removal of metabolic wastes

Diagnosis

- Hct is usually 20–30%.
- Hemoglobin less than 11%
- MCV normal
- Peripheral smear: RBCs are normochromic
- Presence of echinocytes or acanthocytes

Signs and Symptoms

There are many symptoms of anemia of kidney disease. Different patients will experience different combinations of symptoms; and if the anemia is mild, the symptoms may not be noticeable. Some of the symptoms are: Pale skin color, fatigue, irritability, dizziness, weakness, shortness of breath, sore tongue, brittle nails, decreased appetite (especially in children), and frontal headaches.

Guidelines

National Kidney Foundation, The National Kidney Foundation Kidney Disease Outcomes Quality Initiative (NKF KDOQI™). www.kidney.org/professionals/kdoqi/guideline_anemiaHBUpdate/KDOQI_finalPDF.pdf.

Guidelines Summary

- Treatment guidelines for stress treatment are based on hemoglobin (Hb).
- Hb should be between 11–12 mg/dL.
- Hb targets are not intended to apply to the treatment of iron deficiency in patients receiving iron therapy without the use of erythropoiesis-stimulating agents (ESAs).
- ESAs are the drug of choice.
- In dialysis and nondialysis patients with CKD receiving ESA therapy, the Hb target should not be greater than 13.0 g/dL.
  - Hb should not be greater than 13.0 g/dL due to the all-cause mortality and adverse cardiovascular event in patients with CKD and Hb greater than 13.0 g/dL.

Drugs for Anemia of Chronic Renal Disease and Dialysis

Generic	Brand	Dose	Contraindications	Primary Side Effects	Key Monitoring	Pertinent Drug Interactions	Med Pearl
Mechanism of action – induces erythropoiesis by stimulating the division and differentiation of committed erythroid progenitor cells; induces the release of reticulocytes from the bone marrow into the bloodstream							
Epoetin Alfa	Procrit	IV, SQ Initial: 50–100 units/kg 3x wk	• Hb >12 g/dL • Hb increase >1 g/dL per 2-wk time period	• Hypertension • Hypotension • Peripheral edema	• Hb 1–2x wk until maintenance dose established and after dosage changes • Iron stores • Blood pressure	None	Indicated for IDA, sickle-cell disease, autoimmune hemolytic anemia, bleeding, CRF
Darbepoetin alfa	Aranesp	IV, SQ Initial: 0.45 mcg/kg 1x wkly	• Uncontrolled hypertension	• Dizziness • Diarrhea • Infection			Only indicated for patients with chronic renal failure and nonmyeloid malignancies whose anemia is a result of chemotherapy

Storage and Administration Pearls

- Refrigerate vial between 36–46°F.
- Do not freeze or shake.
- Multidose vials, with preservative, are stable for 1 week at room temperature.

Patient Education Pearls

- These medications can be administered only by infusion or injection.
- Frequent blood tests will be needed to determine appropriate dosages.
- Avoid alcohol and do not make significant changes in dietary iron without consulting prescriber.
- Check blood pressure frequently.

PERNICIOUS ANEMIA

Definitions

Pernicious anemia is a type of megaloblastic anemia. Pernicious anemia is a decrease in red blood cells that occurs when the body cannot properly absorb vitamin B12 (cyanocobalamin) from the gastrointestinal tract. Vitamin B12 is necessary for the formation of red blood cells. Megaloblastic anemia is a blood disorder characterized by red blood cells that are larger than normal due to deficiency in folate or cyanocobalamin.

Diagnosis

- Detecting antibodies to intrinsic factor is specific for the diagnosis of pernicious anemia.
- A Schilling test is used to detect antibodies to intrinsic factor.
- Serum vitamin B12 should be measured.
- Serum methylmalonic acid and homocysteine are elevated in pernicious anemia.
- Homocysteine is elevated only in folic acid deficiency.

Signs and Symptoms

- Symptoms similar to iron-deficiency anemia
- May find glossitis, jaundice, and splenomegaly
- Ataxia, paresthesias, confusion, and dementia
- Folate acid deficiency: does not result in neurologic disease

Treatment Summary

- No major guidelines have been recently published on the treatment of pernicious anemia.
- Treatment is directed toward replacing the deficient factor.
- Blood transfusions are rarely required.
- Pernicious anemia is treated with vitamin B12.
- With therapy the reticulocytosis should begin within 1 week, followed by a rising Hb over 6–8 weeks.
- Coexisting iron deficiency is present in one-third of patients and is a common cause of incomplete response to therapy.

Drugs for Pernicious Anemia

Mechanism of action – partial alpha-4B2 nicotinic receptor agonist; prevents nicotine stimulation of mesolimbic dopamine system

Generic	Brand	Dose	Contra-indications	Primary Side Effects	Key Monitoring	Pertinent Drug Interactions	Med Pearl	Top 200
Cyanocobalamin (B12)	Nascobal	• Intranasal: 500 mcg in one nostril wkly • Initial: IM 30 mcg/day for 5–10 days • Maintenance: 100–200 mcg/month	Hypersensitivity to cobalt	• Anxiety • Itching • Diarrhea	• Vitamin B12 • Hematocrit • Reticulocyte count • Folate • Iron	• May decrease the effect of chloramphenicol • Long-term treatment with metformin may decrease the absorption of vitamin B12	• Oral neomycin or aminosalicylic acid may significantly reduce B12 absorption • Hydroxycobalamin is a longer-acting form of vitamin B12	Yes
Folic acid (folate)	Apo-Folic	• Oral, IM, IV, SQ: 0.4 mg/day • Prevention of neural tube: 0.4 mg/day	Hypersensitivity to folic acid	• Allergic reaction • Bronchospasm • Flushing • Malaise • Pruritus • Rash	• Hematocrit • Reticulocyte count • Folate • Iron	Folic acid administration may decrease serum levels of phenytoin	• Phenytoin and other anticonvulsant may inhibit folic acid absorption • Products containing more than 0.8 mg of folic acid are Rx only	Yes

Storage and Administration Pearls

- Cyanocobalamin Injection is clear pink-to-red solution, stable at room temperature.
- Cyanocobalamin must be protected from light.
- Intranasal spray must be stored in the refrigerator and not frozen.

Patient Education Pearls

- Pernicious anemia may require treatment for life.
- Report rashes on extremities or acute persistent diarrhea.

LEARNING POINTS

- Coexisting iron deficiency is present in many forms of anemia and should always be assessed.
- When treating with ESA, Hb should not be greater than 13.0 g/dL due to the all-cause mortality and adverse cardiovascular event in patients with CKD and Hb greater than 13.0 g/dL.
- Iron absorption is enhanced through simultaneous intake of ascorbic acid (i.e., vitamin C).
- Laxatives, stool softeners, and adequate intake of liquids should be regularly recommended to patients taking iron therapy, to alleviate the medication's constipating effects.
- Long-term metformin therapy can decrease the absorption of vitamin B12.

PRACTICE QUESTIONS

1. Which of the following drugs need to be protected from light?

      I. Lasix
     II. Epoetin-alfa
    III. Enalaprilat

  (A) I only
  (B) III only
  (C) I and II only
  (D) II and III only
  (E) I, II, and III

2. Which of the following is NOT a characteristic of pernicious anemia?

  (A) Weakness
  (B) Forgetfulness
  (C) Pica
  (D) Tendency to fall easily
  (E) Treatment includes B12 replacement

3. Which of the following is NOT a treatment for anemia of chronic renal failure?

  (A) Darbepoetin-alfa
  (B) Ferrous sulfate
  (C) Cyanocobalamin
  (D) Erythropoietin
  (E) All of the above

ANSWERS

1. **A**

Lasix (furosemide) is the only drug on this list that needs to be protected from light. Epoetin-alfa (II) should not be frozen or shaken. Enalaprilat (III) is the only IV ACE inhibitor; however, it does not require an amber bag to protect it from light.

2. **C**

Pica, or the craving to eat nonfood substances such as ice or dirt, is characteristic of iron-deficiency anemia but not pernicious anemia. Weakness, forgetfulness, and the tendency to fall easily are all commonly seen symptoms associated with pernicious, or B12 deficiency, anemia. And because pernicious anemia is caused by a decrease in vitamin B12, a common treatment is B12 replacement (E).

3. **C**

Cyanocobalamin is the correct choice. Cyanocobalamin, or B12, is a treatment option in pernicious anemia. In anemia of chronic renal failure, the kidneys are not able to adequately produce red blood cells, so treatment options include drugs that stimulate red blood-cell production. Darbepoetin-alfa (A) and erythropoietin (D) are drugs that stimulate red blood cell production. In addition to the need for red blood cells, these patients also require iron supplementation during erythropoietin therapy, hence the need for ferrous sulfate (B).

Dermatological Disorders

13

This chapter covers the following disease states:

- **Acne**
- **Psoriasis**

 Suggested Study Time: **30 minutes**

ACNE

Definitions

Acne vulgaris is an inflammatory skin disorder that results in comedones, papules, pustules, nodules, or cysts on the face, back or chest. The disorder occurs most commonly in teenagers at or near puberty but can occur at any age.

Diagnosis

Although no strict diagnostic criteria exist, the presence of five or more lesions (of any type) is generally considered sufficient for diagnosis.

Signs and Symptoms

Acne vulgaris lesions appear most commonly on the face but also on the back and chest. The severity of acne vulgaris varies and is based on the types of lesions present. Type I acne is the mildest form and is associated with a mostly noninflammatory presentation of open and closed comedones. Type II acne is a more moderate form with multiple papules present. Type III acne is associated with a more severe form of acne consisting of an inflammatory condition with multiple pustules. Type IV is the most severe form, consisting of inflammatory nodules and cysts that lead to scarring.

Guidelines

Guidelines of care for acne vulgaris management. *J Am Acad Dermatol*, no. 56 (4) (April 2007): 651–63.

www.guideline.gov/summary/summary.aspx?doc_id=10797&nbr=005625&string= acne+AND+vulgaris.

Guideline Summary

- Topical benzoyl peroxide is the first-line therapy recommendation for most mild to moderate forms of acne vulgaris (type I).

- Topical antibiotics and topical retinoids are considered first-line for moderate acne vulgaris (type II) and second-line for mild-moderate (type I).

- Moderate-severe, inflammatory acne (type III) should be treated with topical therapy (benzoyl peroxide, retinoids, or antibiotics) plus oral antibiotics.

- Severe, inflammatory acne (type IV) can be treated with the combination of oral antibiotics and topical therapy but often requires the use of oral isotretinoin therapy.

- Oral isotretinoin is an effective therapy option for the treatment of severe, inflammatory acne, or more moderate forms that have been refractory to other treatment options.

- All females of child-bearing age that have been prescribed isotretinoin must agree to use two forms of contraception during isotretinoin use. Because of the known teratogenic risk associated with isotretinoin therapy, all patients, pharmacies, physicians, and wholesalers must register with the iPLEDGE program. This is an FDA program designed to monitor and decrease the risk of fetal exposure to isotretinoin.

Drugs for Acne

Generic	Brand	Dose & Max	Contraindications	Primary Side Effects	Key Monitoring Parameters	Pertinent Drug Interactions	Med Pearls	Top 200
Topical								
Nonprescription								
Benzoyl peroxide	Many	2.5–10% cream, lotion, gel, wash	Hypersensitivity	Excessive drying, photo-sensitivity, peeling, erythema	Presence of adverse effects, efficacy	Retinoids: combination causes significant irritation	OTC	No
Sulfur	SAStid	3–8% soap				Other topical agents: additive drying	OTC	No
Salicylic acid	Many	0.5–2% wash					OTC	No
Antimicrobials								
Clindamycin	Cleocin T	1% gel, lotion apply BID	Hypersensitivity, ulcerative colitis	Burning, itching, dryness, irritation	Presence of adverse effects, efficacy	Neuromuscular blocking agents		No
Erythromycin	Theramycin Z, Benzamycin, Emgel	2% gel, liquid, ointment, pledgets	Hypersensitivity			None		No
Retinoids								
Tretinoin	Retin-A Renova Avita	0.015–0.1% gel, cream, lotion	Hypersensitivity	Photosensitivity, burning, dryness, erythema, irritation	Presence of adverse effects	Other topical drying agents – additive drying; Other photosensitizing medications	Apply after freshly washed face is completely dry	Yes
Adapalene	Differin	0.1% gel						Yes
Tazarotene	Tazorac	0.05–0.1% gel						No
Alitretinoin	Panretin	0.1% gel						No
Other								
Azelaic acid	Azelex, Finevin	• 15% cream, 20% gel • Apply BID	Hyper-sensitivity	Burning, stinging, tingling, pruritus, photosensitivity	Presence of adverse effects	None		No

Drugs for Acne *(cont'd)*

Generic	Brand	Dose & Max	Contraindications	Primary Side Effects	Key Monitoring Parameters	Pertinent Drug Interactions	Med Pearls	Top 200
Oral								
Antimicrobials								
Tetracycline	• Achromycin • Sumycin	250–3,000 mg daily (divided BID–QID)	Hypersensitivity	Rash, photo-sensitivity, GI upset	Presence of adverse effects	Antacids, PCN, oral contraceptives, anticoagulants	Take 2 hrs before or after meals, avoid calcium containing foods (dairy)	No
Doxycycline	Vibramycin	50–200 mg daily (divided BID)						No
Minocycline	Minocin	50–200 mg daily (divided BID)				As above, and isotretinoin		No
Erythromycin	• E.E.S. • Erythrocin	250–3,000 mg daily (divided BID)	Hypersensitivity; use of terfenadine, astemizole, cisapride	GI upset, diarrhea, nausea, vomiting, abdominal pain	Presence of adverse effects	Terfenadine, astemizole, cisapride: combination of these agents with erythromycin increases the risk of fatal arrhythmia; anticoagulants, lovastatin, digoxin	Significant drug interactions and GI side effects limit use	No
Isotretinoin								
Isotretinoin	Accutane	0.5–2 mg/kg/day (divided BID)	Pregnancy, hypersensitivity	Cheilitis, dry mouth, dry skin, pruritus, erythema, GI upset, headaches, hyperlipidemia, depression (rare)	Periodic lipid panel, presence of adverse effects	Isotretinoin increases concentrations of corticosteroids, phenytoin; and has additive toxicity with vitamin A	• Females must agree to at least two forms of contraception during therapy • Must register in iPLEDGE program	No

Storage and Administration Pearls

- Apply topical acne products only after washing the face and then waiting for the skin to dry completely (approximately 30 minutes).
- Protect tetracycline from light. Tetracycline, doxycycline, and minocycline should be taken 2 hours before or after a meal, and interact with calcium-containing products such as dairy items.

Patient Education Pearls

- Topical agents and antimicrobials increase risk of excessive burning from the sun. Apply sunscreen prior to sun exposure.

PSORIASIS

Definitions

Psoriasis is a chronic inflammatory skin disease associated with silvery scalelike lesions. There are two primary types of psoriasis identified: Type I is diagnosed early in life in patients with a family history, while type II develops later in life and generally has no family history present.

Diagnosis

Diagnosis is based on thorough history and physical and depends primarily on the observation of lesions.

Signs and Symptoms

Sharp, demarcated, erythematous papules and plaques covered with silvery scales is a sign. Affected areas may include the scalp, trunk, back, arms, legs, palms, soles, face, and/or genitalia. Psoriatic arthritis refers to secondary joint inflammation that occurs in patients with psoriasis. The most commonly affected joints are the elbows, wrists, ankles, and knees.

Guidelines

No widely accepted clinical practice guidelines exist for the management of psoriasis. The following represents a summary of available treatment recommendations compiled from multiple primary and tertiary sources.

Summary of Treatment Recommendations

- The goal of therapy is complete resolution of lesions.
- There is significant interpatient variability in response to the available medications. Options for initial treatment include topical agents such as emollients and keratolytics (salicylic acid or sulfur), coal tar, anthralin, calcipotriene, or retinoids.
- Systemic treatment is considered as initial therapy in very severe cases or as second-line therapy in patients that do not respond to topical options. Systemic options include antimetabolite therapy (methotrexate, cyclosporine, tacrolimus), oral corticosteroids, psoralens, immunosuppressants, or retinoids.

Drugs for Psoriasis

Generic	Brand	Dose & Max	Contraindications	Primary Side Effects	Key Monitoring Parameters	Pertinent Drug Interactions	Med Pearls	Top 200
Coal Tar								
Coal tar	• Medotar • Fototar	1–25% ointment, cream, lotion apply 1–4x daily	Hypersensitivity	Photosensitivity	Presence of adverse effects	Other photosensitizing agents	OTC	No
Retinoids								
Tretinoin	• Retin-A • Renova • Avita	0.015–0.1% gel, cream, lotion	See details above					
Adapalene	Differin	0.1% gel						
Tazarotene	Tazorac	0.05–0.1% gel						
Alitretinoin	Panretin	0.1% gel						
Anthralin								
Dithranol	• Anthralin • Psoriatec	0.5–1% cream, apply 1x daily	Hypersensitivity, inflamed eruptions	Discoloration of skin, hair, fabrics, irritation	Presence of adverse effects	Topical steroids	Staining of fabric can be permanent	No
Calcipotriene								
Calcipotriene	Dovonex	0.005% cream, ointment, solution; apply 1–2x daily	Hypersensitivity, hypercalcemia	Burning, itching, skin irritation, drying	Presence of adverse effects	Other topical agents: additive drying		No

Drugs for Psoriasis *(cont'd)*

Generic	Brand	Dose & Max	Contraindications	Primary Side Effects	Key Monitoring Parameters	Pertinent Drug Interactions	Med Pearls	Top 200
Systemic								
Antimetabolites								
Methotrexate (MTX)	None	7.5 mg PO 1x wkly	Hypersensitivity, alcoholic liver disease, pre-existing blood dyscrasias	Leukopenia, nausea, fatigue, chills, fever, hepatotoxicity, photosensitivity	Periodic CBC, liver enzymes	NSAIDs, salicylates, probenecid, phenytoin, sulfonamides increase MTX levels	Necessary to use contraception in female patients (Pregnancy category X)	Yes
Immunosuppressants								
Alefacept	Amevive	15 mg IM wkly	CD4 count <250 cells/mcL, HIV	Lymphopenia, headache, chills, dizziness, myalgias	Periodic WBC count, CD4 count prior to first dose and wkly during 12 wks of therapy	Other immuno-suppressants; live or attenuated vaccines	Alefacept pregnancy registry program for female patients who become pregnant	No
Etanercept	Enbrel	50 mg SQ 2x wkly	Hypersensitivity	Injection site reactions, infections, headache, rash, nausea, neutropenia	Periodic WBC	Risk of blood dyscrasias and infection when combined with anakinra or other immuno-suppressants	Available in prefilled syringes; pregnancy registry for pregnant females on medication	No
Efalizumab	Raptiva	0.7–1 mg/kg SQ wkly	Hypersensitivity	Headache, chills, fever, increased risk of infection, myalgia, thrombocytopenia	Presence of side effects; signs and symptoms of infection, periodic platelet counts	Other immuno-suppressants; live or live attenuated vaccines	Efalizumab pregnancy registry for females who become pregnant	No
Retinoids								
Acitretin	Soriatane	25–50 mg PO daily	Hypersensitivity, impaired hepatic or renal function, use with MTX	Dry skin, alopecia, rash, chelitis, peeling, pruritus	Presence of adverse effects	• Methotrexate: increased risk of hepatitis • Tetracyclines: increased intra-cranial pressure	Law requires medication guide to be given to the patient each time acitretin is dispensed; pregnancy category X	No

Storage and Administration Pearls

- Store out of reach of children.

- Avoid application of topical agents near the eyes.

- Alefacept should be stored in a refrigerator between 2–8°C (36–46°F), protected from light, and retained in drug/diluent pack until time of use.

- Efalizumab (lyophilized powder) must be refrigerated at 2–8°C (36–46°F). Protect the vial from exposure to light. Store in original carton until time of use.

- Etanercept solution must be refrigerated at 2–8°C (36–46°F) and should not be frozen.

Patient Education Pearls

- Wash hands thoroughly after application of topical agents.

- Keep topical agents away from eyes.

LEARNING POINTS

- First-line therapy for mild to moderate acne vulgaris is topical benzoyl peroxide.

- Topical retinoids should not be combined with other topical acne agents due to risk of excessive drying and photosensitivity.

- Oral isotretinoin is reserved for refractory or severe cases of acne vulgaris. Patients, pharmacists, and physicians must register with the FDA iPLEDGE program to use this medication.

- Oral isotretinoin is associated with significant teratogenicity. Females on isotretinoin therapy must agree to use two forms of contraception during the course of therapy.

- Significant interpatient variability exists in the response to psoriasis treatments. Initial therapy generally consists of topic agents such as keratolytics, coal tar, or anthralin.

- Antimetabolite and immunosuppressant therapy carries significantly greater adverse effect risk and therefore should be reserved for severe or refractory cases.

PRACTICE QUESTIONS

1. Which of the following is appropriate initial treatment for type III acne?

    (A) Topical antibiotics and topical retinoids
    (B) Topical antibiotics + oral antibiotics
    (C) Topical benzoyl peroxide
    (D) Oral antibiotics
    (E) Isotretinoins

2. Which of the following psoriasis medications is NOT Pregnancy category X?

        I. Dovonex
        II. Methotrexate
        III. Soriatane

    (A) I only
    (B) III only
    (C) I and II only
    (D) II and III only
    (E) I, II, III

ANSWERS

1. **B**

First-line therapy for type III acne is topical therapy (benzoyl peroxide, retinoids, or antibiotics) plus oral antibiotics. First-line therapy for type I acne is topical benzoyl peroxide (C). First-line therapy for type II acne is topical antibiotics and topical retinoids (A). Oral antibiotics are not used alone (D) without topical agents. Isotretinoins (E) are usually reserved for type IV or other types that are refractory to other treatment options.

2. **A**

Methotrexate (II) is Pregnancy category X and requires the use of contraception when used by females of child-bearing age. This rules out choices (C), (D), and (E). Soriatane (III) is a retinoid that is also Pregnancy category X and requires a medication guide dispensed with each medication, thus eliminating choice (B). Dovonex (I) is calcipotriene and is one of the first-line therapy options for psoriasis. It is not Pregnancy category X (it is pregnancy category C). Therefore, (A) is the answer.

Antidotes

14

The following chapter addresses drugs that are used as antagonist drugs to do one of the following:

- **Reverse the effect of one drug**
- **Prevent toxicity**
- **Treat toxicity**

 Suggested Study Time: **15 minutes**

ANTIDOTES

Definitions

The drugs included in this chapter act in a variety of ways to counter the toxic effects of exogenous and endogenous substances in the body. Therefore, they are used in the management of poisoning and overdosage. Many antidotes are used to protect against the toxicity of drugs such as antineoplastics, and in the management of metabolic disorders such as Wilson's disease, where toxic substances accumulate.

Accidental and deliberate drug overdosage is a common problem seen by ambulance staff and emergency workers. The majority of these episodes of poisoning are dealt with along similar lines with general supportive care, but some require more specific action.

Some antagonists, such as the opioid antagonist naloxone, compete with the poison for receptor sites. Other antagonists, such as atropine, block substances that mediate the effects of the toxin. This may reduce absorption of the toxin from the gastrointestinal tract, inactivate or reduce the activity of the toxin, or increase the toxin's elimination via drugs that affect the metabolism of the toxin.

Some antidotes, such as fomepizole in methyl alcohol poisoning, act by reducing the rate of metabolism to a toxic metabolite. Others, such as methionine and glutathione, promote the formation of inactive metabolites. Acetylcysteine also acts by bypassing the effect of the toxin. On the NAPLEX, antidotes questions can be an easy way to earn points if you learn the correct antidote for the toxicity.

ACUTE POISONING

In the management of suspected acute poisoning, it is often impossible to determine with any certainty the identity of the poison or the size of the dose received. As a result, a common procedure needs to be in place:

- First, call the poison control center: (800) 222–1222.
- Next, take a history of the event and drug, or substance, involved.
    - What mode of poisoning has occurred (i.e., ingestion or inhalation)?
    - When did it happen?
    - Has any treatment occurred yet (i.e., induced vomiting)?

Few poisons have specific antidotes or methods of elimination, and the mainstay of treatment for patients with suspected acute poisoning is therefore supportive and symptomatic therapy; in many cases, nothing further is required. Clinicians should assess the ABCDs: airway, breathing, circulation, dextrose, decontamination. Symptoms of acute poisoning are frequently nonspecific, particularly in the early stages. Maintenance of the airway and ventilation is the most important initial measure; other treatment—for example, for cardiovascular or neurological symptoms—may be added as appropriate.

Some centers also recommend the routine administration of dextrose to all unconscious patients since hypoglycemia may be a cause of unconsciousness, although blood glucose measurements should be obtained first where facilities are immediately available.

Specific antidotes are available for a number of poisons and are the primary treatment where there is a severe poisoning with a known toxin. These antidotes may be life-saving in such cases but their use is not without hazard, and in many situations they are not necessary. These agents are discussed in greater detail in the chart below.

Measures to reduce or prevent the absorption of the poison are widely advocated. For inhalational poisoning, the victim is removed from the source of poisoning. Some toxins, particularly pesticides, may be absorbed through the skin, and clothing should be removed and the skin thoroughly washed to avoid continued absorption. Caustic substances are removed from the skin or eyes with copious irrigation. However, for orally ingested poisons the best method of gastrointestinal decontamination remains controversial; this is addressed in the following sections.

GENERAL ANTIDOTES

Activated Charcoal

Activated charcoal absorbs a wide range of toxins and is often given to reduce absorption within the gastrointestinal tract. A single dose is generally effective, particularly if it is given within 1 hour of ingestion. Delayed use, however, may be beneficial for modified-release preparations or for drugs that slow gastrointestinal transit time, such as those with antimuscarinic properties. Charcoal is generally well tolerated, although vomiting is common, and there is a risk of aspiration if the airway is not adequately protected. Repeated doses may be useful in eliminating some substances even after systemic absorption has occurred.

Active removal of poisons from the stomach by induction of emesis or gastric lavage has been widely used, but there is little evidence to support its role. Emesis should not be induced if the poison is corrosive or petroleum-based, or if the poison is removable by treatment with activated charcoal.

Ipecac

When used appropriately, ipecac is a safe emetic. However, its efficacy in preventing deaths has never been proven, and the routine use of ipecac at home has been questioned.

A recent survey found that increased home use of ipecac was not associated with referral to an emergency department. Additionally, there was no difference in adverse outcome rate between the poison centers that more commonly recommended ipecac compared with those centers that did not. The authors concluded that although their data cannot exclude a benefit of ipecac in a very limited set of poisonings, any benefit remains to be proven.

There are a number of drawbacks to using ipecac. Adverse effects include lethargy, diarrhea, and persistent vomiting. Persistent vomiting can be especially troublesome because it may reduce the efficacy of other orally administered treatments for poisoning, such as activated charcoal, N-acetylcysteine, or agents used for whole-bowel irrigation. Second, ipecac is sometimes given, either without medical advice or based on inappropriate medical advice, when it is not needed (i.e., in the case of ingestion of a nontoxic agent) or when it is contraindicated. Examples of contraindications to ipecac include the following:

- Lack of a gag reflex
- Lethargy
- Seizures
- Following the ingestion of caustic agents, corrosive agents, ammonia, or bleach
- Chronic misuse: May lead to cardiomyopathy

Gastric lavage may occasionally be indicated for ingestion of noncaustic poisons that are not absorbed by activated charcoal, but only if less than 1 hour has elapsed since ingestion. Gastric lavage should not be attempted if the airway is not adequately protected.

Whole-bowel irrigation using a nonabsorbable osmotic agent such as a macrogol has also been used, particularly for substances that pass beyond the stomach before being absorbed (such as iron preparations or enteric-coated or modified-release formulations), but its role is not established.

Antidotes

Toxic Agent	Generic	Brand	Dose	Contra-indications	Primary Side Effects	Key Monitoring	Med Pearl	Top 200
Mechanism of action – pure opioid antagonist that competes and displaces narcotics at opioid receptor sites								
Opioids	Naloxone	Narcan	IV, IM, SQ 0.4 mg q 2–3 min as needed. Repeat dose q 20–60 min	Hypersensitivity	• Tachycardia • Ventricular arrhythmia • Anxiety • Diaphoresis	• Respiratory rate • Heart rate • Blood pressure	Adverse affects can occur secondarily to reversal (withdrawal)	No
Mechanism of action – acts as a competitive antagonist at opioid receptor sites								
Opioids	Nalmefene	Revex	IV, 0.25 mcg/kg followed by 0.25 mcg/kg at 2–5 minute intervals	Hypersensitivity	• Nausea • Tachycardia • Vomiting • Agitation	• Respiratory rate • Sedation • Blood pressure	6-Methylene analog of naltrexone	No
Mechanism of action – acts as a competitive antagonist at opioid receptor sites								
Opioids	Naltrexone	Trexan	• Alcohol dependence • Opioid antidote	• Acute opioid withdrawal • Failure to pass Narcan challenge • Positive urine drug screen	• Syncope • Headache • Arthralgia • Diarrhea	• Narcotic withdrawal • LFT	• Do not give until patient is opioid-free for 7–10 days • Alcohol and opioid dependence • Highest affinity for mu receptors	No
Mechanism of action – competitively inhibits the activity at the benzodiazepine recognition site on the GABA/benzo complex								

Benzodiazepines	Flumazenil	Romazicon	IV, 0.2 mg over 15 sec; repeat until conscious	Patients showing signs of serious cyclic antidepressant overdosage	• Palpitations
					• Hot flashes
					• Tremor
					• Abnormal vision
						Benzo reversal may result in seizures in some patients	• If patient has not responded 5 min after receiving a cumulative dose of 5 mg, the sedation is likely not due to benzodiazepines
							• Reversal affects of nonbenzodiazepines
							  - Zaleplon (Sonata)
							  - Zolpidem (Ambien)
								No

Antidotes *(cont'd)*

Toxic Agent	Generic	Brand	Dose	Contra-indications	Primary Side Effects	Key Monitoring	Med Pearl	Top 200
Mechanism of action – competitively inhibits alcohol dehydrogenase, an enzyme that catalyzes the metabolism of ethanol, methanol, and ethylene glycol								
• Ethanol • Methanol • Ethylene glycol	Fomepizole	Antizol	IV: loading dose 15 mg/kg, followed by 10 mg/kg q 12 hrs x 4 doses	Hypersensitivity	• Headache • Nausea • Metallic taste	• Fomepizole plasma levels should be monitored • Urinary ethylene glycol or methanol levels • Renal function		No
Mechanism of action – inhibits destruction of acetylcholine by acetylcholinesterase which prolongs effects of acetylcholine (anticholinergic drug overdose)								
Anticholinergic drugs	Physostigmine	Eserine	IV, IM, SQ: 0.5–2 mg to start; repeat q 2 min until response	• GI or GU obstruction • Asthma, gangrene, severe cardiovascular disease	• Palpitation • Bradycardia • Restlessness • Seizure	• Heart rate • Respiratory rate		No
Mechanism of action – antigen-binding fragments (Fab) are specific for the treatment of digitalis intoxication								
Digoxin	Digoxin Immune Fab	Digibind	40 mg will bind to 0.5 mcg/mL of digoxin or digitoxin	Sheep products	• Exacerbation of heart failure • Rapid ventricular response	Serum potassium levels	Digoxin levels will greatly increase with digoxin Fab use and are not an accurate determination of body stores	No
Mechanism of action – supplies a free thiol group which binds to and inactivates acrolein, the urotoxic metabolite of ifosfamide and cyclophosphamide								
• Isophosphamide • Cyclophosphamide	Mesna	Mesnex	IV, 60–80% of ifosfamide dose given TID to QID	Thiol compounds	• Bad taste • Vomiting secondary to bad taste • Platelet-count decrease	Urinalysis	Orphan drug: used for the prevention of hemorrhagic cystitis induced by ifosfamide	No

Antidotes *(cont'd)*

Toxic Agent	Generic	Brand	Dose	Contra-indications	Primary Side Effects	Key Monitoring	Med Pearl	Top 200
Mechanism of action – cardioprotective by converting intracellularly to a ring-opened chelating agent that interferes with iron-mediated oxygen free radical generation								
Doxorubicin	Dexrazoxane	Zinecard	IV, 10:1 ratio of dexrazoxane: doxorubicin	Hypersensitivity	Most adverse affects thought to be attributed to chemotherapy	• Adds to myelosuppressive effects • LFTs		No
Mechanism of action – free thiol metabolite is available to bind to and detoxify reactive metabolites of cisplatin								
Cisplatin	Amifostine	Ethyol	IV	Hypersensitivity to amifostine or aminothiol	• Hypotension • Nausea/vomiting	• Blood pressure should be monitored every 5 min during the infusion • Serum calcium levels	Antiemetic medication is recommend prior to and in conjunction with amifostine	No
Mechanism of action – combines with strongly acidic heparin to form a stable complex (salt) neutralizing the anticoagulant activity of both drugs								
Heparin	Protamine	Protamine	Protamine dosage is determined by the dosages of heparin; 1 mg; 90 USP units heparin. Max: 50 mg	Hypersensitivity	• Hypotension • Flushing • Dyspnea	• aPTT • Blood pressure		No
Mechanism of action – promote liver synthesis of clotting factors (II, VII, IX, X) which counteracts the mechanism of warfarin								
Warfarin	Vitamin K (phytonadione)	Mephyton	• Depends on INR and bleeding risk factors; i.e., >9 INR: no significant bleeding: hold warfarin, give vitamin K 5–10 mg, expect INR to be reduced within 24–48 hrs • Hypersensitivity		• Cyanosis • Dizziness	• PT • INR	IM route should be avoided due to hematoma formation	No

Antidotes *(cont'd)*

Toxic Agent	Generic	Brand	Dose	Contra-indications	Primary Side Effects	Key Monitoring	Med Pearl	Top 200
Mechanism of action – reduced form of folic acid: supplies the necessary cofactor blocked by methotrexate								
Methotrexate	Leucovorin	Leucovorin	2–15 mg/day for 3 days or until blood counts are normal	• Pernicious anemia • B12-deficient megaloblastic anemias	• Rash • Anaphylactoid reactions	Plasma methotrexate concentration	• Continue leucovorin until plasma methotrexate level <0.05 mmol/L • Decreased efficacy of cotrimoxazole against *Pneumocystis carinii* pneumonitis	No
Mechanism of action – absorbs toxic substances or irritants, thus inhibiting GI absorption								
Activated Charcoal	Activated Charcoal	Actidose	25–100 g/dose	• Non-intact GI tract • GI perforation	• Hypernatremia • Hypokalemia	• Constipation • Diarrhea	• Sorbitol accelerates bowel evacuation	
Mechanism of action – bind toxic agents in the biliary: forms a nonabsorbable complex with bile acids in the intestine; inhibits enterohepatic reuptake								
Leflunomide	Cholestyramine Resin	• Questran • Questran Light	4 g–24 g/day Administered up to 6x day	• Complete biliary obstruction • Bowel obstruction	• Constipation • Nausea • Stomach pain • Gallstones • Bloating	Serum levels of poison	• Arava (leflunomide) 8 g cholestyramine TID for 1 to 3 days; plasma level should reach <0.02 mg/L	No
Mechanism of action – exact mechanism of acetaminophen toxicity is unknown								
Acetaminophen	Acetylcysteine	• Acetadote • Mucomyst	140 mg/kg followed by 17 doses of 70 mg/kg q 4 hrs	Hypersensitivity	• Drowsiness • Chills • Fever	• AST, ALT • Bilirubin • PT • Serum creatinine	• Therapy should continue until acetaminophen levels are undetectable and there is no evidence of hepatotoxicity • Activated charcoal • 5–10 g:g acetaminophen	No

Storage and Administration Pearls

- Protamine: Refrigerate stable for 2 weeks at room temperature.
- Fomepizole: If solution becomes solid in the vial, warm carefully by running warm water over the vial.
- Naltrexone: Should be stored in the refrigerator. May be kept at room temperature for <7 days prior to use.
- Digoxin immune Fab: Should be refrigerated.
- Activated charcoal: Absorbs gas from air; store in closed container.

Patient Education Pearls

- Patient should stay calm and call the poison control center.
- If patient currently has ipecac in his home, it's better to dispose of it, according to the research.
- Most drugs don't have antidotes, so it's important to take medication as prescribed.

LEARNING POINTS

- It is important to memorize the phone number for the poison control center. The number should also be pasted on every telephone in your pharmacy.
- Storing ipecac in the home in case of acute poisoning is no longer recommended because of limited data suggesting any benefit. It is better to call the poison control center or 911 for advice.
- Few poisons have specific antidotes or methods of elimination; therefore, the mainstay of treatment for patients with suspected acute poisoning is supportive and symptomatic therapy.
- Flumazenil is the antidote for benzodiazepines and is commonly used in the hospital setting.
- Do not confuse Fomepizole and flumazenil. At first glance they may seem similar, but they have completely different uses.
- Protamine is the antidote for heparin, and vitamin K is the antidote for warfarin. Protamine and vitamin K are not interchangeable and have different mechanisms of actions. These two antidotes are used for both inpatient and outpatient treatment.

PRACTICE QUESTIONS

1. Which drug is used to decrease toxicities associated with cisplatin?

   (A) Amifostine
   (B) Physostigmine
   (C) Nalmefene
   (D) Fomepizole
   (E) Leucovorin

2. How many doses of activated charcoal are typically effective?

   (A) 1
   (B) 2
   (C) 3
   (D) 4
   (E) 5

ANSWERS

1. **A**

Amifostine is used to prevent cisplatin toxicities associated with renal toxicity. Physostigmine (B) is used primarily to reverse toxic CNS effects caused by anticholinergic drugs. Nalmefene (C) is used as a partial reversal of opioid drug effects. Fomepizole (D) is used for methanol and ethylene glycol poisoning, and leucovorin (E) is used as an antidote for folic acid antagonist.

2. **A**

Activated charcoal typically requires only a single dose to be effective, particularly if it is given within 1 hour of toxin ingestion.

Gynecologic, Obstetric, and Urologic Disorders

15

This chapter covers the following topics:

- **Contraception**
- **Hormone replacement therapy**
- **Erectile dysfunction**
- **Urinary incontinence**

 Suggested Study Time: **45 minutes**

CONTRACEPTION

Definition

Contraception refers to the prevention of pregnancy and is accomplished pharmacologically through two general mechanisms: (*1*) inhibition of contact between sperm and egg, and (*2*) prevention of implantation of the fertilized egg in the endometrium. Available products most commonly contain estrogen, progestin, or both. The estrogen component suppresses follicle-stimulating hormone (FSH) and prevents the development of a viable follicle. The progestin component contributes to the production of thick cervical mucus and the involution of the endometrium, and blocks ovulation.

Therapy Selection

Available prescription therapies

- Combination estrogen and progestin
  - Monophasic
  - Multiphasic
- Progestin only

- Implantable
- Emergency contraception
  - Start within 72 hours of unprotected intercourse
  - Approved OTC if patient is >18 years of age
  - Plan B
    - » 2 tablets 0.75 mg levonorgestrel (taken q12h x 2 doses)
  - Preven
    - » 0.25 mg levonorgestrel, 0.05 mg ethinyl estradiol (taken q12h x 2 doses)

Advantages and Disadvantages

Table 1.

Product type	Advantages	Disadvantages
Combination products	Long history of superior efficacy; multiple formulations allow opportunity to try multiple-dose combination of estrogen/progestin components in different dosage forms (transdermal patch, oral, multiphasic, continuous); decreased length of menses; decreased incidence of cramping; decreased risk of ectopic pregnancy	Drug interactions present; need for backup contraception with missed pills
Progestin only	Can be used in safely patients that are breastfeeding, are >35 years of age, and/or have systemic lupus erythematosus or intolerable estrogen-related side effects	Slightly less effective; requires even stricter compliance than combinations; higher incidence of breakthrough bleeding; need for backup contraception with missed pills
Implantable	Longer-term efficacy	Not readily reversible; requires insertion at medical office

Adverse Effects Associated with Hormonal Imbalance

Table 2.

Estrogen Excess	Estrogen Deficiency	Progestin Excess	Progestin Deficiency
• Breast tenderness • Cyclic weight gain • Edema • Bloating • Hypertension • Melasma • Migraine • Nausea	• Vasomotor symptoms (hot flushes) • Spotting • Breakthrough bleeding • Libido • Dyspareunia	• Libido • Depression • Fatigue • Weight gain • Acne • Hypomenorrhea • Vaginal candidiasis	• Heavy menstruation • Weight loss • Delayed menses • Spotting • Breakthrough bleeding

Pharmacologic Contraceptives

Hormonal Contraceptives

Oral contraceptives

Monophasic/High-dose estrogen

Generic	Brand	Dose & Max	Contra-indications	Primary Side Effects	Key Monitoring Parameters	Pertinent Drug Interactions	Med Pearls	Top 200
• Ethinyl estradiol/ norgestrel	• Ovral • Ogestrel	50 mcg E. estradiol/ 0.5 mg norgestrel	• Pregnancy • Breast cancer • History of deep vein thrombosis or pulmonary embolism • Lactation (<6 wks postpartum) • Smoker >35 years of age	• Breast tenderness • Increased breast size • Nausea • Edema • Bloating • Cyclic weight gain • Headaches during active pills • Thrombophlebitis (rare) *Estrogen-excess side effects most common*	• Presence of adverse effects • Pregnancy	• Effect of oral contraceptive pill (OCP): • Antibiotics (ampicillin, sulfonamides, tetracycline) • Anticonvulsants (phenytoin, topiramate, barbiturates) • Protease inhibitors • Rifampin *Need backup method of contraception during use and for at least 1 wk after; for chronic therapy with above medications use another form of contraception*	Take 1 tablet daily at the same time of day for 21 days, followed by 7 days of inactive placebo pills	No
• Ethinyl estradiol/ Ethynodiol diacetate	• Demulen 1/50 • Zovia 1/50	50 mcg E. estradiol/1 mg E. diacetate						No
• Ethinyl estradiol/ norethindrone	Ovcon 50	50 mcg E. estradiol/1 mg norethindrone						No
• Mestranol/ norethindrone	• Ortho-Novum 1/50 • Necon 1/50 • Norinyl 1/50	50 mcg Mestranol/ 1 mg norethindrone						No

Pharmacologic Contraceptives *(cont'd)*

Generic	Brand	Dose & Max	Contra-indications	Primary Side Effects	Key Monitoring Parameters	Pertinent Drug Interactions	Med Pearls	Top 200
Monophasic/Low-dose estrogen								
Ethinyl estradiol and levonorgestrel	• Alesse • Aviane • Lessina • Levlite	20 mcg E. estradiol, 0.1 mg levonorgestrel	• Pregnancy • Breast cancer • History of deep vein thrombosis or pulmonary embolism • Lactation (<6 wks postpartum) • Smoker >35 years of age	• Nausea • Vomiting • Breakthrough bleeding • Spotting • Melasma • Headache • Weight change • Edema • Venous thromboembolism • Side effects associated with hormonal imbalance (see Table 2) • Presence of adverse effects • K with drospirenone		• Effect of OCP: • Antibiotics (ampicillin, sulfonamides, tetracycline) • Anticonvulsants (phenytoin, topiramate, barbiturates) • Protease inhibitors • Rifampin *Need backup method of contraception during use and for at least 1 wk after; for chronic therapy with above medications use another form of contraception*		No
	• Levlen • Levora • Nordette • Portia • Seasonale • Lo Ovral • Low-Ogestrel	30 mcg E. estradiol, 0.15 mg levonorgestrel					Seasonale is taken continuously for 84 days with 7 placebo pills; menses only q 3 mos	Yes
Ethinyl estradiol and drospirenone	• Yasmin • Yaz	30 mcg E. estradiol, 3 mg drospirenone					Decreased duration of menses	Yes

Pharmacologic Contraceptives *(cont'd)*

Generic	Brand	Dose & Max	Contra-indications	Primary Side Effects	Key Monitoring Parameters	Pertinent Drug Interactions	Med Pearls	Top 200
Ethinyl estradiol and norgestrel	• Apri • Deogen • Ortho-Cept	30 mcg E. estradiol, 0.3 mg norgestrel						Yes
Ethinyl estradiol and norethindrone acetate	• Loestrin 21 1/20 • Loestrin Fe 1/20 • Microgestin Fe 1/20	20 mcg E. estradiol, 1 mg n. acetate						Yes
Ethinyl estradiol and norethindrone	Ovcon 35	35 mcg E. estradiol, 0.4 mg norethindrone						No
	• Brevicon • Modicon • Neocon 0.5/35 • Nortrel 0.5/35	35 mcg E. estradiol, 0.5 mg norethindrone						Yes
	• Necon 1/35 • Norinyl 1/35 • Nortrel 1/35 • Ortho-Novum 1/35	35 mcg E. estradiol, 1 mg norethindrone						Yes
Ethinyl estradiol and desogestrel	Kariva	10–20 mcg E. estradiol, 0.15 mg desogestrel						No
	Mircette	10–20 mcg E. estradiol, 0.15 mg desogestrel						No
Ethinyl estradiol and norgestimate	• Ortho cyclen • Sprintec • MonoNessa • Previfem	35 mcg E. estradiol, 0.25 mg norgestimate						Yes

Pharmacologic Contraceptives *(cont'd)*

Generic	Brand	Dose & Max	Contra-indications	Primary Side Effects	Key Monitoring Parameters	Pertinent Drug Interactions	Med Pearls	Top 200
Biphasic								
Ethinyl estradiol and norethindrone	• Ortho-Novum 10/11 • Necon 10/11	35 mcg E. estradiol, 0.5–1 mg norethindrone	• Pregnancy • Breast cancer • History of deep vein thrombosis or pulmonary embolism • Lactation (<6 wks postpartum) • Smoker >35 years of age	• Nausea • Vomiting • Breakthrough bleeding • Spotting • Melasma • Headache • Weight change • Edema • Venous thromboembolism • Side effects associated with hormonal imbalance (see Table 2)	• Presence of adverse effects • Pregnancy	• Effect of OCP: • Antibiotics (ampicillin, sulfonamides, tetracycline) • Anticonvulsants (phenytoin, topiramate, barbiturates) • Protease inhibitors • Rifampin *Need backup method of contraception during use and for at least 1 wk after; for chronic therapy with above medications use another form of contraception*	• Created to decrease overall hormone exposure • High incidence of breakthrough bleeding	No

Pharmacologic Contraceptives *(cont'd)*

Generic	Brand	Dose & Max	Contra-indications	Primary Side Effects	Key Monitoring Parameters	Pertinent Drug Interactions	Med Pearls	Top 200
Triphasic								
Ethinyl estradiol and norethindrone	• Tri-Norinyl • Necon 7/7/7 • Ortho-Novum 7/7/7 • Estrostep 21 • Estrostep Fe	35mcg e. estradiol, 0.5–1 mg norethindrone	• Pregnancy • Breast cancer • History of deep vein thrombosis or pulmonary embolism • Lactation (<6 wks postpartum) • Smoker >35 years of age	• Nausea • Vomiting • Breakthrough bleeding • Spotting • Melasma • Headache • Weight change • Edema • Venous thrombo-embolism • Side effects associated with hormonal imbalance (see Table 2)	• Presence of adverse effects • Pregnancy	Effect of OCP: • Antibiotics (ampicillin, sulfonamides, tetracycline) • Anticonvulsants (phenytoin, topiramate, barbiturates) • Protease inhibitors • Rifampin *Need backup method of contraception during use and for at least 1 wk after. For chronic therapy with above medications use another form of contraception.*	• Many triphasics approved for treatment of acne as well • More difficult to deal with missed pills • Decreases overall hormone exposure	Yes
Ethinyl estradiol and desogestrel	Cyclessa							No
Ethinyl estradiol and norgestimate	• Trinessa • Ortho-TriCyclen • Orth-TriCyclen Lo							Yes
Ethinyl estradiol and levonorgestrel	• Enpresse • Tri-Levlen • Triphasil • Trivora							Yes
Transdermal								
Ethinyl estradiol and norelgestromin	Ortho Evra	20 mcg E. estradiol and 0.15 mg norelgestromin	• Pregnancy • Breast cancer • History of deep vein thrombosis or pulmonary embolism • Lactation (<6 wks postpartum) • Smoker >35 years of age	• Nausea • Vomiting • Breakthrough bleeding • Spotting • Melasma • Headache • Weight change • Edema • Venous thrombo-embolism • Side effects associated with hormonal imbalance (see Table 2)	• Presence of adverse effects • Pregnancy	Same as OCP	• Safe with usual activities • Do not apply lotion to site of application • Improved compliance over oral	Yes

Pharmacologic Contraceptives *(cont'd)*

Generic	Brand	Dose & Max	Contra-indications	Primary Side Effects	Key Monitoring Parameters	Pertinent Drug Interactions	Med Pearls	Top 200
Other								
Ethinyl estradiol and etonogestrel	NuvaRing	• 0.015 mg E. estradiol and 0.12 mg etonogestrel released daily • Inserted by patient intravaginally q4 wks (active for 3 wks)	Negative pregnancy test needed for initiation	Same as OCP (systemic absorption occurs)	Same as OCP (systemic absorption occurs)	Same as OCP (systemic absorption occurs)	• May be removed before intercourse • Not to be used >4 mos after dispensed	Yes
Progestin-only contraceptives								
Oral								
Norethindrone	• Ortho Micronor • Errin • Nor-QD • Nora-BE • Camila	0.35 mg daily	Negative pregnancy test prior to initiation	• Libido Depression • Fatigue • Weight gain • Acne • Hypomenorrhea	Presence of side effects	None	Can be used in breast-feeding women, those >35 who smoke, and those at risk of CHD	No
Norgestrel	Ovrette	0.075 mg daily						No
Parenteral								
Medroxy-progesterone	Depo-Provera	150 mg/mL IM q 12 wks	• Must have negative pregnancy test to start therapy or to continue therapy if >14 wks since last injection • Breast cancer • Liver disease	• Weight gain • Decreased bone mineral density • Acne • Delayed return of fertility after discontinuation	Bone mineral density	None	• Supplement calcium and vitamin D due to potential bone loss • Do not use for >2 years unless unable to use other forms of contraception • No risk of thrombo-embolism	No

Pharmacologic Contraceptives *(cont'd)*

Implantable/Intrauterine

Generic	Brand	Dose & Max	Contra-indications	Primary Side Effects	Key Monitoring Parameters	Pertinent Drug Interactions	Med Pearls	Top 200
Levonorgestrel	Norplant	• Subdermal implant in upper arm • Replace q3–5 yrs	• History or high risk of pelvic inflammatory disease (PID) or ectopic pregnancy • Breast cancer	• Spotting • Breakthrough bleeding • Amenorrhea • Mastalgia • Headache • Abdominal pain • PID	• Presence of side effects • Pregnancy	None	• Not available as new therapy, but some women may still have • Lasts 3–5 years	No
Levonorgestrel	Mirena	• 20 mcg released daily • Intrauterine	• Abnormal uterine bleeding • High risk for STDs (multiple sexual partners • Uterine or cervical cancer				Remains in place for up to 5 years	No
Progesterone	Progestasert	Intrauterine	• Acute cervicitis or vaginitis • Postpartum endometriosis				Remains in place for 1 year	No
Etonogestrel	Implanon	• 68 mg subdermal implant in upper arm • Replace q3–5 yrs	History or high risk of pelvic inflammatory disease or ectopic pregnancy	• Amenorrhea • Infrequent menses • Weight gain			Not studied in women >130% IBW	No

Non-hormonal

Generic	Brand	Dose & Max	Contra-indications	Primary Side Effects	Key Monitoring Parameters	Pertinent Drug Interactions	Med Pearls	Top 200
Copper–T380	ParaGard	Intrauterine placement for up to 10 yrs.	History or high risk of pelvic inflammatory disease or ectopic pregnancy	Heavy bleeding, cramping	None	None	Can remain in place for up to 8–10 yrs with efficacy	No

Storage and Administration Pearls

- Store at controlled room temperature 20–25°C (68–77°F) in a dry area, protected from direct light.
- After use, discard NuvaRing away from children or pets.

Patient Education Pearls

- Hormonal contraceptives do not prevent the transmission of sexually transmitted infections.
- Efficacy is high with strict adherence to therapy schedule.
- Establish a regular time to take OCP, preferably as a part of daily routine, such as brushing teeth.
- Plan a backup contraceptive method.
- Smoking with oral contraceptives poses significant risks and should be avoided.
- Contact physician immediately if any of the following occur:
  - Abdominal pain
  - Chest pain (severe), shortness of breath
  - Headache (severe), dizziness, weakness, or numbness
  - Eye problems (vision loss or blurring), speech problems
  - Severe leg pain (calf or thigh)
- Specific instructions for missed doses:

Doses Missed	Instructions for Patient
1	Take missed dose immediately and next dose at regular time
2 (during first 2 wks)	Take two doses daily for the next 2 days, then resume taking
2 (during third wk)	Sunday start: Take one dose daily until Sunday, dispose of current pack, then begin next pack without placebo pills. Backup method required for 7 days. Other: Dispose of current pack and begin new pack. Backup method required for 7 days.
3 or more	

HORMONE REPLACEMENT THERAPY

Definitions

- Menopause is the cessation of menses after the loss of ovarian follicular activity.
- Perimenopause refers to the period of time immediately prior to menopause and the 1 year following menopause onset.

Diagnosis

Diagnosis is made when amenorrhea occurs for a minimum of 12 consecutive months.

Signs and Symptoms

Symptoms are related primarily to lack of estrogen and include vaginal dryness, vaginal atrophy, hot flushes, and night sweats. Other potential symptoms include arthralgia, depression, migraine, mood swings, myalgia, and insomnia.

Guidelines

Estrogen and progestogen use in peri- and postmenopausal women: March 2007 position statement of the North American Menopause Society. *Menopause*, no. 14 (2) (January 2007): 168–82. www.guideline.gov/summary/summary.aspx?doc_id=10712&nbr=005575&string=hormone+AND+replacement.

Guideline Summary

- All women should undergo careful evaluation prior to initiation of hormone replacement therapy (HRT), including comprehensive history and physical, mammography, and, potentially, bone densitometry.
- The primary indication for HRT is vasomotor symptoms of hot flushes and night sweats.
- Local vaginal therapy is recommended when vaginal symptoms are the only complaint.
- Prevention of osteoporosis with HRT should be considered only for women with a very strong risk of osteoporosis and in whom other available therapies are not options.
- In women who are receiving HRT and who have an intact uterus, progestin is indicated as a means of reducing the risk of endometrial hyperplasia and cancer that exists with unopposed estrogen use in these patients.
- There is insufficient evidence of efficacy and evidence of safety concerns with the prolonged use of HRT. Therefore, at present, HRT is not recommended for use for any of the following indications: Cardiovascular disease, stroke prevention, hyperlipidemia, or dementia prevention.
- The Women's Health Initiative (WHI) indicated increased risks of venous thromboembolism, stroke, coronary disease, and breast cancer in women who receive HRT for an extended period of time.
- The current recommendation is to use HRT at the lowest effective dose for the shortest possible duration.

Hormone Replacement Therapy

Generic	Brand	Dose & Max mg (frequency)	Contraindications	Primary Side Effects	Key Monitoring Parameters	Med Pearls	Top 200
Oral preparations							
Estrogens							
Conjugated estrogens	Premarin	0.3–2.5 mg daily	• Abnormal bleeding • Breast cancer • History of DVT or PE • Pregnancy • Estrogen-dependent tumor • CVA or MI in past year • Thromboembolic disease	• Nausea • Fluid retention • Bloating • Headaches • Mood changes • Breast tenderness • Increased risk of VTE, stroke, MI, breast cancer	Presence of side effects (especially vaginal bleeding or symptoms of VTE, stroke, or MI)	• Most studied • No generic equivalent • Should not be abruptly discontinued; taper	Yes
Synthetic conjugated estrogen	Cenestin	0.3–1.25 mg daily				• Long half-life	No
Micronized estradiol	• Estradiol • Estrace • Gynodiol	0.5–2 mg daily				• Most potent hepatic effects • Should not be abruptly discontinued; taper	Yes
Estrone sulfate	• Estropipate • Ortho-Est • Ogen	0.625–5 mg daily					No
Esterified estrogens	• Estratab • Menest	0.3–2.5 mg daily				Should not be abruptly discontinued; taper	No
Progestins							
Medroxyprogesterone	Provera	2–10 mg daily		• Decreased libido • Cramping • Mood changes • Bloating • Nausea • Depression • Headache	Presence of adverse effects		Yes
Micronized progestin	Prometrium	100–200 mg daily				Primary use in patients with adverse effects associated with synthetic estrogens	Yes

Hormone Replacement Therapy *(cont'd)*

Generic	Brand	Dose & Max mg (frequency)	Contraindications	Primary Side Effects	Key Monitoring Parameters	Med Pearls	Top 200
Combination oral preparations							
Conjugated equine estrogens and medroxyprogesterone	Prempro	0.3–0.625 mg estrogen/1.5–2.5 mg progestin	• Abnormal bleeding • Breast cancer • History of DVT or PE • Pregnancy • Estrogen–dependent tumor • CVA or MI in past year • Thromboembolic disease	• Nausea • Fluid retention • Bloating • Headaches • Mood changes • Breast tenderness • Increased risk of VTE • Stroke • MI • Breast cancer	Presence of side effects (especially vaginal bleeding or symptoms of VTE, stroke, or MI)		Yes
Conjugated equine estrogens and medroxyprogesterone	Premphase	0.625 mg/0 mg x14 days then 0.625/5 mg x14 days					No
Estradiol and drospirenone	Angelique	1/0.5 mg					No
Ethinyl estradiol and norethindrone acetate	FemHRT	2.5–5 mcg estrogen/0.5–1.0 mg progestin					No
Estradiol and norethindrone acetate	Activella	0.5–1.0 mcg estrogen/0.1–0.5 mg progestin					No
Estradiol and norgestimate	Prefest	1 mg/0 x15 days then 1/0.09 mg x15 days					No
Transdermal and topical preparations							
17β Estradiol transdermal	• Estraderm • Vivelle • Climara • Alora • Esclim	• 25–50 mcg/ 24 hours • Applied 1–2x wk	• Abnormal bleeding • Breast cancer • History of DVT or PE • Pregnancy • Estrogen–dependent tumor • CVA or MI in past year • Thromboembolic disease	• Skin irritation • Nausea • Fluid retention • Bloating • Headaches • Mood changes • Breast tenderness • Increased risk of VTE • Stroke • MI • Breast cancer	Presence of side effects (especially vaginal bleeding or symptoms of VTE, stroke, or MI)	• Limited hepatic effects • Useful in patients with GI disturbances • Adverse effects less common in general	Yes
17β Reservoir	Estraderm	0.025–0.1 mg (2x/wk)					No
17β Gel	• Estrogel (Qday) • Elestrin (Qday) • Divigel (Qday)	0.2–1 mg daily					No
17β Topical emulsion	Estrasorb (2 pkt q day)	0.05 mg daily					No
17β Transdermal spray	Evamist (initial: 1 spray q day, may increase to 2–3 sprays/day)	0.021 mg/spray					No

Hormone Replacement Therapy *(cont'd)*

Generic	Brand	Dose & Max mg (frequency)	Contraindications	Primary Side Effects	Key Monitoring Parameters	Med Pearls	Top 200
Vaginal preparations							
Conjugated estrogen cream	Premarin	1.25 mg applied vaginally from 1–2x wkly to daily	• Abnormal bleeding • Breast cancer • History of DVT or PE • Pregnancy • Estrogen-dependent tumor • CVA or MI in past year • Thromboembolic disease	Systemic side effects possible but rare	• Presence of adverse effects • Efficacy	• Used in cases of vaginal symptoms only • Effective for stress incontinence	Yes
Estrone cream	Neo-estrone cream	1 mg/g					No
Estradiol ring	Estring	7.5 mcg/d x 90 days				Long-term use associated with endometrial hyperplasia	No
	Femring	5 mcg/d x 90 days					No
17β Cream	Estrace cream	2–4 g/d x 2–4 wk, 1 g/d x 1–3 wk				• Used in cases of vaginal symptoms only • Effective for stress incontinence	No
Estradiol tablet	Vagifem	2 x 25 mcg/wk					No

Drug Interactions

	Interacting Drug(s)	Result
Estrogen	CYP450 3A4 inducers: barbiturates, carbamazepine, rifampin, St. John's wort	↓ Effect of estrogen
	Hydantoins, thyroid hormone, anticoagulants (oral)	↓ Effect of interacting drug
	CYP450 3A4 inhibitors: azole antifungals, macrolide antibiotics, ritonavir, grapefruit juice, atorvastatin	↑ Effect of estrogen
	Corticosteroids, tricyclic antidepressants (potential increased toxicity)	↑ Effect of interacting drug
Progestin	Aminoglutethimide, rifampin	↓ Effect of progestin

Storage and Administration Pearls

- Store at controlled room temperature in a dry location.
- Dispose of patches in a safe place inaccessible to children or pets.

Patient Education Pearls

- Potential risks of HRT should be discussed thoroughly with every patient.
- Adverse effects may be decreased if a low dose is used for a short period of time.
- Contact physician promptly for any of the following: Abnormal vaginal bleeding, abdominal pain or tenderness, speech or visual disturbance, breast lumps, numbness in extremities, severe headache, vomiting, sharp pain in leg or chest, shortness of breath.

ERECTILE DYSFUNCTION

Definition

Erectile dysfunction (ED) is often referred to as impotence and is defined as the inability to achieve a penile erection suitable for sexual intercourse.

Diagnosis

Diagnostic workup of ED includes an assessment of the severity of the dysfunction, a complete history and physical, a review of medications, a physical examination, and selected laboratory tests (serum glucose, lipid profile, thyroid). Each component of the evaluation is used to rule out potential reversible causes of the ED.

Signs and Symptoms

The inability to achieve or maintain an adequate erection is the hallmark symptom; however, symptoms such as depression and anxiety are also commonly associated with ED.

Guidelines

Erectile Dysfunction Guideline Update Panel. The management of erectile dysfunction: an update. Linthicum (MD): American Urologic Association Education and Research, Inc.; 2006 May. www.guideline.gov/summary/summary.aspx?doc_id=10018&nbr=0053 32&string=erectile+AND+dysfunction.

Guidelines Summary

- Initial treatment for most patients will consist of therapy with a phosphodiesterase-5 (PDE5) inhibitor because these agents are known to be efficacious and are minimally invasive.
- PDE5 inhibitors are contraindicated in patients who are currently taking organic nitrates, due to a risk of significant, dangerous hypotension when these agents are used concomitantly.
- If a patient does not respond to therapy with a PDE5 inhibitor, alternate therapy options should be considered, including a different PDE5 inhibitor, alprostadil intra-urethral suppositories, intracavernous injection, vacuum constriction devices, and penile prostheses.

Drugs for Erectile Dysfunction

Mechanism of action – Phosphodiesterase-5 (PDE5) inhibitors: enhance the activity of nitric oxide by inhibiting an enzyme (PDE5) responsible for its degradation; enhanced nitric oxide allows relaxed smooth muscles and increased vasodilation and blood flow to the penis following stimulation

Generic	Brand	Dose & Max	Contra-indications	Primary Side Effects	Key Monitoring Parameters	Pertinent Drug Interactions	Med Pearls	Top 200
Oral								
Sildenafil	Viagra	• 25–100 mg PRN 0.5–4 hrs prior to sexual activity. • Max: 1x daily	• Use with nitrates (continuous or intermittent) • Hypersensitivity • Nitric oxide donors	• Hypotension • Headache • Flushing • Dyspepsia • Priapism (not common)	• Efficacy • Presence of adverse effects • Blood pressure	• *Nitrates:* • *Combination results in potentially fatal hypotension. Avoid concomitant use within at least 24 hours.* • Alpha-blockers: Potential significant reduction in blood pressure Combination should be avoided if possible, or lowest does of each agent used with close monitoring PDE5 inhibitors are metabolized by CYP450 3A4; therefore, inhibitors and inducers of this enzyme will affect PDE5 inhibitor levels accordingly	Erection occurs only after physical and psychological stimulation	Yes
Tadalafil	Cialis	2.5–20 mg PRN prior to sexual activity; or 2.5–5 mg PO 1x daily						Yes
Vardenafil	Levitra	2.5–20 mg PRN ~ 1 hr prior to sexual activity						Yes
Topical								
Testosterone transdermal patch	• Testoderm • Testoderm-TTS • Androderm	2.6–6 mg patch applied daily	• Hypersensitivity • Carcinoma of the breast or prostate	• Elevated liver enzymes • Hyperlipidemia • Depression • Aggression	• Periodic liver function • PSA • Lipid panels	Increases the effects of anticoagulants and cyclosporine	Only useful in ED due to hypogonadism	No
Testosterone gel	AndroGel 1%	5–10 g daily						No

Drugs for Erectile Dysfunction *(cont'd)*

Generic	Brand	Dose & Max	Contra-indications	Primary Side Effects	Key Monitoring Parameters	Pertinent Drug Interactions	Med Pearls	Top 200
Intramuscular								
Testosterone	• Depo-testosterone (cypionate) • Delatestryl (enanthate)	200–400 mg q 2–4 wks	• Hypersensitivity • Carcinoma of the breast or prostate	• Elevated liver enzymes • Hyperlipidemia • Depression • Aggression	• Periodic liver function • PSA • Lipid panels	Increases the effects of anticoagulants and cyclosporine	Only useful in ED due to hypogonadism	No
Intraurethral								
Alprostadil	Muse	125–1,000 µg pellets 5–10 min before intercourse	• Hypersensitivity • Urethral stricture • Chronic urethritis	• Urethral pain • Burning • Priapism • Hypotension	• Presence of adverse effects • Efficacy • Blood pressure periodically	None	Duration of effect is 30–60 min	No
Intracavernosal								
Alprostadil	• Caverjec • Edex	1–40 mcg 5–20 min before intercourse	• Hypersensitivity • Sickle-cell trait • Multiple myeloma • Leukemia	• Pain at injection site • Erythema • Priapism • Hypotension	• Presence of adverse effects • Efficacy • Blood pressure periodically	None	Self-injection training should be done in physician's office	No

Storage and Administration Pearls

- Sildenafil should be taken at least 30 minutes prior to sexual activity and can be taken, at earliest, 4 hours prior.
- Vardenafil should be taken approximately 1 hour prior to anticipated activity.
- Tadalafil can either be taken prior to activity or as a scheduled daily dose.
- Alprostadil intraurethral: Store unopened foil pouches in a refrigerator at 2–8°C (36–46°F). Do not expose alprostadil urethral suppository to temperatures above 30°C (86°F). Alprostadil urethral suppository may be kept at room temperature (below 30°C [86°F]) for up to 14 days prior to use.
- Alprostadil intracavernosal: Prepare the solution immediately before use. Do not administer unless solution is clear. Do not add any drugs or other solutions to this solution. Discard any unused solution remaining in the cartridge.

Patient Education Pearls

- Testoderm is applied to the scrotum, whereas Testoderm TTS is applied to the arm, back, abdomen, or thigh.
- Testosterone gel is applied to shoulders, arms, or abdomen.
- Males using testosterone products should not allow direct contact between the testosterone product and a pregnant female, as teratogenic effects are possible.

URINARY INCONTINENCE

Definitions

This is a condition associated with the involuntary loss of urine. There are multiple subtypes of urinary incontinence differentiated by etiology. The major classifications are: (1) urethral underactivity (stress incontinence), (2) bladder overactivity (urge incontinence), and (3) urethral overactivity/bladder underactivity (overflow incontinence).

Diagnosis

Diagnosis is based primarily on patient complaints and a thorough history and physical.

Signs and Symptoms

Symptoms of stress incontinence include the loss of small amounts of urine during activities such as sneezing, coughing, laughing, or running. Symptoms of urge incontinence include urinary urgency and frequency that may be associated with the loss of large or small amounts of urine. Overflow incontinence is associated with the loss of a large amount of urine which may be accompanied by symptoms of frequency, nocturia, hesitancy, or weak urinary stream.

Guidelines

Because a nationally recognized guideline for the treatment of urinary incontinence does not currently exist, the following represents general recommendations for treatment of the various subtypes based on multiple primary and tertiary resources.

Summary of Treatment Recommendations

- General
  - Nonpharmacological therapy is important as either monotherapy or an adjunct to pharmacotherapy. Options such as Kegel exercises and scheduled voiding are common.
- Stress incontinence
  - Options for treatment include topical estrogen, alpha agonists, and tricyclic antidepressants. Alpha agonists carry the risk of elevating blood pressure and heart rate, and will be used only with caution in patients with pre-existing hypertension or heart conditions.
- Urge incontinence
  - Options for the treatment of urge incontinence include anticholinergic medications and imipramine.
- Overflow incontinence
  - Treatment options are varied based upon the determined etiology. Since many cases of overflow incontinence are secondary to benign prostatic hyperplasia (BPH), the treatment of choice includes either an alpha antagonist (terazosin, prazosin, doxazosin), a selective alpha 1A antagonist (tamsulosin), or a 5α reductase inhibitor (finasteride or dutasteride).
  - Alpha antagonists are the agents of choice in most cases of BPH. The use of a selective agent is most commonly indicated in patients who experience orthostatic hypotension with the nonselective agents. 5α Reductase inhibitors are reserved for patients with significantly enlarged prostates (50–60 g).

Drugs for Urinary Incontinence

Generic	Brand	Dose & Max	Contra-indications	Primary Side Effects	Key Monitoring Parameters	Pertinent Drug Interactions	Med Pearls	Top 200
Mechanism of action – Topical vaginal estrogen preparations: used in the treatment of stress incontinence (first-line) and urge incontinence (third-line); see hormone replacement therapy drug chart above for more detailed information								
Mechanism of action – Tricyclic antidepressants: imipramine and desipramine are the most commonly used in incontinence; used primarily in urge incontinence and stress incontinence; see drug charts in psychiatric disorders chapter for detailed information								
Anticholinergic agents								
• Oxybutynin • Syrup	Ditropan	2.5–5 mg PO TID–QID	• Urinary retention • Gastric retention • Narrow-angle glaucoma	• Dry mouth • Dry eyes • Constipation • Urinary retention • Somnolence • Blurred vision • Increased intra-ocular pressure	Presence of adverse effects	Additive effects with other anticholinergic medications	Side effects less common with extended-release version and transdermal	Yes
• Extended-release	Ditropan XL	5–30 mg PO daily						
• Transdermal	Oxytrol	3.9 mg/day apply 2x/wk						
Tolterodine	Detrol	1–2 mg PO daily					Side effects less common with extended-release	Yes
Extended-release	Detrol LA	2–4 mg PO 1x/ day						
Darifenacin	Enablex	7.5–15 mg PO daily				• CYP450 3A4 inhibitors increase levels • Additive effects with other anticholinergic medications	Do not exceed 7.5 mg daily in combo with enzyme inhibitors	Yes
Solifenacin	Vesicare	5–10 mg PO daily						Yes
Alpha agonists								
Pseudoephedrine	Sudafed, many	• 30–60 mg PO q 4–6 hours PRN • Max: 240 mg/24 hrs	• MAOI therapy • Hypersensitivity • Uncontrolled HTN	• Increased blood pressure • Increased heart rate	• Blood pressure and heart rate periodically • Blood sugar if diabetic	MAO inhibitors	• Increases blood pressure and heart rate	No
Phenylephrine	Many	10–20 mg q 4 hrs PRN		• Increased blood sugar • Irritability • Insomnia			• Use with caution in HTN or pre-existing cardiac conditions	No

Drugs for Urinary Incontinence (cont'd)

Generic	Brand	Dose & Max	Contra-indications	Primary Side Effects	Key Monitoring Parameters	Pertinent Drug Interactions	Med Pearls	Top 200
Alpha antagonists								
Doxazosin	Cardura	1–8 mg PO daily (HS)	Hypersensitivity	• Hypotension • Orthostasis • Syncope • Dizziness	• Blood pressure • Presence of orthostasis • Efficacy	• Phosphodiesterase inhibitors: combination may result in dangerous hypotension • Additive BP lowering with other antihypertensives	Dosed at HS to prevent dizziness/falls during the day	Yes
Terazosin	Hytrin	1–10 mg PO daily (HS)						Yes
Prazosin	Minipress	2–10 mg daily PO (BID–TID)					Not used often due to need for multiple daily dosing	No
Selective Alpha 1A antagonists								
Tamsulosin	Flomax	0.4 mg 1x daily	Hypersensitivity	Headache, dizziness, orthostasis	• Presence of side effects • Efficacy • Periodic BP	Cimetidine increases tamsulosin levels	Expensive relative to nonselective agents	No
Alfuzosin	Uroxatral	10 mg PO daily	• Hypersensitivity • Moderate to severe hepatic disease	• Dizziness • Fatigue • Headache • Potential for hypotension (rare)	• Presence of side effects • Efficacy • Periodic blood pressure	Levels with CYP3A4 inhibitors: ketoconazole, itraconazole, and ritonavir	• Hepatically eliminated • Tablets are extended-release; do not crush or chew	No
5α Reductase Inhibitors								
Finasteride	Proscar	5 mg PO daily	• Female sex • Hypersensitivity	• Decreased libido • Erectile dysfunction • Gynecomastia	• Obtain PSA prior to therapy initiation • Agents can decrease PSA, thereby decreasing utility to detect cancer	None	• Should not be handled by pregnant women—teratogenic potential • Onset of effect can be up to 6 mos	No
Dutasteride	Avodart	0.5 mg PO daily	• Female sex • Hypersensitivity			• Metabolized by CYP450 3A4 • Unknown but suspected interactions with potent inhibitors and inducers		No

Storage and Administration Pearls

- Store all medications at room temperature and out of the reach of children.
- Alpha-blockers should be taken at bedtime to avoid side effects of syncope and orthostasis while awake.

Patient Education Pearls

- If receiving an alpha-blocker, rise slowly from seated position to avoid potential dizziness associated with the medication.
- If receiving an alpha reductase inhibitor, know that reaching full benefit of this medication may take up to 6 months. An adequate trial should be allowed.
- Anticholinergic medications may make patient drowsy and experience dry mouth, dry eyes, blurred vision, or constipation.

LEARNING POINTS

- Oral contraceptives are highly effective when taken appropriately. Pharmacists should be able to educate patients on potential adverse effects, appropriate administration, and missed-dose instructions.
- Many varieties of contraception exist. It is important to identify adverse effects related to estrogen and progestin components in order to determine the most appropriate therapy change if a patient experiences adverse effects.
- Postmenopausal hormone replacement therapy is primarily indicated in patients with vasomotor symptoms. Because of results from large clinical trials, HRT is not indicated for the prevention of heart disease, for dementia, or as first-line therapy for osteoporosis.
- Progestin therapy should be used in patients who are on HRT and have an intact uterus.
- Although multiple therapies exist for the treatment of erectile dysfunction, phosphodiesterase inhibitors are the most commonly used agents. PDE5 inhibitors have significant drug interactions with nitrates and alpha-blockers.
- There are several subtypes of urinary incontinence, and therapy should be individualized on the basis of the identified etiology. Anticholinergic agents are among the most commonly used and may result in unpleasant side effects of dry mouth, dry eyes, constipation, and somnolence.

PRACTICE QUESTIONS

1. Which of the following is most accurate regarding the coadministration of sildenafil and nitroglycerin?

   (A) There is no drug interaction between the two medications.

   (B) There is a minor drug interaction between the two medications. The patient should be counseled to monitor for signs and symptoms of the interaction.

   (C) There is a major drug interaction between these two agents, but they can be safely coadministered as long as doses are separated by at least 1 hour.

   (D) There is a major drug interaction between sildenafil and some forms of nitroglycerin. The specific formulation of nitroglycerin should be determined before the medications are taken.

   (E) There is a major, potentially life-threatening drug interaction between the two agents. Coadministration should be strictly avoided.

2. Which of the following is a progestin-only contraceptive?

   I. Ovcon-50
   II. NuvaRing
   III. Ovrette

   (A) I only
   (B) III only
   (C) I and II only
   (D) II and III only
   (E) I, II, III

3. In which of the following clinical scenarios would hormone replacement therapy be contraindicated?

   (A) Breast cancer
   (B) Obesity
   (C) Stage III CKD
   (D) Diabetes mellitus
   (E) History of hysterectomy

4. Which of the following is the correct trade name for tadalafil?

   (A) Viagra
   (B) Levitra
   (C) Cialis
   (D) Caverject
   (E) Proscar

ANSWERS

1. **E**

There is a major, life-threatening drug interaction between these two medications. When coadministered, the two agents can result in a life-threatening drop in blood pressure. All forms of nitroglycerin carry this risk, and coadministration should be avoided for *at least* 24 hours.

2. **B**

Ovrette is a progestin-only oral contraceptive. Ovcon is a high-dose estrogen combination oral contraceptive. NuvaRing is a vaginal system with both estrogen and progestin components.

3. **A**

Hormone replacement therapy is contraindicated in patients with breast cancer due to the potential to exacerbate tumor growth. Obesity, kidney disease, and diabetes are not contraindications to hormone replacement therapy. Patients with a history of hysterectomy may take unopposed estrogen but do not need progestin.

4. **C**

Cialis is the trade name for tadalafil. Viagra is the trade name for sildenafil, Levitra is the trade name for vardenafil, Caverject is the trade name for alprostadil, and Proscar is the trade name for finasteride.

Clinical Lab Tests

16

 Suggested Study Time: **20 minutes**

Clinical lab tests are very important to pharmacists in that they are commonly used to measure the safety and efficacy of medications. It is imperative that a pharmacist have a working knowledge of the most commonly used clinical lab tests in order to be able to recommend testing when necessary, and to interpret the results obtained. Education of the patient regarding clinical lab tests may also be a role of the pharmacist in some instances.

ELECTROLYTES AND MINERALS

Among the most common laboratory tests, electrolyte concentrations are used to detect and assess many medical conditions and are measured most commonly as part of a basic metabolic panel, or chem 7.

Substance	Normal Reference Range	Most Common Uses/Comments
Sodium	136–145 mEq/L	• May detect hypo- or hypernatremia • Used to monitor serum osmolality to determine total body water balance
Potassium	3.5–5.0 mEq/L	• May detect hypo- or hyperkalemia • Used primarily to monitor safety of medications and renal function
Chloride	96–106 mEq/L	• May detect hypo- or hyperchloremia • Used in evaluation of acid-based balance and to monitor for safety of medications
Magnesium	1.5–2.2 mEq/L	• May detect hypo- or hypermagnesemia
Calcium	8.5–10.8 mg/dL	• May detect hypo- or hypercalcemia • Used to monitor renal osteodystrophy
Phosphate	2.6–4.5 mg/dL	• May detect hypo- or hyperphosphatemia • Monitored along with calcium for renal osteodystrophy

RENAL

The kidneys are the body's major filter of toxins. Thus, the renal system plays a large role in the maintenance of physiological homeostasis. The kidneys also serve the role of producing and activating substances that have an impact on red–blood-cell production, blood pressure regulation, and mineral metabolism.

The following represent the most commonly used lab assays for evaluation of renal function. Urinary sodium, potassium, and chloride as well as hematologic assays and electrolytes may also be used in the assessment.

Substance	Normal Reference Range	Comments
Serum creatinine (sCr)	0.7–1.4 mg/dL	• Excretion of creatinine closely estimates the glomerular filtration rate (GFR) • Elevated serum creatinine is indicative of decreased GFR • Serum creatinine is used in the Cockroft-Gault equation to calculate CrCl • May be inaccurate in the very elderly due to decreased muscle mass
Creatinine clearance (CrCl)	90–140 mL/min	• Estimate of GFR • Can be measured over 24 hours or calculated using serum creatinine and ideal body weight
Blood urea nitrogen (BUN)	8–20 mg/dL	• Used along with other labs to monitor hydration, renal function, protein tolerance, catabolism • Most commonly used in BUN:sCr ratio to determine hydration status and renal function
BUN:sCr	1:1–20:1	• >20:1 indicates dehydration in most patients
Urine microalbumin	<30 mg:g creatinine	• Microscopic protein that escapes into the urine when significant glomerular injury is present • Most commonly used to identify nephropathy in patients with diabetes

HEPATIC

The functions of the liver are numerous and varied. Some of the primary functions include the synthesis of bilirubin, coagulation factors, and albumin; amino acid and carbohydrate metabolism; and cholesterol synthesis. Along with these activities, the liver is also the primary site of metabolism for the majority of drugs and hormones. Hepatic assays are important in assessing the overall liver function and also in monitoring the safety of many medications.

The following represent the most commonly used lab assays for the assessment of hepatic function. Viral antigens and antibodies are not reviewed in this chapter.

Substance	Normal Reference Range	Comments
Albumin	3.5–5 g/dL	• Reflects liver's synthetic ability, nutritional status, and hydration; if low, should be factored into serum drug concentrations of highly protein bound drugs such as phenytoin
Total protein	5.5–8.3 g/dL	• Represents estimated sum of albumin and globulin measurements
Prothrombin time (PT)	10–13 seconds	• Represents the time needed for a series of events in coagulation cascade to occur • Helps to determine synthetic ability of liver; if elevated, indicates potential decreased production of clotting factors
Alkaline phosphatase (ALP)	Varies with assay used	• Used to detect hepatocellular injury but is not specific, so should be combined with other tests
Aspartate aminotransferase (AST)	8–42 IU/L	• Aminotransferases are the most frequently used assays in monitoring hepatic disease and are sensitive indicators of hepatic injury • Elevations indicate injury • Used often to monitor potential hepatic damage of medications
Alanine aminotransferase (ALT)	3–30 IU/L	
Total bilirubin	0.3–1 mg/dL	• Elevations may indicate hepatocellular injury, but test is not sensitive
Ammonia	30–70 µg/dL	• Elevations indicate an inability of the liver to remove ammonia from the blood • Used to identify hepatic encephalopathy
Amylase	44–128 IU/L	• Most commonly used to diagnose acute pancreatitis
Lipase	<1.5 U/mL	• Most commonly used in the late diagnosis of acute pancreatitis (3–4 days postonset)

ENDOCRINE

Disorders of the endocrine system most commonly result from the deficiency or excess of a hormone. These hormones act as regulators within the body by stimulating or inhibiting biological responses. The most common endocrine disorder is diabetes mellitus (DM), which is discussed in detail in a previous chapter. Thyroid disorders are also common.

The assays listed below represent the most commonly used measurements to monitor diabetes and thyroid disorders, and the medications used to treat these disease states.

Substance	Normal Reference Range	Comments
Fasting plasma glucose (FPG)	70–100 mg/dL	• Most commonly used assay for diagnosis of DM; must be repeated on another day to confirm diagnosis • Patients may also self-monitor this value • Used for disease-state monitoring and adjustment of medication
2-Hour postprandial glucose	100–140 mg/dL	• May be measured as part of an oral glucose tolerance test (OGTT) or by the patient at home • Used for disease-state monitoring and adjustment of medication
A1c	4–6%	• Represents blood sugar over an approximate 90-day time frame • Most common lab test to monitor glycemic control in DM • May be inaccurate in cases of severe anemia • Not used in diagnosis of DM • Although 4–6% is normal range, <6.5–7% is the goal for a patient with DM • A1c correlation to plasma glucose: {TABLE}
Free thyroxine (T4)	0.8–1.5 ng/dL	• Measures unbound T4 and is the most accurate representation of thyroid activity
Thyroid-stimulating hormone (TSH)	0.25–6.7 µU/mL	• Low levels indicate hyperthyroid state; high levels indicate hypothyroid state • Used to monitor thyroid supplementation and need for dose adjustments

A1c correlation table (within A1c row):

A1c%	Mean Plasma Glucose (mg/dL)
6	135
7	170
8	205
9	240
10	275
11	310
12	345

CARDIOLOGY

Laboratory tests are used both to detect and to monitor cardiac disorders. Because cardiovascular disease is the leading cause of death, it is imperative that pharmacists have a working knowledge of the markers used to evaluate these conditions.

The following measurements represent the most commonly used lab assays to detect acute cardiac conditions and to monitor chronic cardiac risk.

Substance	Normal Reference Range	Comments
Total cholesterol	<200 mg/dL	• Does not require that the patient fast but is most commonly measured as part of a complete fasting lipid panel • Not as useful as LDL and HDL in determining cardiovascular risk
Low-density lipoproteins (LDL)	Patient dependent-goals <160 mg/dL	• Highly atherogenic, known as "bad" cholesterol, used as the primary marker of cardiovascular risk • Higher values correlate with higher risk • Most often calculated rather than measured: LDL = Total cholesterol − HDL − Trigs/5 • Calculation inaccurate if triglycerides >400 mg/dL
High-density lipoproteins (HDL)	>40 mg/dL	• Antiatherogenic lipoprotein known as "good" cholesterol • Higher values associated with decreased cardiovascular risk
Triglycerides (Trigs)	<150 mg/dL	• High levels associated with cardiovascular risk • Very high levels associated with increased risk of pancreatitis
Troponin I	<1.5 ng/mL	• Elevated levels used to diagnose acute myocardial infarction (MI) • Elevation seen within 3–12 hrs and remain elevated for 5–10 days (I) or 5–14 days (T)
Troponin T	<0.1 ng/mL	
Creatine kinase–MB (CK–MB)	<12 IU/L	• Used to diagnose acute MI • Specific for cardiac tissue • Rises 3–12 hrs after onset and stays elevated for 2–3 days
B-type natriuretic peptide (BNP)	<100 pg/mL	• Secreted in response to cardiac stretching • Used to monitor heart failure

HEMATOLOGY

The complete blood count (CBC) is among the most commonly ordered lab tests. The indices described below make up the CBC and are used to detect and monitor anemias and other hematologic disorders.

Indices	Normal Reference Range	Comments
Red blood cells (RBC)	Males: 4.5–5.9 x 10^{12} cells/L Females: 4.1–5.1 x 10^{12} cells/L	• May be elevated in smokers
Hemoglobin (Hgb)	Males: 14–17.5 g/dL Females: 12.6–15.3 g/dL	• Indicates oxygen-carrying capacity of blood
Hematocrit (Hct)	Males: 42–50% Females: 36–45%	• Percentage of blood made up by erythrocytes; approximately 3 times Hgb.
Mean cell volume (MCV)	80–96 fL/cell	• Hematocrit/RBC • Decreased in iron deficiency • Increased in vitamin B12 and folate deficiency
Mean cell hemoglobin concentration (MCHC)	33.4–35.5 g/dL	• Hgb/Hct • Decreased in iron deficiency
Reticulocyte count	0.5–2.5% of RBCs	• Reticulocytes are immature erythrocytes • Increased in blood loss (acute) • Decreased in iron deficiency and B12 and folate deficiency
RBC distribution width (RDW)	11.5–14.5%	• Variation in red blood cells • Increased in iron deficiency
White blood cells (WBC)	4.4–11 cells/μL	• Made up of granulocytes and lymphocytes • Elevated in infection
Platelet count	150,000–450,000/μL	• Important measure of coagulation

PRACTICE QUESTIONS

1. Which of the following lab tests is NOT used to monitor hepatic function?

    (A) Total protein
    (B) Ammonia
    (C) Prothrombin time
    (D) Alkaline phosphatase
    (E) Microalbumin

ANSWERS

1. **E**

There are many tests used for the assessment of hepatic function. Total protein (A) represents the estimated sum of albumin and globulin that are produced by the liver. Ammonia (B) is removed from the blood by the liver, and elevations indicate the liver is not able to remove it. The prothrombin time (C) helps determine the liver's ability to make clotting factors under normal circumstances (without anticoagulant therapy). Alkaline phosphatase (D) is used to detect hepatocellular injury and is often combined with AST/ALT. Microalbumin (E) is actually a test of the kidneys and is elevated when glomerular injury is present. Therefore, (E) is correct.

Over-the-Counter Medications

17

This chapter covers the following drug classes:

- **Top 10 herbals and supplement**
- **Decongestants**
- **Antihistamines and proton pump inhibitors**
- **Cough suppressants**
- **Antidiarrheals**
- **Constipation medications**
- **Athlete's foot medications**

The text also provides an overview of basic treatment for common ailments treatable by pharmacists. This chapter also makes recommendations as to when self-treatment is not appropriate.

 Suggested Study Time: **75 minutes**

TOP 10 HERBALS AND SUPPLEMENTS

Definitions

As they are being interviewed, asking patients about herbals and supplements is an important assessment measure. Data suggest that 1 in every 5 adults in the United States reports having used a natural product at least once in the previous 12 months.

The Dietary Supplement Health and Education Act of 1994 categorizes herbals, vitamins, protein bars, and shakes as dietary supplements. As a result, manufacturers are not required to demonstrate safety, purity, or efficacy of supplements. Labeling must include the FDA statement: "This product was not evaluated by FDA, not intended to diagnose, treat, cure or prevent disease products and cannot have specific claims on labels." The use of phrases such as, "helps boost, support, enhance" are acceptable, though they essentially mislead the public and generate the need for healthcare assistance. It is important that you recommend only products that have undergone a standardization assurance.

Common Usage

- Saw palmetto
  - Used in men to improve symptoms of benign prostatic hyperplasia (BPH)
  - Effects of saw palmetto are comparable to symptomatic improvements
- Glucosamine and chondroitin
  - Used widely for treating osteoarthritis and joint structure support
  - Glucosamine: A precursor molecule important for maintaining elasticity, strength, and resiliency of the cartilage in articular (movable) joints
- Fish oils or omega-3 fatty acids
  - Used primarily for hypertriglyceridemia
  - Contain eicosapentaenoic acid (EPA) and docosahexaenoic acid (DHA), and are believed to be efficient in many people
- St. John's wort
  - Used for mild to moderate depression
  - Used in Europe for centuries for mild to moderate depression and its efficacy is comparable with tricyclic antidepressants; one study suggests it is no more effective than a placebo or sertraline in moderate to severe depression; it should not be used with other SSRIs.
- CoEnzyme Q10
  - Used for cardiovascular diseases, including angina, heart failure, and hypertension, and may help with myalgias due to statin therapy
- Melatonin
  - Used for insomnia, particularly when adjusting to shift-work cycles or jet lag
  - Naturally secreted from the pineal gland and appears to be the sleep-regulating hormone of the body; adults experience about a 37% decline in daily melatonin output between 20 and 70 years of age
- Echinacea
  - Used as an immune stimulant
  - Has been studied extensively in the area of flu and cold prevention/treatment
- Black cohosh
  - Used for women's health problems, especially postmenopausal symptom relief and painful menses

- Ginger
  - Used primarily for motion sickness, dyspepsia, and nausea
  - Lacks sedative affects of other antinausea treatments
  - Has been studied in pregnant women at less than 17 weeks' gestation

Over-the-Counter Medications

Generic	Brand	Dose & Max Mg (frequency)	Contra-indications	Primary Side Effects	Key Monitoring Parameters	Pertinent Drug Interactions	Med Pearls
Mechanism of action – inhibits production of dihydrotestosterone (DHT), inhibits receptor binding, and accelerates the metabolism of DHT							
Serenoa repens	Saw palmetto	Prostrate: 160 mg BID	Pregnancy or lactation	Transient nausea, vomiting, and GI distress	Improvements in BPH symptoms	• Oral contraception • Estrogens • Finasteride and dutasteride • Warfarin	• Standardized to contain at least 80–90% fatty acid and sterol per dose • Decreases prostate size, but does not alter PSA levels
Mechanism of action – glucosamine is an amino-sugar that is naturally produced and is a key substrate in the synthesis of macromolecules for connective tissues; chondroitin absorbs water, adding to cartilage thickness, and is found in natural physiologic connective tissue; inhibits synovial enzymes that may contribute to cartilage destruction							
Glucosamine/Chondroitin	Osteo-BioFlex	• Gluc: 500 mg TID • Chon: 400 mg TID	• Gluc: allergy to shellfish • Chon: Hx of bleeding	• GI discomfort • Increased glucose • Increased bleeding time	• Arthritis pain • Glucose • Aspirin • Warfarin	Gluc: insulin and oral diabetes medications	Chon: discontinue 14 days before dental procedure
Omega-3 Fatty Acids	Fish Oils	Triglycerides 500–3,000 mg/day	• Active bleeding • Hx of anticoagulants	• GI upset • loose stools • nausea • decrease glucose • lower blood pressure	• Hypoglycemia • Blood pressure	• Warfarin • Aspirin • Antiplatelet agents	Mainly for treatment of triglycerides
Mechanism of action – increases concentrations of serotonin in the CNS and may have some MAO inhibition affects							
Hypericum perforatum	St. John's wort	300 mg TID	• Pregnancy • Severe depression • MAO-I contra-indications	Nausea and vomiting	• Depression symptoms • INR if on warfarin	• CYP450 • 3A4 inhibitor • Cyclosporine, azoles, statins • Digoxin, lithium, thyroid meds, anything that affects serotonin	• Standardized to contain 0.3–0.5% hypericin • Min of 4–6 wks of therapy is recommended before results seen
Mechanism of action – involved in ATP generation and serves as a lipid-soluble antioxidant providing protection against free-radical damage within the mitochondria							
Ubiquinone	CoEnzyme Q10	20–300 mg/day	• Concurrent use with doxorubicin	Abdominal discomfort, headache, nausea, and vomiting	Bleeding time	Warfarin	

Over-the-Counter Medications *(cont'd)*

Mechanism of action – supplements the naturally deficient concentrations of melatonin

Generic	Brand	Dose & Max Mg (frequency)	Contra-indications	Primary Side Effects	Key Monitoring Parameters	Pertinent Drug Interactions	Med Pearls

Melatonin	Melatonin	1–5 mg q HS	Caution with warfarin	Morning sedation or drowsiness	INR with warfarin use	• CYP450 1A2 inhibitor
						  • Theophylline
						  • Caffeine
						  • Clozapine 2C9
						• Warfarin
							Drugs that deplete vitamin B6 may inhibit the ability of the body to synthesize melatonin

Mechanism of action – may stimulate white blood cell function, including cell-mediated immunity

Echinacea purpurea/ angustifolia	Echinacea	50–1,000 mg TID on day 1, then 250 mg QID	• Use for more than 10 days in acute infections
			• Immunosuppressed patients
			• Pregnancy
					• Electrolytes
					• Improvements in symptoms
						• CYP450 3A4 inhibitor
						  • Cyclosporine
						  • Tacrolimus, sirolimus
						  • Methotrexate
						  • Corticosteroids
							• Standardized to contain 4% echinacosides or esters
							• Prophylaxis therapy should be 3 wks on, 1 wk off

Mechanism of action – contains phytoestrogens, which mimic estrogen

Cimicifuga racemosa	Black cohosh	20–40 mg BID	• Hx of estrogen-dependent tumors • Endometrial cancer • Pregnancy	• Nausea, vomiting • Hypotension • Headaches	• Blood pressure • Serum hormones at baseline and 6 mos	• Oral contraceptives • HRT • NSAIDs • anticoagulants	Standardized to 1 mg triterpene glycosides, calculated as 27-deoxyactein per dose

Mechanism of action – has local affects at the GI tract and in the CNS

Zingiber officinale	Ginger	250 mg TID with food	Active bleeding	Very few side effects	Increased bleeding time	• Warfarin • Aspirin	Standardized to contain 4% volatile oils or 5% total pungent compounds

DECONGESTANTS

Definitions

Vasoconstrictive agents serve multiple roles in patient care including hemorrhoids, hypotension, ocular procedures and redness, and nasal congestion. Decongestants are the mainstay of therapy for colds and play an important role with allergic rhinitis. Nasal congestion can be treated with topical or oral adrenergic-agonist decongestants. This agonist effect causes vasoconstriction, which reduces the vascular blood supply to the sinuses, relieving intranasal pressure and reducing mucosal edema and mucus production. Decongestants are indicated for temporary relief of nasal congestion and cough associated with postnasal drip. They are no longer approved for sinusitis. Most recently, the FDA does not recommend OTC medications for children under the age of 2 years and includes decongestants because of the increased risk of death.

Signs and Symptoms

- Common cold
  - Sore throat; nasal congestion; rhinorrhea; sneezing; common, low-grade fever; chills; headache; malaise; myalgia; cough
- Postnasal drip
  - Continued mucus accumulation in the back of the nose and throat leading to or giving the sensation of mucus dripping downward from the back of the nose

Guidelines

Handbook of Nonprescription Drugs: An Interactive Approach to Self-Care, 15th Edition, 2006.

Guidelines Summary

- Once the patient is excluded from the following bullet points, a pharmacist may appropriately recommend a decongestant.
  - Fever >101.5°F
  - Chest pain
  - Shortness of breath
  - Hypertension, arrhythmias, insomnia, and anxiety
  - Worsening of symptoms or development of additional symptoms during self-treatment
  - Concurrent underlying chronic cardiopulmonary disease
  - AIDS or chronic immunosuppressant therapy
  - Frail patients of advanced age
  - Children less than 2 years of age
  - Current medications such as MAOIs
- Topical decongestants should not be recommended for longer than 3-5 days due to the risk of rhinitis medicamentosa, a condition of rebound nasal congestion brought on by overuse of intranasal vasoconstrictive medications.

Decongestants

Oral Decongestants

Mechanism of action – alpha-adrenergic stimulator with weak beta-adrenergic activity

Generic	Brand	Dose & Max Mg (frequency)	Contra-indications	Primary Side Effects	Key Monitoring Parameters	Pertinent Drug Interactions	Med Pearls
Phenylephrine	• Neo-synephrine • Numerous others	• Topical: 1–2 sprays q4 hrs • Oral: 10–20 mg q4 hrs	• Hypertension • Ventricular tachycardia	• Reflex bradycardia • Restlessness • Hypertension • Tremor	• Blood pressure • Pulse • Anxiety	• MAO inhibitors • TCAs and methyldopa may enhance vasopressor effect	Avoid using with, or within 14 days of, MAO inhibitor therapy
Pseudoephedrine	• Sudafed • Numerous others	Oral: 240 mg/24 hrs	• Narrow-angle glaucoma • MAO inhibitor therapy within 14 days				

Topical Decongestants

Generic	Brand	Dose & Max Mg (frequency)	Contra-indications	Primary Side Effects	Key Monitoring Parameters	Pertinent Drug Interactions	Med Pearls
Oxymetazoline	• Afrin • Numerous others	• Intranasal: 2–3 sprays BID • Ophthalmic: 1–2 drops q6 hrs	• Hypersensitivity • Narrow-angle glaucoma	• Hypertension • Palpitation • Stinging	• Rebound congestion • Blood pressure	MAO inhibitors	Not recommended for longer than 3–5 days
Naphazoline	Naphcon	• Nasal: 1–2 drops q6 hrs • Ophthalmic: 1–2 drops q6 hrs				• MAO inhibitors • TCAs and methyldopa may enhance vasopressor effect	

ANTIHISTAMINES AND PROTON PUMP INHIBITORS

Definitions

Antihistamines can be used for multiple roles in patient care, including contact dermatitis, allergic rhinitis, common colds, insomnia, heartburn, and nausea and vomiting.

Three histamine receptors have been identified: Stimulation of histamine-1 receptors produces sneezing, pruritus, and mucus production. Histamine-2 receptors result in stomach acid production. Histamine-3 receptors are located in the brain and control the synthesis and release of histamine.

Antihistamines are classified into two categories: First-generation and second-generation. Second-generation antihistamines are nonsedating because they do not cross the blood-brain barrier.

Signs and Symptoms

- Contact dermatitis: Papules, vesicles, erythema, crusting, and oozing
- Allergic rhinitis: Nasal stuffiness, rhinorrhea usually clear, pruritus of nose, sneezing, watering eyes, nasal drainage
- Common colds: Nasal stuffiness, sneezing, scratchy throat, cough, hoarseness, headache, fever
- Insomnia: Difficulty initiating sleep at usual time and/or wakefulness during usual sleep cycle, daytime tiredness
- Heartburn: Stomach and chest pain, choking with swallowing, relief with solids or liquids

Guidelines

Handbook of Nonprescription Drugs: An Interactive Approach to Self-Care, 15th Edition, 2006.

Guidelines Summary

- Contact dermatitis
  - Identify the cause: chemical, acids, solvent, fragrances, metals, poison ivy, etc.
  - Clean the area with mild soap and water.
  - Refer patient to physician if the rash causes edema or invades the eyelids, external genitalia, anus, or massive areas of the body.
  - Treatment includes topical treatment with hydrocortisone, bicarbonate pastes, and antihistamines.

- Allergic rhinitis and common cold
  - Once the patient is excluded from the following, treatment recommendations can occur:
    - » Symptoms of otitis media or sinusitis
    - » Symptoms of lower respiratory tract infection
    - » History of nonallergic rhinitis
- Insomnia
  - Transient or short-term insomnia but no underlying problems are okay to self-treat.
  - Discuss good sleep hygiene practices—no caffeine after 5 P.M., no exercise in the evening.
  - If diphenhydramine is recommended, it should be taken at bedtime only as needed.
  - Patients who complain of continuing insomnia after 14 days of treatment should be referred to a physician.
- Heartburn
  - Patient must be assessed for the following issues prior to self-treatment:
    - » Frequent heartburn for more than 3 months
    - » Heartburn while taking H2RA or PPI or after initiating either one for 2 weeks
    - » Nocturnal heartburn
    - » Difficulty swallowing solid foods
    - » Vomiting up blood or black material; or black, tarry stools
    - » Chronic hoarseness, wheezing, coughing, choking
    - » Unexplained weight loss
    - » Pregnancy and nursing mothers
  - If the patient is a candidate, any of the following treatments are available— including antacids, which provide rapid relief versus the oral tablets, which have a slower onset of action.

Antihistamines

Generic	Brand	Dose & Max Mg (frequency)	Contra-indications	Primary Side Effects	Key Monitoring Parameters	Pertinent Drug Interactions	Med Pearls
First-Generation Histamine H1 Antagonist							
Mechanism of action – competes with histamine for H1 receptor sites on effector cells in the gastrointestinal tract, blood vessels, and respiratory tract							
Clemastine	Tavist	• 1.34 mg TID • Max: 8.04 mg/day	Narrow-angle glaucoma	• Sedation • Anticholinergic • Dry mouth • Constipation • Blurred vision • Urinary retention	Mental alertness	May increase gastric degradation of levodopa	
Chlorpheniramine	Chlor-Trimeton	• 4 mg q4–6 hrs • Max: 24 mg/day					
Brompheniramine	Dimetapp Numerous others	1–2 tabs admin BID	• Hypersensitivity • MAO-I within 14 days				
Diphenhydramine	Benadryl Sominex	• Allergic: 25–50 mg q6–8 hrs • Max: 400 mg/day • Insomnia: 50 mg HS	Acute asthma			• Acetylcholinesterase inhibitors • 2D6 substrates codeine, tramadol	
Doxylamine	Unisom	50 mg q HS	Hypersensitivity				
Second-Generation Histamine H1 Antagonist							
Mechanism of action – long-acting tricyclic antihistamine with selectivity at H1-receptor antagonistic properties; less blood–brain barrier penetration							
Loratadine	Claritin	10 mg/day	Hypersensitivity	• Some sedation • Headache • Dizziness	• Relief of symptoms • Some sedation • Anticholinergic effects	Increased toxicity with CNS depressants and anticholinergics	
Cetirizine	Zyrtec	5–10 mg/day					

Antihistamines *(cont'd)*

Histamine H2 antagonist

Mechanism of action – competitive inhibition of histamine at H2 receptors of the gastric parietal cells, resulting in reduced gastric acid secretion

Generic	Brand	Dose & Max Mg (frequency)	Contra-indications	Primary Side Effects	Key Monitoring Parameters	Pertinent Drug Interactions	Med Pearls
Cimetidine	Tagament	400 mg/day (OTC)	• Hypersensitivity	• Gynecomastia • Increased LFTs • Stevens-Johnson syndrome	• LFTs • Scr • CBC • Gastric pH • GI bleeding	• CYP450 • 2D6, 1A2, 2C19	• Shorter half-life • Renal adjustment required
Ranitidine	Zantac-OTC	Tabs: 75 mg or 150 mg BID		• Arrhythmias • Dizziness • Leukopenia • Aplastic anemia		• CYP450 • Inhibits 1A2, 2D6	Renal adjustment required
Famotidine	• Pepcid AC • Pepcid Complete	OTC: 10–20 mg BID		LFTs		May increase serum levels of -azoles	• Renal adjustment required • Pepcid Complete contains calcium carbonate, magnesium
Nizatidine	Axid AR	75 mg BID		Thrombocytopenia		• CYP450 • Inhibits 3A4	Renal adjustment required

Mechanism of action – proton pump inhibitor; suppresses gastric basal and stimulated acid secretion by inhibiting the parietal cell H+/K ATP pump

Generic	Brand	Dose & Max Mg (frequency)	Contra-indications	Primary Side Effects	Key Monitoring Parameters	Pertinent Drug Interactions	Med Pearls
Omeprazole	Prilosec OTC	20 mg/day	Hypersensitivity	Increased LFTs		• CYP450 • Inhibits: 1A2, 2C9, 2C19, 2D6, 3A4 • Induces: 1A2	Treatment up to 14 days

COUGH SUPPRESSANTS

Definitions

A cough is caused by irritants or stimuli stimulating receptors located throughout the respiratory tract. The larynx is more sensitive than the trachea and bronchi. When activated, the receptors send signals through the brain-stem reflex pathway, the voluntary cerebral cortex pathway, or both. The signals eventually end up in the "cough center" of the medulla oblongata. The overall objective is to expel the irritant or stimuli.

Diagnosis

- A cough can be classified in the following ways:
  - Acute: duration less than 3 weeks
    - » Most commonly caused by a virus
  - Subacute: duration greater than 3 to 8 weeks
    - » Caused by infection, bacterial sinusitis, asthma
  - Chronic – duration longer than 8 weeks
    - » Smoking, post nasal drip, asthma, and GERD
- Angiotensin-converting enzymes cause a dry cough in 20% or more of treated patients.
- Systemic and ophthalmic B-adrenergic blockers may cause cough in COPD patients.

Signs and Symptoms

- Productive
  - A wet or "chesty" cough, which expels secretions from the lower respiratory tract.
  - Secretions may be clear, purulent, discolored, or malodorous.
- Nonproductive
  - Serves no useful physiologic purpose.
  - Nonproductive coughs are caused by viral respiratory tract infections, atypical bacteria, GERD, cardiac disease, and some medications.

Guidelines

Handbook of Nonprescription Drugs: An Interactive Approach to Self-Care, 15th Edition, 2006.

Guidelines Summary

- The primary goal of treating a cough is to reduce the number and severity of cough episodes.
- Codeine and dextromethorphan are the drugs of choice for nonproductive cough.
- Diphenhydramine is a better choice for coughs associated with allergies but is highly sedating.
  - Consider Claritin and/or Zyrtec, as there is less sedation.
- Guaifenesin is marketed only as an expectorant and should not be used to treat effectively productive coughs.
- Patients should be excluded from self-treatment if they have any of the following:

Cough with thick yellow sputum or green phlegm	Fever >101.5°F	Unintended weight loss
Drenching nighttime sweats	Hemoptysis	History of asthma, COPD, CHF
Foreign-object aspiration	Cough greater than 7 days	Cough worsens during self-treatment

Cough Suppresants

Generic	Brand	Dose & Max Mg (frequency)	Contra-indications	Primary Side Effects	Key Monitoring Parameters	Pertinent Drug Interactions	Med Pearls
Mechanism of action – serves as antitussive agent by depressing the medullary cough center							
Dextromethorphan	• Robitussin • Delsym • Several others	• Cough: 10–20 mg q4 hrs or 30 mg q6–8 hrs • Extended-release: 60 mg BID • Max: 120 mg/day	Do not use within 2 wks of an MAO inhibitor	• Abdominal discomfort • Coma • Constipation • Dizziness • Respiratory depression		• CYP450 • Inhibits 2D6Q	• Withdrawn from OTC market for children under age 2 • Chemically related to morphine; lacks narcotic properties except in overdose
Mechanism of action – expectorant; irritates the gastric mucosa and stimulates respiratory tract secretions, thereby increasing fluid volumes and decreasing mucous viscosity							
Guaifenesin	• Mucinex • Several other combination products	• IR: 200–400 mg q4 hrs • ER: 600–1,200 mg BID • Max: 2.4 g/day	Hypersensitivity	• Dizziness • Kidney stone formation		None	More effective with water intake
Mechanism of action – causes cough suppression by direct central action in the medulla; produces CNS depression							
Codeine phosphate		• 10–20 mg q 4–6 hrs • Max: 120 mg/day	Pregnancy	• Nausea and vomiting • Constipation • Sedation	• LFTs • CNS depression	• CYP450 • 2D6 inhibitor • Alcohol	10% of a codeine dose is demethylated in the liver to form morphine

ANTIDIARRHEALS

Definitions

Diarrhea is defined as an abnormal increase in stool frequency or liquidity. Each individual has a different frequency, which is affected by many variables. The typical range of stool frequency can be three times per day to once every 2 days. More than three bowel movements per day is considered to be abnormal.

Diagnosis

- Diarrhea is defined and characterized by more than three bowel movements in 1 day.
- Diarrhea may be acute, persistent, or chronic in nature.
- Acute diarrhea is defined as an episode of less than 14 days' duration.
- Persistent diarrhea is diarrhea of 14-day to 4-week duration.
- Chronic diarrhea lasts more than 4 weeks.

Signs & Symptoms

- Abdominal pain, cramping, and frequency are signs.
- Stool is approximately 75% water and 25% solid material.
- Stool contains unabsorbed food residue and minerals, bacteria, desquamated epithelial cells.

Guidelines

Handbook of Nonprescription Drugs: An Interactive Approach to Self-Care, 15th Edition, 2006.

Guidelines Summary

- Acute diarrhea can be managed with fluids, electrolyte replacement, dietary interventions, and nonprescription drug treatment.
- Persistent and chronic diarrhea requires medical care, and patients are not candidates for self-treatment if this is present.
- Patients should be excluded from self-treatment if any of the following apply:
  - <6 months of age
  - Severe dehydration
  - >6 months of age with persistent high fevers greater than 102.2°F
  - Blood, mucus, or pus in the stool
  - Protracted vomiting, severe abdominal pain
  - Pregnancy
  - Chronic or persistent diarrhea

Antidiarrheals

Generic	Brand	Dose & Max Mg (frequency)	Contra-indications	Primary Side Effects	Key Monitoring Parameters	Pertinent Drug Interactions	Med Pearls
Mechanism of action – decreases pain through inhibition of central cyclo-oxygenase, which in turn inhibits prostaglandin synthesis							
Loperamide	Imodium	Initial: 4 mg, followed by 2 mg after each loose stool, up to 16 mg/day	• Abdominal pain without diarrhea • Children <2 yrs • Primary tx for acute dysentery, acute ulcerative colitis, and other colitis	• Constipation • Abdominal cramping • Abdominal distention	• CNS depression • Urinary retention • Paralytic ileus • Monitor for dehydration	• CYP450 • 2B6 substrate • May decrease levels of saquinavir	Toxicity can be treated with 100 g activated charcoal through nasogastric tube, and Naloxone
Mechanism of action – inhibits both antisecretory and antimicrobial and antiviral action; provides some anti-inflammatory action							
Bismuth	Kaopectate Pepto-Bismol	524 mg q 30 min to 1 hr PRN; up to 8 doses/24 hrs	• Influenza or chickenpox due to risk of Reye's syndrome • Hx of GI bleed • Pregnancy: third trimester	• Discoloration of tongue and feces (grayish) • Impaction of feces • Hearing loss, tinnitus		May decrease level and/or effects of tetracycline derivatives	
Mechanism of action – helps re-establish normal intestinal flora; suppresses the growth of potentially pathogenic microorganisms by producing lactic acid, which favors the establishment of an aciduric flora							
Lactobacillus	• Culturelle • Lactinex	• Culturelle: 1 caplet QD or BID • Lactinex: 4 tabs 3–4x daily	Hypersensitivity	Flatulence	Improvement	None	Lactinex must be stored in refrigerator

CONSTIPATION MEDICATIONS

Definitions

Chronic constipation is a symptom-based disorder, characterized by unsatisfactory defecation resulting from difficult stool passage and/or infrequent defecation. The ROME III classification defines constipation as a functional bowel disorder that presents with a persistently difficult, infrequent, or seemingly incomplete defection, and that does not meet the criteria for irritable bowel syndrome. Constipation occurs often and is considered a gastrointestinal disorder with changes in frequency, size, consistency, and ease of stool passage. Patients will describe constipation as: (*1*) Straining to have a stool; (*2*) the passage of hard, dry stool; (*3*) the passage of small stools; (*4*) feelings of incomplete bowel evacuation; and/or (*5*) bloating. It increases as the patient ages in both men and women.

Constipation is a frequent compliant during pregnancy. It can be caused by medication (e.g., anticholinergics, analgesics, benzos, sucralfate, calcium channel blockers), menopause, dehydration, psychological condition (depression), and more.

Diagnosis

- There are three clinical subgroups of constipation:
  - Normal transit constipation
    - » Most common form—59%
  - Slow transit constipation
    - » Accounts for 13%—delayed colonic transit
  - Pelvic floor dysfunction
  - Combination syndrome
- Less frequency of stooling than the "normal" 3–5 times/week
- Harder stool than "normal"
- Smaller stools than "normal"
- Colonoscopy if age >50, alarm signs, or additional symptoms present

Signs and Symptoms

- Lack of passing a bowel movement
- Very hard stools, lumpy stools
- Need for performing manual maneuvers to pass stools
- Anorexia, dull headache, low back pain, abdominal distention

Guidelines

American Gastroenterological Association Medical Position Statement: Guidelines on Constipation. *Gastroenterology*, no. 119 (2000): 1761–1778.

Guidelines Summary

- Educate patient about high fiber and increased hydration in diet.
- Lifestyle modifications:
  - Encourage patients to avoid postponing defecation.
  - Monitor bowel habits with a daily diary.
  - Encourage patients to maintain moderate exercise.
- Patients should be excluded from self-treatment if they have any of the following:
  - Marked abdominal pain or significant distention or cramping
  - Marked or unexplained flatulence
  - Fever
  - Nausea and/or vomiting
  - Paraplegia or quadriplegia
  - Daily laxative use
  - Unexplained changes in bowel habits and/or weight loss
  - Bowel symptoms that persist for 2 weeks
  - History of irritable bowel disease
- Pharmacology begins with bulk-forming agents, proceeds to osmotic laxatives.
- If these options are not helpful, stimulant laxatives should be considered.
- Enemas, suppositories, and lubricants are also available as options.

Drugs for Constipation

Generic	Brand	Dose & Max Mg (frequency)	Contraindications	Primary Side Effects	Key Monitoring Parameters	Pertinent Drug Interactions	Med Pearls	Top 200
Mechanism of action – bulk-forming by absorbing water in the intestine to form a viscous liquid that promotes peristalsis								
Psyllium	Metamucil	1 tbsp TID 2–6 caps TID 1–2 wafers TID	• Fecal impaction • GI obstruction	• Abdominal cramps • Diarrhea	• Improvement • Diarrhea	• Warfarin • Digitalis • Diuretics	• Affects absorption of other meds • Take with full glass of water	Yes
Calcium polycarbophil	FiberCon	2–4 tabs QD						
Methylcellulose	Citrucel	1–2 caps 6x/day 1 scoop TID						
Mechanism of action – osmotic agent that causes water retention in the stool								
Polyethylene glycol 3350	MiraLax	17 g in 8 oz of water QD	• GI obstruction	• Abdominal cramps • Diarrhea • Bloating	• Improvement • Diarrhea	None	Can reconstitute with 8 oz of water, juice, cola, or tea	
Mechanism of action – stimulates peristalsis by directly irritating the smooth muscle of the intestine								
Senna	Senokot	2 tabs QD to 4 tab BID	• Fecal impaction • GI obstruction	• Abdominal cramps • Diarrhea • Bloating	• Improvement • Diarrhea	None		
Bisacodyl	Dulcolax	5–15 mg QD				Milk and antacids may decrease the effect of bisacodyl		
Mechanism of action – reduces surface tension of the oil-water interface of the stool, resulting in enhanced incorporation of water and fat and allowing for stool softening								
Docusate sodium	Colace	100 mg BID	• Concomitant with mineral • Fecal impaction • GI obstruction	• Intestinal obstruction • Diarrhea • Cramping	• Improvement • Diarrhea	None	Take with full glass of water	
Docusate calcium	Surlak	240 mg QD						
Mechanism of action – promotes bowel evacuation by causing osmotic retention of fluid which distends the colon with increased peristaltic activity								
Magnesium hydroxide	Phillips Milk of Magnesia	1–2 tbsp QD or BID	Hypersensitivity	Diarrhea	• Improvement • Diarrhea		Caution with impaired renal function	
Mechanism of action – eases passage of stool by decreasing water absorption and lubricating the intestines								
Mineral oil	Fleet	1–2 tbsp at bedtime	• Colostomy • Ileostomy • Appendicitis • Ulcerative colitis	• Abdominal cramps • Diarrhea • Bloating		May impair absorption of fat-soluble vitamins (A, D, K, E)	Aspiration is possible, especially in elderly population	

ATHLETE'S FOOT MEDICATIONS

Definitions

Athlete's foot is a fungal infection called tinea pedis. The infection can range from mild itching to a severe inflammatory process characterized by fissuring, crusting, and discoloration of skin.

Diagnosis

- Typically found in the lateral toe webs
- Can then spread to the sole or instep of the foot

Signs and Symptoms

- Fissuring and scaling
- Maceration in the interdigital spaces
- Malodor
- Stinging and burning sensation

Guidelines

Handbook of Nonprescription Drugs: An Interactive Approach to Self-Care, 15th Edition, 2006.

Guidelines Summary

- Patients should be excluded from self-treatment if they have any of the following:
  - Causative factor unclear
  - Nails or scalp involved
  - Face, mucous membranes, or genitalia involved
  - Signs and symptoms of possible secondary bacterial infection
  - Excessive and continuous exudation, fever, malaise
- Apply a thin layer of medication to affected area for 2 weeks, even after the signs and symptoms disappear.

Athlete's Foot Medications

Generic	Brand	Dose & Max Mg (frequency)	Contraindications	Primary Side Effects	Key Monitoring Parameters	Pertinent Drug Interactions	Med Pearls
Mechanism of action – squalene epoxidase inhibitor resulting in deficiency of ergosterol within the fungal cell							
Butenafine	• Lotrimin Ultra • Mentax	Apply QD	Hypersensitivity	• Burning • Contact dermatitis • Erythema • Irritation • Stinging	Clinical signs of improvement	Minimal systemic absorption	• *E. floccosum* • *T. mentagrophytes* • *T. rubrum*
Terbinafine	Lamisil	Apply QD					
Mechanism of action – binds to phospholipids in the fungal cell membrane, altering cell wall permeability and resulting in loss of intracellular elements							
Clotrimazole	Lotrimin AF 1%	Cream; apply BID	Hypersensitivity	• Burning • Contact dermatitis • Erythema • Itching	Clinical signs of improvement	Minimal systemic absorption	• *E. floccosum* • *T. mentagrophytes* • *T. rubrum* • *Candida albicans*
Miconazole	Micatin	Apply BID x 4 wks					
Mechanism of action – distorts the hyphae and stunts mycelial growth in susceptible fungi							
Tolnaftate	Tinactin	Spray: BID	Hypersensitivity	• Burning • Contact dermatitis • Erythema • Itching	Clinical signs of improvement	Minimal systemic absorption	• *E. floccosum* • *T. mentagrophytes* • *T. rubrum*

LEARNING POINTS

- The Dietary Supplement Health and Education Act of 1994 categorizes herbals, vitamins, protein bars, and shakes as dietary supplements. As a result, manufacturers are not required to demonstrate safety, purity, or efficacy of supplements.

- Decongestants are the mainstay of therapy for colds and play an important role with allergic rhinitis.

- Angiotensin-converting enzymes cause a dry cough in 20% or more of treated patients.

- Having more than three bowel movements per day is considered to be abnormal.

- Constipation can be caused by medications (anticholinergics, analgesics, benzos, sucralfate, calcium channel blockers, and more), menopause, dehydration, psychologic condition, depression, and more.

- When treating athlete's foot, a 2-week treatment period is typically required.

PRACTICE QUESTIONS

1. Which of the following would NOT be the case with levothyroxine administration?

    (A) Insulin level should be increased due to hyperglycemic effect.
    (B) Ciprofloxacin causes decreased absorption.
    (C) Calcium and antacids cause decreased absorption.
    (D) Iron causes increased absorption.
    (E) Both (A) and (D) are correct.

ANSWERS

1. **D**

Iron causes a decrease, not an increase, in the absorption of levothyroxine, so (D) is correct. Levothyroxine causes a hyperglycemic effect, and insulin doses should be increased accordingly (A). Ciprofloxacin, calcium, and antacids all cause a decrease in the absorption of levothyroxine (B and C). Patients should be advised to take levothyroxine on an empty stomach, preferably before the first meal to avoid drug interactions.

Part Three

Pharmaceutical Sciences, Mathematics, and Biostatistics

Pharmaceutics

18

 Suggested Study Time: **1.5 hours**

Pharmaceutics encompasses a number of disciplines, including dosage form design, biopharmaceutics, and pharmacokinetics. This chapter focuses on dosage form design (drug dosage forms, and the physical and chemical properties that allow these products to be manufactured).

A key concept to keep in mind is that patients don't simply take drugs, they take dosage forms: The active ingredient is not the only substance involved.

PHYSICAL PHARMACY

Physical pharmacy is a branch of pharmaceutics that deals principally with the physical and chemical properties of drugs. It is a highly mathematical subject, but the Board exam is not concerned with these aspects except as they relate to chemical kinetics. As you study, focus mainly on how specific properties of drugs make particular types of formulations more or less suitable. A simple example would be antibiotic suspensions that arrive at the pharmacy in dry powder form. The reason for this is that many antibiotics are chemically unstable in liquid formulations; if the water is added only at the time of dispensing, the drug will remain effective long enough for the patient to finish the bottle. If the product were manufactured as a liquid, the drug would be degraded by the time the bottle was processed, shipped, and stored in the pharmacy prior to dispensing.

Preformulation

Preformulation is an important stage of drug development where the pharmaceutical company characterizes many of the physico-chemical properties of the drug. Preformulation allows the company to make the best decisions about how to formulate the drug into a usable dosage form.

Solubility and Lipophilicity

Drugs must be in solution before they can be absorbed by the body. Drugs must possess at least some aqueous solubility in order to be effective; poorly soluble compounds show incomplete and unpredictable absorption. However, at least some lipophilicity must also be present, as drugs must be able to pass through biological membranes in order to reach their sites of action. Salts or esters of drugs may be formed to increase or decrease the solubility, depending on the characteristics needed in a particular case. For example, the benzathine salt of penicillin G has a very low solubility, which causes the drug to dissolve slowly after injection, which prolongs the duration of action.

Dissolution rate is improved by decreasing particle size, which increases the surface area of the drug that comes into contact with the body fluids. A more in-depth treatment of factors that influence dissolution rate and absorption is contained in the biopharmaceutics chapter.

Ionization Behavior

Ionization behavior is one of the most important factors in drug development. It applies only if a drug is an electrolyte; when such a drug goes into solution, a fraction of the molecules dissociate into ions (i.e., charged compounds). The proportion of ionized to un-ionized drug is very important because the two behave very differently in the body:

- Ionized drug: More soluble, but cannot cross body membranes
- Un-ionized drug: Less soluble, but can cross body membranes

Remember: Until the drug is absorbed across the body membranes it cannot get to the site of action, but it needs to go into solution before that can happen. The equilibrium between the more soluble ionized form and the more absorbable un-ionized form of the drug is crucial.

The Henderson-Hasselbalch equation (below) can be used to calculate exact ratios of ionized to un-ionized drug, but the following table will give you a rough estimate of the ionization behavior of weak acids and bases when comparing pH of absorption site to the pKa. In most cases, you will be able to obtain a sufficiently accurate answer by using the table instead of the actual equation, saving valuable exam time.

$$pH = pKa + \log \frac{[base]}{[acid]}$$

Ionization Behavior of Weak Acids and Bases

	Acid	**Base**
pH > pKa	More ionized	More un-ionized
pH = pKa	Equal	Equal
pH < pKa	More un-ionized	More ionized
Note that for pH more than 2 units away from pKa, expect complete ionization/un-ionization.		

Salts are often preferred over the weak acid or base because they dissolve more quickly, are more stable on storage, and are easier to crystallize and handle during processing. Different salt forms may have very different properties, and pharmaceutical companies may intentionally modify drugs into more useful salts for a given purpose. Calcium salts, for example, show wide variation in absorption and possible efficacy.

A final note on acid/base determinations: It is impossible to tell if a drug is an acid or a base by looking only at the pKa. Some acids have higher pKa (phenytoin = 8.3) than do some bases (morphine = 8.0). You can tell if a drug is an acid or base, however, by what type of salt it forms. Weak acids form sodium, calcium, potassium, or other cationic salts; weak bases form hydrochloride or other anionic salts.

Stability

Physical, chemical, and microbiological stability are all very important in preformulation studies. While physical instability does not generally result in decreased drug concentration, it can lead to problems with dose uniformity and pharmaceutical elegance (for instance, the mottled appearance that can develop in tablets over time, or the formation of a nonsuspendable sediment in a liquid dosage form). Polymorphism and anhydrous-to-hydrate conversions can be considered types of physical instability and are discussed in greater detail in the following section.

Chemical instability does result in loss of drug or excipient molecules. This can lead to either undertreatment, when a patient does not receive the full dose intended, or toxicity from toxic degradation products. In some cases, chemical instability can lead to microbiological instability if a preservative degrades and can no longer protect the formulation from bacterial or fungal overgrowth. The main types of degradation that occur in drug products are:

- Hydrolysis: Occurs in presence of water; typically no change in formulation appearance
- Oxidation: Occurs in presence of atmospheric oxygen; often results in insoluble precipitates or colored compounds

- Photochemical decomposition: Occurs on exposure to light; often results in colored compounds

Temperature, humidity, and light often hasten the degradation process, and drug companies use this fact to perform accelerated stability testing and to assign product expiration dates. Finished products must retain 90% of the labeled dose during their shelf life, so studies are performed at extreme storage conditions, and mathematical equations are used to estimate the degradation rate constants at normal conditions. A good estimate, however, is that every 10°C rise in temperature doubles the rate constant.

Most drugs degrade by either zero- or first-order kinetics (see "Rate and Half-Life Equations table, below). Drugs following zero-order degradation have a constant degradation rate that is independent of the drug concentration. First-order degradation, however, is concentration-dependent—the amount of drug degrading per unit of time is not constant. Suspensions degrade by pseudo–zero order kinetics, because only the drug molecules that are actually in solution can degrade. The concentration of drug in solution is in equilibrium with that in suspension, and the concentration of drug in solution is maintained at a constant level; suspended particles go into solution to replace the degraded drug. This continues as long as some solid is still present.

Rate and Half-Life Equations

Order	Rate Equation		Half-Life Equation
Zero	$C = C_0 - k_0 t$		$t_{1/2} = 0.5 \dfrac{C_0}{k_0}$
First	$\log C = \log C_0 - \dfrac{k_0 t}{2.303}$	$C = C_0 e^{-kt}$	$t_{1/2} = \dfrac{\ln 2}{k_1} = \dfrac{0.693}{k_1}$

Solid-State Properties

Because most drugs are given as solid-dosage forms, many properties specific to the solid state are important in pharmacy.

Crystallization

Solids are present in crystalline or amorphous forms, or as a combination of the two. Crystalline forms show fixed geometric patterns, whereas the atoms in amorphous solids are randomly placed (as they would be in a liquid). The most important things to remember about crystalline versus amorphous solids for the purposes of this test are as follows:

- Crystalline solids have definite melting points, whereas amorphous solids melt over a range of temperature.

- Amorphous solids are more soluble than the corresponding crystalline forms.
- Solids tend to revert to the more stable crystalline form on storage.

Solvates are crystalline structures that contain trapped solvent; when the solvent is water, they are called hydrates. Typically, hydrates are less soluble than their anhydrous counterparts, whereas solvates are more soluble.

Polymorphism

Polymorphs are one of several crystalline structures that have the same chemical formula. The properties they exhibit can vary substantially, however, and this leads to pharmaceutical companies patenting different polymorphic forms based on variations in solubility, bioavailability, solid-state stability, or processing behavior (such as improved powder flow or tablet compaction).

Metastable polymorphs will revert to the most stable form over time; in some instances, however, the metastable form might have more favorable properties than the stable form, e.g., better solubility. In those cases, even though it is not the most stable form, it may be the best one to market, provided the stability is at least acceptable.

The classic example of excipient polymorphism is cocoa butter, which is often used in suppository and troche formulations. Four polymorphs exist; only the β form is stable. When cocoa butter is heated above 34°C, some of the β form converts to unstable polymorphs. The unstable polymorphs are liquid at room temperature. The cocoa butter is never able to remain solid outside of the refrigerator in those cases. This explains why chocolate or cocoa butter that has been overheated does not fully solidify when cooled.

Another pharmacy-related example is ritonavir (Norvir®), a protease inhibitor used to treat HIV. Initially, it was thought to exist in only one polymorphic form, with relatively poor aqueous solubility. It was marketed in a soft gelatin capsule, which contained an ethanol/water cosolvent system. After drug approval, several batches failed quality control tests. It was discovered that a second polymorphic form with even lower solubility had formed, causing the drug to precipitate out of the cosolvent system. The product had to be reformulated to include Cremophor™ (polyethoxylated castor oil) as a solubilizing agent.

Rheology

Rheology is the science of flow properties, especially important when discussing liquid and semisolid dosage forms. During manufacturing, rheology is important when mixing and packaging materials. Once the products reach the consumer, the rheology affects the removal of the product from its container, whether by pouring, extruding from a tube, or passing through a syringe needle.

Viscosity and fluidity are two common terms associated with rheology. Viscosity refers to the resistance offered when part of the liquid flows past another part; fluidity is essentially the opposite. Viscous liquids are thick and slow-moving; fluid liquids are thin and flow more readily.

Rheological behavior is divided into two main types: Newtonian flow and non-Newtonian flow. Newtonian materials do not change viscosity with changes in stirring speed; they do, however, become less viscous when heated. True solutions and pure liquid compounds such as water and oil are examples of Newtonian materials. Non-Newtonian materials do change viscosity when stirring speed changes. Three types of non-Newtonian behavior exist: Dilatant, plastic, and pseudoplastic. Dilatant materials become more viscous when stirred more rapidly, which can cause manufacturing equipment to malfunction. Plastic and pseudoplastic materials become more fluid when stirred. Plastic flow is best illustrated by a nonpharmacy example: Tomato catsup. It doesn't pour until shaken enough for contacts between adjacent particles to be broken but then acts much like a Newtonian material. Concentrated suspensions show similar behavior. Pseudoplastic flow differs in that flow can start immediately on stirring or shaking; the harder the bottle is shaken, the more fluid the material becomes. Polymer solutions often exhibit pseudoplastic flow.

Thixotropic products are a special case and are actually the ideal situation for pharmaceutical suspensions. They are viscous at rest but become fluid when shaken. Because of this, the suspension settles only slowly, but the liquid pours easily when shaken. After shaking stops, thixotropic products gradually become viscous again. Both plastic and pseudoplastic materials can show thixotropic behavior.

Testing

Numerous quality-assurance tests exist for dosage forms, though only four will be discussed here. These four are used to test tablets and sometimes capsules.

Disintegration testing is performed by placing tablets into mesh-bottomed cylinders that are immersed in a solution and agitated at a specified rate. The tablets are considered to have disintegrated when the particles are small enough to fall through the mesh screen. It is not a good measure of in vivo behavior, but is a frequently used quality-control measure for tablets.

A better measure of in vivo behavior is dissolution testing. Here, the tablets or capsules are immersed in appropriate dissolution liquids (typically, simulated gastric fluid) and samples are taken at specific time points to determine how much of the drug has gone into solution. While this test is still not a true predictor of in vivo behavior—because it does not demonstrate absorption—it is an improvement over disintegration testing, as the drug must go into solution with body fluids before being absorbed.

Friability and hardness testing evaluate the ability of tablets to withstand manufacturing, packaging, and shipping. Hardness testing measures the force required to cause a tablet to break, and friability testing measures what percentage weight of a tablet is lost after it is tumbled for a specified amount of time in a friabilator. Tablets that are too soft or fragile will suffer too much damage during manufacturing and shipping to be useful, even if they have excellent dissolution and absorption behavior.

PHARMACEUTICAL DOSAGE FORMS

What things need to be considered when a drug company designs a dosage form for a particular drug? Some of the primary considerations are:

- Nature of the illness
- Manner in which the illness is treated
- Age of the patient
- Condition of the patient
- Stability of the drug

Suppose a patient suffers from motion sickness and is getting ready to go on a cruise. Would a tablet be the best dosage form in which his antinausea medication should be formulated? Probably not, as there is a risk that he could vomit and lose the medication before it had a chance to be absorbed by the body. For this reason, scopolamine is formulated into transdermal patches for motion sickness.

Some drugs can be used to treat different conditions based on their formulation and route of administration. An example is the antifungal product terbinafine (Lamisil®). It is given as cream for surface conditions such as athlete's foot, and as tablets for more deep-seated fungal infections of the toenails and fingernails.

Age of the patient plays a large role in development of dosage forms. Young children and the elderly are much more likely than adults and teenagers are to have difficulty swallowing. Therefore, most medications for small children are marketed as easy-to-swallow dosage forms such as liquids and chewable or rapid-dissolve tablets. Other groups of patients may also lack the ability and willingness to swallow. Patients with psychiatric conditions will often refuse to swallow medication, and rapid-dissolve formulations or injections may be required to ensure that they receive treatment. Severely debilitated or comatose patients cannot swallow and may receive medicine through nasogastric tubes or by injection.

Oral Delivery: Solids

Solid dosage forms are the most commonly prescribed—over 80% of dosage forms are tablets or capsules. These products are convenient for the patient and are the preferred route for giving nonemergency medications. Some benefits of solid dosage forms are that they are already divided into accurate doses and are easy to handle. Taste is generally less of an issue than with liquid dosage forms and can be masked by coating the product, as long as the dosage is not designed to be chewed or dissolved in the mouth.

Solid products, however, are not perfect. If a very rapid response is needed, traditional tablets and capsules are not the best option because they take time to dissolve and become absorbed by the body. If formulated improperly, the absorption of the active ingredient(s) may be irregular or incomplete.

Traditional Release

The simplest type of solid dosage form is the powder. Powders taken orally have a few advantages: They are absorbed more rapidly than tablets and capsules because they do not have to undergo a disintegration step, they are easier to swallow than large tablets and capsules, and they are more chemically stable than liquids. It is easier to give large doses of drug in a powder than in a tablet. One gram of drug plus excipients is much easier to stir into water and swallow than it would be if formulated into a tablet.

On the other hand, it is very difficult to mask the taste or smell of unpleasant drugs when they are given in powder form. They are also highly inconvenient to handle and, if provided in bulk containers (such as Metamucil®), may be subject to dose inaccuracy. Therefore, potent drugs should not be given as powders. If a drug is hygroscopic, it also should not be formulated into a powder dosage form as it will pick up too much moisture from the air. Finally, contrary to expectations, powders can be more expensive to produce than other solid dosage forms; there is a fairly substantial risk of explosion when working with large quantities of powder, and special handling equipment may be necessary to offset this risk.

Granules have many of the same advantages and disadvantages as powders. The primary difference between the two substances is that granules are prepared agglomerations of smaller particles. They behave as single particles but are irregularly shaped and have a larger particle size than the associated powders. Granules therefore flow better than powders and are more easily wetted by fluids, whether in manufacturing, in administration of the drug, or in the body. A simple example of the differences in properties of granulated versus powdered solids is sugar. Granulated (common table) sugar flows much more readily and dissolves easily in coffee or other liquids. Powdered sugar tends to clump, not flow freely, and dissolve slowly.

Granules are used more as a component of tablets and capsules than they are as dosage forms in their own right. They can be made by wet or dry methods. Wet granulation involves forming a dough of powder and liquid, pressing that dough through a mesh screen to form appropriately sized particles, and drying. In dry granulation, dry powders are compacted together, without the presence of liquid, into ribbons or oversized tablets that are then ground to size.

Capsules are a much more frequently dispensed type of solid dosage form and contain drug and excipients enclosed inside a gelatin, starch, or cellulose shell. They, like tablets, have many advantages over powders and granules. Since capsules are essentially unit-of-use products, they have excellent dose accuracy and the ability to mask the taste and smell of unpleasant drugs. They are also easy to administer, as the active ingredient does not need to be measured out. It is also easy to formulate products with multiple active ingredients. One advantage that capsules have over tablets is that they can be extemporaneously prepared in the pharmacy in instances where the prescriber requests a nonstandard dose of drug.

Capsules do have some disadvantages. They are permeable to moisture and may not be a suitable dosage form for moisture-sensitive drugs. They are also not suitable for water- or alcohol-based preparations, as those bases would dissolve the capsule shell. Some liquids, however, can be dispensed in capsules. Oil or nonaqueous water-miscible liquids such as polyethylene glycol (PEG) 400 can be used to dissolve or suspend drugs and vitamins that are then placed into soft gelatin capsules. Finally, gelatin may be inappropriate for certain patient populations who wish to avoid animal (particularly pork-based) products. In those cases, vegetarian capsule shells made of starch or cellulose may be substituted. Many dietary supplements and herbal products are manufactured in such capsules for this reason.

Tablets are the most frequently prescribed dosage form and are preferred for many reasons. In addition to the advantages they share with capsules, they are easy to make in a variety of shapes and colors, aiding in product identification. They are also inexpensive and quick to produce, especially when compared to most other dosage forms.

In order to make a drug into a tablet, however, the drug needs to be compressible. In other words, when force is placed on the powders in tableting equipment, they must be able to stick together sufficiently to make a durable tablet. Not all powders possess this property. If only small amounts of noncompressible active ingredient are needed, a compressible diluent can be used. Failing that, some materials can be granulated to improve compressibility. This does not work in all cases; if the material remains noncompressible, it may be best to formulate the product as a capsule instead of a tablet.

Types of Immediate-Release Tablets

Type of Tablet	Key Features	Example
Compressed	All ingredients contained in a single layer; designed to be swallowed whole; may or may not be coated	Various
Multi-compressed	Contain separate layers of drug, for various reasons (incompatibility of drugs, immediate- plus extended-release in the same tablet, etc.)	Mucinex® (guaifenesin)
Chewable	Disintegrate rapidly when chewed; usually mannitol-based (pleasant mouth feel, sweet taste)	Children's vitamins Dilantin Infatabs® (phenytoin)
Buccal	Dissolved in cheek cavity; may be designed to erode slowly or quickly	Fentora™ (fentanyl)
Sublingual	Dissolve under the tongue; erode quickly and are absorbed rapidly	Nitroglycerin tablets
Effervescent	Contain drug that dissolves rapidly after adding to water; results in carbonated liquid that masks taste	Alka Seltzer®

Many immediate-release tablets are coated. This process can help mask unpleasant tastes and odors, as well as improve the appearance of the tablet, protect the drug from the atmosphere, and allow it to be swallowed more easily. The two types of coating used for immediate-release products are sugar and film coatings. Sugar coating produces a very attractive tablet that is typically much larger than the uncoated product, due to the several layers of sugar, color, flavor, and waterproofing shellac added. The process is very time-consuming, and batch variations are common in the coated tablets. The coatings are applied manually in coating pans, not mechanically, by highly skilled personnel. Film coatings are much thinner, and leave a coat of opaque, colored polymer on the surface of the tablet. Although they are customarily machine-applied, requiring less skill in application, many coating defects are possible:

- Picking and peeling: Film fragments flake from the tablet surface
- Orange-peel effect: Coating leaves rough surface on the tablet
- Mottling: Coating has uneven color distribution
- Bridging: Score lines or logos present on tablet are filled in by coating
- Erosion: Coating solution is in contact with tablet for too long and disfigures the core

Extended Release

Extended-release oral products maintain more constant blood levels than do immediate-release products. Because of this, patients can take the drugs less often (once or twice a day instead of up to four times), which improves adherence. Adverse effects are usually fewer and less severe, as the concentration of the drug in the blood does not vary as widely from peak and trough as much as with immediate-release products. There is a risk of dose-dumping, however, especially if the patient chews the medicine instead of swallowing it whole.

Drugs that are best suited for extended release are usually given in fairly small doses, as the practical limit for the amount of drug to be contained in an individual tablet or capsule is 500 mg. The drug should also not have either a particularly fast or slow rate of absorption: Drugs that absorb too quickly require too large a dose, and drugs that absorb slowly are inherently long-acting, and an extended-release formulation is not needed. Because of the risk of dose-dumping, the drug should have a good margin of safety and be uniformly absorbed from the GI tract. Different methods of achieving extended release are given in the table below.

Types of Extended-Release Tablets and Coatings

Type of Tablet		Key Features	Example
Enteric coat		Coating remains intact until drug reaches small intestine; can protect drug from stomach acid and enzymes, or stomach from irritating drugs	Enteric-coated aspirin
Diffusion-controlled reservoir system		Beads or pellets are coated with polymer that releases drug at varying speeds; may involve several release rates	Theo-Dur® (theophylline)
Diffusion-controlled matrix system		Drug is mixed into an inert plastic matrix; drug dissolves and leaves matrix	
	Wax	Remains intact in GI tract and is eliminated in feces; inform patient that this is normal	Desoxyn Gradumet® (methamphetamine)
	Hydrophilic	Water causes matrix to swell; drug diffuses through gel layer, and may also be released as matrix erodes	Slo-Niacin® (niacin)
Dissolution-controlled system		Rate of release affected by dissolution and tablet or bead erosion (some hydrophilic matrices fall into this category as well as diffusion-controlled)	Cardizem CD® (diltiazem)
Ion-exchange resin		pH conditions of GI tract cause drug to be released from resin	Ionamin® (phentermine resin)
Osmotically controlled system		Tablet pulls water into system, then releases drug at controlled rate by osmotic pressure; tablet shell eliminated in feces	Glucotrol XL® (glipizide)
Complex formation		Drug is combined with other agents, forming a slowly soluble chemical complex	Rynatan allergy products

Rapid Release

Rapid-release products are becoming more important, particularly in the OTC industry. Because they can be taken without water, they are convenient for the patient, and they have a rapid onset of action. Some of the products are very soft, however, and they may require expensive protective packaging.

Types of Rapid-Release Solid Dosage Forms

Type of Product	Key Features	Example
Tablets	Product can contain large doses of drug	Claritin RediTabs
Strips	Dissolves before sick children can spit it out; cannot put large doses of drug into product	Triaminic Thin Strips
Lollipops	Absorbed through buccal mucosa	Fentanyl Actiq®

Oral Delivery: Liquids

Oral liquid dosage forms have the same advantages as other oral products, with the additional advantage of being easy to swallow for small children and others who cannot easily swallow solid dosage forms. Several disadvantages exist as well. Liquids are less portable and convenient than solids. Incorrect doses are much more likely, as patients or caregivers could measure using an inappropriate measuring device (i.e., not all spoons are standard size), and product may be spilled before being consumed. Also, taste can be a large issue, as more of the drug will reach a patient's taste buds than with the same drug in a tablet or capsule.

Solvents

Water is the most common solvent for pharmaceutical products; purified water prepared by distillation, reverse osmosis, or ion-exchange treatment is acceptable for oral use. Other commonly used solvents include ethyl alcohol, glycerin, sorbitol, propylene glycol, and some edible oils. Typically, solvents other than water are included to improve solubility and, in some cases, add sweetness to the final product (glycerin, sorbitol, and propylene glycol). Only small amounts of sorbitol and glycerin should be present in a given dose of liquid, however, as they may act as osmotic laxatives in higher quantities.

Types of Liquids

Single-phase liquid dosage forms are all variants of the solution. One or more soluble substances are dissolved in one or more solvents, including water. Therefore, the drug(s) must be water-soluble and stable in aqueous solution. The presence of other excipients in varying amounts results in the following designations:

Types of Single-Phase Liquid Dosage Forms

Type of Product	Key Features	Examples
Syrups	• Contain sugar or sugar substitutes • Little or no alcohol • Thickeners improve mouth feel and physically conceal the drug from taste buds • Taste pleasant; often used with children	• Various cough/cold preparations
Elixirs	• By definition alcoholic, but some non-alcoholic commercial products are mislabeled as elixirs • Slightly sweet; artificial sweetener usually used since sucrose is not very soluble in alcohol • Less viscous than syrups	• Diphenhydramine • Phenobarbital • Digoxin
Tinctures	• 15–80% alcohol • Usually consist of drug extracted from plant material • Unpleasant taste; not commonly used today	• Laudanum (opium tincture; 1,000 mg morphine/100 mL) • Paregoric (camphorated opium tincture; 40 mg morphine/100 mL)
Spirits	• Alcoholic solutions of aromatic or volatile substances • High concentration of alcohol • Active ingredient may precipitate out when added to aqueous preparations	• Flavoring agents
Aromatic waters	• Aqueous solutions of volatile oils • Very dilute	• Flavoring and perfuming agents
Fluid extracts	• Similar to, but more potent than, tinctures • Used as drug source, not as dosage form	

Multiphase liquids are more complicated than single-phase liquids. They still possess most of the advantages and disadvantages of other liquid-dosage forms but have the additional disadvantage of being nonhomogenous. Because of this, suspensions and emulsions should always have "Shake Well" labels attached.

Suspensions are multiphase products that contain finely divided solid particles distributed through the liquid phase. They can be used on the skin, used in the ear or eye, or given by IM or SQ injection, but are most commonly given by mouth. Some advantages exist over single-phase liquids: Drugs that have an unpleasant flavor are preferred as suspensions, since the drug does not interact with the taste buds as much when it is not dissolved. Also, drugs that have poor stability in water do not degrade as readily in suspension as they do in solution.

The primary concern with making suspensions is to have a particle size that is small enough to remain suspended in the dispersion medium of choice while not being so small that the particles start to attract each other and form clumps that will not resuspend. This can be achieved by two techniques, used separately or in combination: Use of structured vehicles and controlled flocculation.

- Structured vehicles: Increase viscosity and slow the sedimentation of suspended particles. Natural and synthetic polymer solutions are often used (cellulose gels, acacia, bentonite).
- Controlled flocculation: Add materials that promote loose aggregation of suspended particles, but that keep their surfaces apart, by charge or interaction of polymer chains. Settle, but loosely, and resuspend easily.

Emulsions are dispersions that consist of nonmiscible liquids. The dispersed phase is also called the internal phase, and the dispersion medium is called the external phase. These products are very thermodynamically unstable and require an emulsifying agent to keep them combined properly. A good nonpharmacy example is mayonnaise. Lemon juice or vinegar serves as the external phase, and the lecithin from the egg yolk emulsifies the product so that the oil that is added does not separate out.

Only oil-in-water (O/W) emulsions are used for oral dosage forms, as water needs to be in the external phase to be palatable to the patient; otherwise, all the patient would taste would be the oil in the outer portion of the product. Topical products can be either O/W or W/O. When prepared in the pharmacy, emulsions are made by rapid stirring in a mortar and pestle, shaking in a bottle (though only with reasonably thin oils), or using a hand blender, or by heating the phases separately and then mixing them. Three types of emulsifiers are used, depending on the product being made:

- Surfactants: Contain hydrophilic and hydrophobic portions, which remain at the interface of the oil and water phases to stabilize the product. Often used in combination.
- Hydrophilic colloids: Water-soluble polymers that form a film around oil droplets in O/W emulsions. Tend to increase viscosity of the product.
- Finely divided solids: Form a film of particles around the droplets of the dispersed phase, but allow interaction with the dispersion medium as well.

The exact quantity of surfactant needed can be determined by the hydrophilic-lipophilic balance (HLB) system. Surfactants and the ingredients to be emulsified have been assigned experimentally determined HLB numbers, and the exact amount of emulsifier needed can be determined algebraically if a formula has not already been determined.

Topical Delivery

Topical products are used for three primary reasons: To protect injured areas of the skin from the environment, to hydrate the skin, and to apply medication to the skin for local effect. In some cases, drug may reach the blood supply and be systemically absorbed; this is not desired with topical delivery. Systemic absorption of a drug applied to the skin is known as transdermal drug delivery and is discussed later in this chapter.

Powders and liquids are used as topical delivery systems, though not as frequently as semisolid preparations. Of the types of liquids mentioned in the oral delivery section, solutions, suspensions, and emulsions may all be used topically. Two external-use–only liquid products are:

- Liniments: Alcoholic solutions used to irritate the skin and relieve more deep-seated pain or discomfort (Heet®, Absorbine Jr®), or oleaginous emulsions used as emollients or protective agents. Liniments are applied by rubbing and are not suitable for application to bruised or broken skin.

- Collodions: Contain pyroxylin in an alcohol/ether base that evaporates, leaving an occlusive film on the skin; used to hold edges of incised wounds together.

Ointment Bases

Five types of ointment bases exist:

- Hydrocarbon/oleaginous: Greasy, petroleum-based products used for emollient effect (Vaseline®, petrolatum)

- Anhydrous absorption: Greasy products that form W/O emulsions when aqueous solutions are added; can be used to incorporate solutions into an otherwise lipophilic base (hydrophilic petrolatum, anhydrous lanolin)

- W/O emulsion: Similar to anhydrous absorption bases, but already contain some water (hydrous lanolin, cold cream)

- O/W emulsion (water-removable): Creamy emulsions that are easily washed from the skin; may be diluted with water to form lotions (hydrophilic ointment, Lubriderm®)

- Water-soluble: Greaseless, water-washable bases containing no oleaginous compounds; cannot add large amounts of water or will soften too much (polyethylene glycol ointment)

Particular bases are chosen on the basis of the desired rate of drug release, stability of the drug in the base, the need for an occlusive barrier, and ability to wash the ointment easily from the skin. When preparing ointments in a pharmacy, if a levigating agent is needed, it should be compatible with the type of ointment base used. For instance, mineral oil will mix well with any ointment base containing hydrocarbons (all except water-soluble bases). Water-miscible liquids such as glycerin and PEG will be more appropriate when using bases that contain water, such as water-soluble or emulsion bases. If solutions need to be incorporated into an ointment base, acceptable options are anhydrous absorption base or either type of emulsion base.

Other topical product definitions are:

- **Creams:** Terminology often used to describe emulsion bases; soft, cosmetically acceptable topical products

- **Pastes:** Very thick semisolids containing at least 20% solids by weight
- **Gels:** Jelly-like dispersions that are water-soluble, water-washable, and greaseless

Rectal, Vaginal, and Urethral Delivery

Rectal, vaginal, and urethral dosage forms such as suppositories and enemas are less frequently prescribed than many other types of dosage form, but they do have an important place in certain types of therapy. They can be useful for local therapy in rectal or vaginal conditions, or when protecting susceptible drugs from GI tract degradation or first-pass metabolism.

Rectal conditions amenable to local therapy with suppositories, enemas, or other rectally administered dosage forms include hemorrhoids, rectal itching, ulcerative colitis, and constipation.

Rectal suppositories can also be used to administer drug for systemic absorption. Usually, this is done when the patient cannot or will not take medication by mouth. Infants, small children, and severely debilitated patients cannot easily swallow. Patients with severe nausea (as a symptom of a condition such as gastroenteritis or migraine, or as a side effect of chemotherapy or anesthesia) cannot hold down oral anti-emetics long enough for the medication to take effect; several medications (chlorpromazine, prochlorperazine, and trimethobenzamide) are given rectally to avoid this problem.

Vaginal dosing, including suppositories, creams, and other dosage forms, is usually used for local effect, either for treatment of local infections (clindamycin and -azole antifungals) or for contraception (nonoxynol-9). Hormone replacement may also be administered via vaginal cream or suppository, and will have local effects on the vaginal mucosa. Systemic absorption may be seen with higher estrogen doses.

Urethral suppositories are seldom seen. Alprostadil was approved in 1997 for use in impotence (as Muse® urethral suppository) but is not commonly used now that oral medications are available and more readily acceptable to patients.

The most common bases used in suppositories are fatty bases similar to cocoa butter that melt at body temperature, and water-soluble bases such as polyethylene glycol and glycerinated gelatin bases that dissolve slowly in body fluids. Fatty bases are more soothing but do not mix well with body fluids and have a tendency to leak from body orifices. For this reason, they are not suitable for vaginal or urethral delivery. Water-soluble bases can be irritating to the mucosa because they take up water from the area. They are frequently used for vaginal or urethral delivery, but seldom for rectal. Different bases release drugs differently based on the water/oil partition coefficient of the base and of the drug. Lipophilic drugs are released slowly from oleaginous bases but more quickly from water-soluble bases. Hydrophilic drugs, on the other hand, are released extremely quickly from fatty bases but more slowly from water-soluble bases.

Pulmonary Delivery

The lung is an increasingly popular delivery site and is no longer reserved only for pulmonary conditions. The lungs possess a large surface area for drug absorption and a good blood supply that bypasses first-pass metabolism. Even though the first inhaled insulin (Exubera®) was a market failure, it proved that large-molecule drugs could be delivered effectively via the lung for systemic use. Continued improvement in delivery devices should cause the field of pulmonary delivery to grow rapidly.

Metered-Dose Inhalers

Metered-dose inhalers (MDI) are primarily used to deliver medications for the treatment of asthma and chronic obstructive pulmonary disease (COPD): Bronchodilators, steroids, and mast cell stabilizers. While MDIs are portable and able to deliver precise quantities of potent drugs, many patients have difficulty using them properly. MDIs have undergone rapid changes in the last few years, due in part to federal legislation restricting the use of chlorofluorocarbon (CFC) propellants due to their link to ozone depletion. Beginning in 2009, medical device exemptions will no longer be allowed for these propellants, so companies have redesigned their products as either hydrofluoroalkane (HFA) propellant devices or dry-powder inhalers. Significant engineering challenges were involved in converting products to use these new delivery devices.

Dry-Powder Inhalers

Dry-powder inhalers (DPIs) avoid some of the difficulties with metered-dose inhalers: They are generally easier for patients to use correctly, since the device can be primed before use and the patient does not have to coordinate breath with device actuation. Ease of use, however, depends significantly on the particular type of device. One study indicated that 92% of patients learned to use the Diskus™ device correctly, whereas only 74% were able to learn proper use of the Turbohaler™.

The Diskus is a classic example of the discrete-dose style of DPI. Individual doses are contained in foil packets, protecting them from humidity and allowing for dose consistency if the device is dropped. Some discrete-dose devices are single-dose units, and the drug is added when the device is ready to be actuated (Rotahaler™, Aerosilizer™, Handihaler™); this is often a necessity if a drug is heat-sensitive and must be kept refrigerated until use, such as Spiriva® (tiotropium bromide). The Twisthaler™, on the other hand, is an example of a reservoir device. All of the doses are contained in a central compartment; and if the device is dropped or exposed to humidity, all doses are affected. Of currently marketed products, only the Twisthaler and Flexhaler™ are reservoir devices.

Nebulizers

Nebulizers allow the drug to be delivered directly to the lung in high concentration and without the use of propellant. They are particularly useful for uncoordinated or unabled patients, including those who are intubated. Two types exist: Jet and ultrasonic. Jet nebulizers can be used with either solutions or suspensions, and operate by the Bernoulli principle: Compressed air from the machine flows at high speed over the medicated liquid, atomizing it and carrying it to the patient. Ultrasonic nebulizers can only be used with solutions. Ultrasonic nebulizers use the vibrations of high-frequency sound waves to move liquid from the machine through the face mask. Vibrations are timed to coincide with inhalation, so less medication is lost than with the jet nebulizers.

Nasal Delivery

Nasal delivery shares many of the advantages of pulmonary delivery: Drugs that are inactivated by the GI tract or that undergo first-pass metabolism are protected, and large-molecule drugs can be absorbed across the nasal mucosa. The nose has a dense vasculature, which aids in absorption. Viscosity enhancers and mucoadhesives are often included in the formulations to increase residence time, as nasal drainage can be a problem. In addition to the many drugs available via nasal delivery (e.g., oxytocin, desmopressin, calcitonin, and butorphanol tartrate), the route shows promise for vaccine delivery, with FluMist™ being the first approved example.

The most commonly used nasal products are saline solutions for dry nasal mucosa, nasal decongestants, and intranasal steroids. Nasal decongestants are adrenergic agents that constrict the nasal vasculature, shrinking the nasal mucosa and to making breathing easier. Overuse can lead to a phenomenon called rhinitis medicamentosa (rebound congestion), so patients should be cautioned to use the products only as directed and for no longer than 3 to 5 days. Intranasal steroids are commonly prescribed for allergic rhinitis; they may be administered in pump spray containers or as metered-dose aerosols.

Parenteral Delivery

Injectable products have many advantages over other dosage forms but also have more potential complications. No drug is lost to first-pass metabolism or acid- or enzyme-mediated degradation in the GI tract, which makes injection a particularly useful route for protein drug delivery. The rate of delivery can be accurately controlled; and drug, nutrients, and fluids can be given when other routes cannot be used. However, injectable drugs must be prepared and administered by highly trained personnel and cannot be retrieved once given. Additionally, the products must be sterile, free from undesired particulate matter, and pyrogen-free.

Sterilization Methods Used in Industry

Method	How Does It Work?	Advantages	Disadvantages	Products Sterilized by This Method
Steam sterilization	Heat coagulates and kills microorganisms	• Method of choice when applicable • Lower heat than dry-heat sterilization	• Cannot use with heat- or moisture-sensitive drugs • Autoclave can have cools spots	• Aqueous solutions in closed containers • Surgical instruments • Glassware
Dry heat sterilization	Heat coagulates and kills microorganisms	• Useful for moisture-sensitive material	• Cannot use with heat-sensitive drugs • Autoclave can have cool spots	• Glassware • Surgical equipment • Oleaginous materials • Powders • Moisture-sensitive material
Filtration	Bacteria and particulate matter are physically removed by membrane filters	• Inexpensive	• Technique failure • Membrane defects • Drug can absorb to membrane	• Small volumes of thin liquid • Heat-sensitive liquid formulations
Ionizing radiation	Gamma radiation mutates and kills bacteria		• Expensive setup	• Sterilizing plastic medical devices
Gas sterilization	Ethylene and propylene oxide gases alkylate microbial protein	• Good for heat- and moisture-sensitive materials	• Possibility of toxic residue • Explosion hazard • Expensive setup • Cannot penetrate glass to sterilize material in sealed containers	• Heat-sensitive material • Moisture-sensitive material • Medical and surgical equipment wrapped in plastic

Multiple-dose injectable products must contain preservative in order to ensure that the product remains sterile after the initial use. Large-volume, single-use products, however, cannot contain preservative, as the amount required to reach an effective concentration would lead to preservative-related toxicity. In addition to sterilization and preservation intended to decrease the likelihood of microbial growth in the product, steps must be taken to ensure that pyrogens (lipopolysaccharides from gram-negative bacterial cell walls that cause high fever, hypertension, and chills) are not present.

The main routes of injectable delivery are intravenous (IV), subcutaneous (SQ), and intramuscular (IM). Intravenous products must be solutions or O/W emulsions (e.g., Intralipid®, a component of total parenteral nutrition), as particulate matter could lead to phlebitis and other complications. SQ and IM injections may be solutions or emulsions; however, they may also be suspensions, which exhibit slower absorption since the drug must go into solution in the tissue before being absorbed into the bloodstream. In the case of some injectable suspensions, such as the contraceptive Depo-Provera® (medroxyprogesterone acetate), release of medication can continue for several months, improving patient convenience. Some products are given by other injectable routes: Allergy tuberculosis testing is handled by intradermal injection; hydrocortisone is frequently injected directly into the joint (intra-articular) in arthritic patients; anesthesia is often injected into the epidural space (around the nerve roots of the spine); and anesthetics, some drugs used to treat meningitis, and some chemotherapy agents are injected into the intrathecal (subarachnoid) space (into the cerebrospinal fluid) to bypass the blood-brain barrier.

Ocular and Otic Delivery

Drug delivery to the eye is complicated by two factors: Drug loss due to blinking and lacrimal drainage, and poor drug penetration through the corneal membrane. Polymers are typically used as viscosity enhancers to prolong retention time and reduce lacrimal drainage; some, such as hyaluronic acid, have mild adhesive properties that prolong retention time even further. Drop size reduction can also serve to improve ocular availability; only about 10 μL of fluid remains in the conjunctival cul-de-sac after blinking, so dose volumes larger than this lead to waste.

Drug penetration into the eye can be improved by creating a prodrug that is more lipophilic than the original compound. It is then converted to the active substance by enzymes in the body.

Most ocular products are solutions, but suspensions, ointments, and gels may also be used. These dosage forms prolong drug contact with the eye and may be preferable in some situations. Drug contact may also be prolonged by the use of an ophthalmic insert (Pilocarpine Ocusert® system); these small inserts are placed in the cul-de-sac of the eye and release the drug over a 7-day period, improving patient adherence with glaucoma therapy.

Ocular products must be sterile when dispensed, and all multidose products must contain preservative. This helps prevent serious ocular infections, which can lead to corneal ulcers and blindness.

Otic products are generally solutions or suspensions, which frequently contain glycerin or propylene glycol to increase viscosity and maximize contact between the product and the ear canal. The hygroscopic nature of these solvents also helps them draw moisture out of the tissues, which can reduce inflammation and decrease the amount of moisture available for any microorganisms to grow. Most otic products fall into one of the following categories:

- Anti-infective and anti-inflammatory products: May contain analgesics and local anesthetics to reduce pain associated with otitis externa or otitis media

- Ear-wax removal agents: Contain surfactants (which emulsifies ear wax) or peroxides (which release oxygen and disrupt the integrity of the ear wax), allowing easy removal

Transdermal Delivery

Transdermal delivery differs from topical delivery in that the drug is intended for systemic use. The drug molecules must therefore be small enough to penetrate the stratum corneum and reach the general circulation. Some transdermal ointments (nitroglycerin ointment) exist, but most products are available as transdermal delivery systems (patches).

Patches

Transdermal patches attach to the skin with adhesive and contain the drug either in a polymer matrix or in a drug reservoir covered by a rate-controlling membrane. An excess of drug is typically present to ensure that a concentration gradient exists, causing drug to exit the patch and enter the skin passively. Patches provide more uniform blood levels than conventional release products and can improve patient compliance since, depending on the drug, they can be worn for 1 to 7 days. GI absorption problems and first-pass metabolism are avoided. A wide range of drugs are now available in patches, including nitroglycerin, nicotine, and hormones (for birth control or hormone replacement therapy).

Ultrasound

Drug can be transported across skin by mixing it with a coupling agent and using ultrasonic energy to disrupt the stratum corneum and increase penetrability. This method of delivery is not common, but high-dose hydrocortisone can be delivered in this fashion.

Iontophoresis

This method of transdermal delivery is not widely used but is gaining popularity. It involves delivery of charged compounds across the skin by applying an electrical current. Since the skin is disrupted, larger molecules may pass than is possible with transdermal patches. Local anesthesia (Numby Stuff) and fentanyl (IONSYS) are available in small iontophoretic patches, and the method is being investigated to deliver protein drugs.

LEARNING POINTS

- A drug cannot work until it is absorbed. It cannot be absorbed until it is dissolved.

- Ionized, hydrophilic drugs dissolve more readily; un-ionized, lipophilic drugs are absorbed more easily.

- Focus on why a particular dosage form might work better for a particular condition or with a particular drug.

- Consider nonoral routes for drugs that undergo extensive first-pass metabolism.

- At this time, protein drugs can be given only by injectable or pulmonary routes. There is future potential with nasal delivery.

PRACTICE QUESTIONS

1. Which of the following dosage forms must be sterile?

   (A) Ophthalmic suspension
   (B) Oral suspension
   (C) Topical suspension
   (D) Suspension for rectal administration
   (E) Otic suspension

2. A 15-year old patient with ADHD who had been stable on a dose of 10 mg BID of Focalin is transitioning to Focalin XR 20 mg QD. After 2 weeks, he returns to the doctor complaining of distractedness during school and a jittery feeling in the morning an hour or two after taking his medication. When asked how he is taking his medication, he states that due to difficulty swallowing he has been opening the capsules of Focalin XR and mixing them with chunky applesauce, which he chews before swallowing. How do you explain the patient's current symptoms?

   (A) The new dose of Focalin XR is too high and should be reduced.
   (B) The patient is experiencing dose-dumping because he is opening the capsules.
   (C) The patient is experiencing dose-dumping because he is chewing the capsule contents with the applesauce.
   (D) The severity of the patient's ADHD has increased and he is suffering from a new-onset anxiety disorder.
   (E) The patient is experiencing dose-dumping because the capsule contents are interacting with the applesauce.

3. What environmental advantage do HFA inhalers have over CFC inhalers?

   (A) They contain less packaging.
   (B) They are less likely to lead to ozone depletion.
   (C) They do not contain mercury.
   (D) They are a pump spray instead of an aerosol spray.
   (E) They do not use petroleum-based mineral oil as an emulsifier.

ANSWERS

1. **A**

All ophthalmic dosage forms must be sterile, and either packaged in single-dose containers or formulated to contain a preservative. Sterility is not required for any of the other routes, as the drug is being applied either to an epithelial surface (topical, otic) or to the GI mucosa (oral, rectal). These surfaces are not sterile in their natural state, and dosage forms applied to them need not be sterile.

2. **C**

Focalin XR derives its extended-release properties from a coating on the beads contained within the capsule. It is therefore appropriate to open the capsule and consume the contents with food or in liquid; applesauce is specifically mentioned in the manufacturer instructions as appropriate. However, crushing or chewing the beads destroys the coating, causing dose-dumping. The patient's jitteriness in the morning and inattention later in the day are symptomatic of too high a dose being absorbed in the morning, and too little medication remaining in his system later in the day.

3. **B**

HFA inhalers were designed to replace CFC inhalers, which are being phased out due to the Montreal Protocol and the effect of CFCs on ozone depletion. HFA inhalers are similar in size to CFC inhalers. Neither type of product contains the other excipients mentioned in the question.

Biopharmaceutics

19

 Suggested Study Time: **2–3 hours**

Biopharmaceutics deals with the relationship between the physico-chemical properties of a drug; the dosage form in which the drug is available; and its route of administration, with the rate and extent of its absorption and elimination from the body. It is the science that links together traditional pharmaceutics (physical pharmacy and dosage form design) with pharmacokinetics. The acronym LADME (liberation, absorption, distribution, metabolism, and excretion) is often used to describe the main processes addressed by biopharmaceutics.

DRUG LIBERATION AND ABSORPTION

A key concept to remember is that drugs are administered as dosage forms, not individual chemicals. Once taken, they must first be liberated from the dosage form in question and absorbed into the bloodstream before they become available in the systemic circulation. The exception is intravenously administered drugs, as they are delivered directly into the systemic circulation.

Liberation from a dosage form can be as simple as powder from a capsule being released from the capsule shell after ingestion, or as complicated as the slow release of drug from a tablet or transdermal patch matrix. Oral compressed tablets are the most commonly dispensed dosage form; in this case, liberation of the drug requires disintegration of the tablet into smaller drug particles that then undergo dissolution.

If the drug is not already in solution within the dosage form (as in an oral syrup or elixir), it must first undergo dissolution. Undissolved drug particles cannot cross biological membranes and are therefore trapped at their location of administration. For oral dosage forms, this means the GI tract; any drug not absorbed is lost in the feces. In the case of an eyedrop given in suspension form, the drug particles remain on the corneal surface until the drug either dissolves and passes through the corneal membrane or is lost via lacrimal drainage. Similarly, topical products remain on the skin surface, and intramuscular and subcutaneous injections remain in the tissues until the drug is dissolved in the body fluids.

The rate and extent to which the drug contained in the dosage forms described above is absorbed into the systemic circulation is the bioavailability. This property plays a very important role in the biopharmaceutics and pharmacokinetics of drugs. The liberation and dissolution of a drug can be affected by processing factors and excipients, which can in turn affect bioavailability. Other factors affecting bioavailability are addressed later in this chapter.

One physico-chemical property that can affect bioavailability is particle size. Decreasing the particle size of a drug formulation increases the surface area, which leads to more rapid dissolution. This is an important factor for drugs with low water solubility; finely milling or micronizing drugs such as griseofulvin and nitrofurantoin can dramatically improve their oral bioavailability.

Many excipients can affect product bioavailability. Some examples are listed in the table below.

Excipients That Affect Product Bioavailability

Excipient Category	Examples	Effect on Drug Particles	Effect on Bioavailability
Disintegrants	Starch, microcrystalline cellulose	Breaks tablet into smaller particles, increases dissolution	Possible increase
Surfactants	Tweens, Spans	Low concentration: Decrease surface tension and increase dissolution rate	Possible increase
		High concentration: Form micelles with drug inside, decrease dissolution	Possible decrease
Lubricants	Magnesium stearate	Has tendency to waterproof particles in large concentration, making them less soluble	Possible decrease

Drug Transport Across Membranes

There are several ways for drugs to cross body membranes that you should be aware of: Passive diffusion, carrier-mediated transport, endocytosis, and drug efflux. In passive diffusion, the drug crosses cell membranes based on a concentration gradient, moving from regions of higher concentration to areas of (relatively) lower concentration. For this mechanism to be practical, the drug must be small enough to be absorbed across cells and lipid-soluble enough to interact with the cell membranes. The rate of transport is described by Fick's first law of diffusion:

$$\frac{dC}{dt} = \frac{DA(C_s - C)}{h}$$

While it is unlikely that the exam will require you to perform calculations based on this equation, you should be familiar with the items that affect it: The concentration gradient (CS-C), the thickness of the membrane being crossed (h), the surface area of the membrane (A), and the diffusion coefficient of the drug (D).

As would be expected, drugs diffuse more slowly through thicker membranes. Body locations with larger surface area tend to promote faster diffusion, as there is more available membrane through which the drug molecule can diffuse. The small intestine is thus a prime location for drug absorption, as the surface area is very large due to the presence of villi and microvilli.

Another key factor to remember is that the GI membranes are more permeable to drug in the un-ionized form. Solubility of weakly acidic drugs therefore increases as the drug moves from the stomach to the intestines; solubility of weakly basic drugs decreases. Because of this, poorly soluble, weakly basic drugs may be poorly absorbed if taken with drugs that reduce gastric acid secretion. Ketoconazole and dipyridamole both exhibit reduced rate and extent of absorption when taken with H_2 blockers such as cimetidine or with proton pump inhibitors such as omeprazole.

Not all drugs are absorbed by passive diffusion; many undergo carrier-mediated transport processes. Active transport, which requires input of energy and occurs against a concentration gradient, is the most common type. Unlike passive diffusion, the process can be saturated or competitively inhibited by chemically similar substrates. Many drugs are transported via transport systems designed to move amino acids and vitamins across cell walls (see table below). Some drugs undergo simultaneous passive diffusion and active transport.

Active Transport Mechanisms for Drugs in the Body

Transporter	Drugs Transported
Peptide	• Penicillins • Cephalosporins • ACE inhibitors
Nucleoside	• Anticancer/antiviral nucleosides
Amino acid	• L-dopa • Methyldopa

Facilitated diffusion is another carrier-mediated transport process; it differs from active transport in that it occurs only from high to low concentrations. As with active transport, the transporter may bind to structurally similar inhibitors, which will decrease the transport rate of the drug. If the inhibitor is present in high concentration, the transporter may become saturated. Furosemide, morphine, and dopamine are examples of drugs that undergo facilitated diffusion.

Macromolecules are most likely to cross cell membranes by endocytosis, a process in which substances are transported across cell membranes by formation of vesicles. Most endocytosis is receptor-mediated; nonreceptor-mediated endocytosis is called either phagocytosis (engulfment of solid particles) or pinocytosis (engulfment of liquid), and is often seen in the gastrointestinal tract and lungs. Protein and peptide drugs such as insulin, erythropoietin, and growth hormone are transported in this fashion. Polio and other oral vaccines are absorbed from the GI tract by phagocytosis, a specific type of endocytosis that is not receptor mediated.

The final method of drug transport with which you should be concerned is drug efflux. In this case, transporters pump drugs and other substances out of cells rather than into them. P-glycoprotein is the key efflux protein, and is linked to multidrug resistance in tumor cells. In this case, resistance occurs because the transporter pumps drug back out of the tumor before it can accumulate to an effective concentration. In addition, p-glycoprotein can reduce net absorption (and hence bioavailability) of other drugs by routing them out of the plasma and back into the lumen of the GI tract. Digoxin, steroids, and immunosuppressive agents are just a few of the drugs that can be affected in this way.

Barriers to Drug Absorption

Several factors can affect drug absorption. Not only must the drug dissolve initially, it must stay in solution during the absorption process itself. The pH of the GI tract varies significantly, and a drug that is in solution at the low pH of the stomach may be less soluble in the higher pH of the small intestine. Food intake can affect absorption and bioavailability in a variety of ways, including increasing the pH in the stomach, which can in turn affect drug dissolution and absorption (increasing dissolution and absorption for weak acids, and decreasing both for weak bases). Chemical stability may be affected as well, which can in turn lower the amount of drug available for absorption.

Food-Related Absorption and Bioavailability Variations

Process	Explanation	Examples
Food-drug complexation	Can bind and make drug insoluble; prevent absorption	Tetracycline complexes with calcium and iron in food and supplements
Alteration of pH	Food acts as buffer in stomach; increases pH	• Increases dissolution (and subsequent absorption) of weak acids • Decreases dissolution of weak bases
Gastric emptying	Foods (especially fatty ones) and some drugs slow gastric emptying and delay drug onset	
Gastric acid secretions	• Pepsin may increase drug metabolism • Bile salts increase dissolution of poorly soluble drugs, but can form complexes with other drugs	Bile acid-drug complexes: Neomycin, kanamycin, nystatin
Competition for specialized absorption mechanisms	Competitive inhibition of drugs by nutrients with similar chemical structures	
Increased volume and viscosity of GI contents	Presence of food can lead to: • Slower drug dissolution • Slower diffusion of dissolved drug from GI tract	
Food-induced changes in first-pass metabolism	Increased bioavailability due to inhibited cytochrome P450 (primarily CYP3A)	Grapefruit juice ingestions lead to increased bioavailability of: • Cyclosporin • Saquinavir • Verapamil
Food-induced changes in blood flow	• Giving some drugs with food increases bioavailability due to increased blood flow to the GI tract and liver following a meal • A larger fraction of drug escapes first-pass metabolism because the enzyme system becomes overwhelmed	Drugs with metabolism sensitive to rate of presentation to liver: • Propranolol • Hydralazine

DRUG DISTRIBUTION

Once in the bloodstream, some drug may be bound to the plasma proteins while the remainder remains unbound. A key point to remember is that only drug that is unbound can pass out of the plasma to reach the site of action. The amount of drug that is bound to plasma protein is in dynamic equilibrium with the amount that is not.

Volume of Distribution

In the average 70-kg (~155-lb) patient, blood volume is approximately 5 L and total body water is about 40 L. After absorption, a drug will distribute into the body fluids; since the total amount of drug placed into the body is known and the concentration of drug in the body can be measured, the volume of fluid through which the drug seems to have distributed can be determined. This volume is referred to as the *apparent* volume of distribution, because it is not a physical volume. Rather, it is a calculated number, dependent on physicochemical properties of the drug, which helps compare the behavior of different drugs.

$$V_d = \frac{dose}{C_p}$$ when dose = IV bolus and C_p is measured immediately after injection

Different types of drugs show very different apparent volumes of distribution:

- Macromolecules: Too large to distribute into the capillaries; V_d will equal plasma volume of individual (about 3 L)
- Small polar drugs: Not lipophilic enough to enter intracellular fluid; V_d will equal plasma + interstitial fluid volume (about 12 L)
- Small lipophilic drugs: Can diffuse into cells; V_d will equal total body water (about 40 L)

Plasma Protein Binding

The above examples all assume that the drug does not bind to plasma proteins. Most drugs do, however, exhibit protein binding, and this greatly affects their volume of distribution. Proteins are large molecules that cannot leave the capillaries; therefore, the drug-protein complex remains in the plasma. However, since the concentration of protein-bound drug is not usually measured, protein binding will cause a decrease in the free plasma concentration of the drug, increasing the apparent volume of distribution. As protein binding is reversible, equilibrium exists between bound and free drug. As free drug distributes out of the bloodstream, bound drug is released from plasma proteins to maintain the equilibrium.

Although plasma proteins are relatively nonspecific in their binding behavior, the different proteins do tend to bind to different types of drug:

- Albumin: Weak acids
- α_1-acid glycoprotein: Weak bases
- Lipoproteins: Basic and neutral drugs
- Globulins: Steroids, vitamins, metal ions

Dosing a highly protein-bound drug based only on physiological volumes (plasma volume, interstitial volume, or total body water) may not produce a high enough concentration at the site of drug action to yield adequate pharmacological response. Therefore, a higher dose may need to be given. The protein-drug complex may also act as a drug reservoir, prolonging action in the body. These factors must be considered when determining dose and dosing frequency. Certain disease states can alter the levels of plasma proteins significantly enough to require drug dose adjustments. Additionally, if a patient is receiving several drugs that all bind to the same plasma protein, one drug may displace another, leading to higher-than-expected drug concentrations and possible toxicity. This is most important in drugs that are more than 95% bound, particularly if they have a narrow therapeutic index. Warfarin (99% bound) is an excellent example of this.

Some Disease States and Physiological Conditions That Affect Plasma Protein Concentration

Decrease plasma protein concentration	• Liver disease • Trauma (albumin) • Surgery (albumin) • Burns • Renal failure (albumin) • Hyperthyroidism • Age (neonate, geriatric) • Pregnancy
Increase plasma protein concentration	• Hypothyroidism • Schizophrenia • Rheumatoid arthritis • Renal failure (α_1-acid glycoprotein) • Trauma (α_1-acid glycoprotein) • Surgery (α_1-acid glycoprotein)

DRUG METABOLISM

Drugs are eliminated from the body by two processes: Metabolism and excretion. Metabolism, also referred to as biotransformation, leads to the chemical conversion of drug to active or inactive compounds called metabolites. These metabolites are generally more polar (and hence more water-soluble) than the parent drugs. This allows the metabolites to be more efficiently cleared in the urine. Not all drugs undergo metabolism.

Metabolism is most likely to occur in organs that contain high levels of enzymes. Many microsomal enzymes, including the cytochrome P450 (CYP450) mixed-function oxidases, are found in the liver, which is the primary site of biotransformation. Metabolizing enzymes are found in many other locations of the body, and significant biotransformation of some drugs can occur in the intestinal tract, kidney, and brain. Drugs administered via nasal, pulmonary, or dermal routes often also show significant biotransformation in the nasal tissue, lung, or skin.

One concern with oral delivery of certain drugs is presystemic, or first-pass, metabolism. Because the venous outflow of the gastrointestinal tract travels directly to the liver via the portal vein, drugs administered via the gastrointestinal tract are susceptible to hepatic metabolism before they reach the systemic circulation. Bioavailability is decreased, so the drug must be given either in a higher dose or by a delivery route that bypasses the gastrointestinal tract. Nitroglycerin, for example, is almost completely degraded by first-pass metabolism and is therefore usually formulated as sublingual tablets or spray, or transdermal ointment or patches. Oral extended-release capsules are also available and are believed to work by saturating the hepatic enzymes responsible for metabolism and by producing metabolites that possess some activity.

Phase I Reactions

Metabolism is classified into Phase I and Phase II reactions. In many cases, a drug may undergo metabolism by competing pathways, leading to multiple metabolites. The metabolites may in turn undergo metabolism. Some of these metabolites may possess therapeutic activity. Some medications are deliberately administered as inactive prodrugs, and the therapeutic component results from the metabolism of the prodrug. Formulating a medication as a prodrug can improve its pharmaceutical, pharmacodynamic, or pharmacokinetic properties.

Phase I reactions are so named because they generally occur before Phase II reactions. They are nonsynthetic and introduce or expose a functional group. The primary types of Phase I reactions are oxidation, reduction, and hydrolysis. Oxidation is the most common type of metabolism, and many of these reactions are catalyzed by enzymes in the CYP superfamily.

Phase II Reactions

Phase II reactions are synthetic reactions. They are often called conjugation reactions, as a reactive group on the drug is attached to a polar molecule or group originating inside the body. This generally leads to a polar, water-soluble metabolite. While most drugs undergo Phase I metabolism prior to Phase II, this is not required provided the drug already possesses one or more reactive groups.

Examples of Phase II reactions are listed in the table below, with glucuronidation being the most common example. Since these reactions involve enzymes, the reactions may be capacity limited. If the concentration of drug approaches or exceeds the metabolic capacity of the enzyme, nonlinear drug metabolism may be observed.

Two types of conjugation reactions (methylation and acetylation) lead to metabolites that are less polar, and therefore less soluble, than the original compound. Less soluble metabolites will have extended elimination half-lives. This can extend the duration of action in cases where an active metabolite is formed, such as *N*-acetylprocainamide. Toxicity may also occur from increased blood or tissue levels of toxic metabolites. For example, at high concentrations the acetylated metabolites of sulfonamides can precipitate in the kidney tubules and lead to kidney damage and crystalluria.

Phase II Reactions

Type of Phase II Reaction	Drugs Metabolized by This Route
Glucuronidation	• Chloramphenicol • Meprobamate • Morphine
Sulfation	• Acetaminophen • Estradiol • Methyldopa • Minoxidil
Amino acid conjugation	• Salicylic acid
Acetylation	• Isoniazid • Procainamide • Sulfonamides • Hydralazine
Methylation	• Catecholamines • Niacinamide • Thiouracil
Glutathione conjugation	• Chlorambucil

Factors Affecting Biotransformation

Several factors can affect metabolizing enzyme activity in the body. Disease state, age, gender, or chemical and nutritional exposure to a variety of substances can lead to enzyme inhibition or enzyme induction. Genetic variability also plays a role. Drug–drug interactions are a common result of the metabolic process, as most marketed drugs are metabolized by multiple pathways, and drugs that inhibit or induce enzyme activity can affect the metabolism of many other drugs.

Enzyme Inhibition

Enzyme inhibition describes the situation when an enzyme is prevented from binding with its substrate. The substrate is therefore unable to be properly metabolized, and plasma levels rise, possibly to toxic levels. In cases where a prodrug must be activated by metabolism, enzyme inhibition may limit, delay, or prevent drug activity. Enzyme inhibitors can act by competitive or noncompetitive means.

Drugs that are metabolized by the same metabolic pathways frequently act as competitive inhibitors to each other. Drug metabolites, herbal products, and foods can also act as enzyme inhibitors. Compounds containing imidazole, pyridine, or quinolone groups in particular are often found to be enzyme inhibitors. The table below contains an incomplete list of common enzyme inhibitors.

One of the most widely known drug–food interactions results from enzyme inhibition. Grapefruit juice is an inhibitor of CYP3A, the isozyme responsible for metabolism of a host of drugs, including macrolide antibiotics, benzodiazepines, calcium channel blockers, and HIV protease inhibitors. While a single portion is unlikely to lead to problems, patients receiving drugs metabolized by this isozyme should be cautioned to avoid grapefruit juice.

Drugs Involved in Inhibition of Metabolic Enzymes

Calcium channel blockers	• Diltiazem • Verapamil
Macrolide antibiotics	• Erythromycin
Quinolone antibiotics	• Ciprofloxacin • Ofloxacin
Imidazole antifungals	• Ketoconazole • Fluconazole • Lansoprazole • Miconazole
Metronidazole	
Omeprazole	
Cimetidine	

Enzyme Induction

Enzyme induction is essentially the opposite of enzyme inhibition. Enzyme inducers stimulate enzyme activity, which leads to decreased plasma levels of the enzyme's targets. In most cases, this means a decrease in both activity and adverse effects. If active or toxic metabolites are produced, however, drug activity and toxic effects may be increased. A number of commonly prescribed drugs induce metabolic enzymes, as do ethanol, tobacco, marijuana, and certain herbal products, most notably St. John's wort. This can lead to clinically significant drug interactions. For example, triazolam is extensively metabolized by CYP3A4. St. John's wort, rifampin, and several seizure medications (carbamazepine, phenytoin, and phenobarbital) induce this isozyme. Using any of these agents with triazolam or other drugs metabolized by 3A4 will lead to significantly reduced plasma concentrations and therapeutic effect.

Some drugs undergo a phenomenon called auto-induction, wherein they stimulate their own metabolism. Carbamazepine is a key example of a drug of this type. Due to auto-induction, long-term administration of carbamazepine can lead to decreased blood levels and therapeutic activity.

Drugs Involved in Induction of Metabolic Enzymes

Seizure medications	• Carbamazepine • Phenytoin • Phenobarbital • Secobarbital
Tuberculosis medications	• Rifampin • Isoniazid
Prednisone	
Omeprazole	
Modafinil	

Genetic Variability

Genetic polymorphisms lead to a number of metabolism-related issues. "Fast" and "slow" metabolizers exist for particular drugs. Dosage adjustments must be made in order to avoid subtherapeutic consequences or toxic effects, depending on the population into which a patient falls.

CYP enzymes in particular possess a high level of polymorphism. The table below lists select drugs metabolized by the most common CYP enzymes. CYP2D6 in particular can be problematic, as individuals can be classed as poor, intermediate, extensive, and ultra-rapid metabolizers. The percentage of poor metabolizers varies somewhat by ancestry, comprising approximately 5–10% of Caucasians, 4% of Blacks, and 1% of Asians. One of the drugs metabolized by CYP2D6 is codeine; in this case, poor metabolizers receive less benefit from the drug, as codeine must be metabolized into morphine to take effect. Pharmacists should be aware of this variability, since poor metabolizers may be falsely labeled as drug-seekers when in fact codeine is an ineffective analgesic for them. These patients should instead be placed on analgesics not activated by CYP2D6, such as morphine itself.

Common Drugs Metabolized by This Pathway

CYP Class	Common CYP Enzymes
1A2	• Caffeine • Theophylline
3A4	• Macrolide antibiotics • Calcium channel blockers • Benzodiazepines – Alprazolam – Midazolam – Triazolam • HIV protease inhibitors
2C9	• Glipizide • Warfarin • Phenytoin
2C19	• Omeprazole • Diazepam
2D6	• Select opioids – Codeine – Dextromethorphan – Hydrocodone – Oxycodone • Fluoxetine • Haloperidol • Tricyclic antidepressants

Glucose-6-phosphate dehydrogenase is an enzyme with over 300 reported polymorphic variants, leading to individuals possessing low, normal, or increased levels of the enzyme. As this enzyme protects red blood cells from oxidative stress, deficiency in combination with certain environmental or pharmacological stresses—such as eating fava beans or taking certain drugs—can lead to life-threatening hemolytic anemia. Prevalence of this deficiency is highest among those of African, Asian, and Mediterranean ancestry, with more severe variants occurring in Mediterranean populations. The high gene frequency in certain populations is believed to be related to its protective effect against malaria.

Substances to Be Avoided in Glucose-6-Phosphate Dehydrogenase Deficiency

- Oxidant drugs
  - Primaquine
  - Chloroquine
- Sulfonamides
- Quinolones
- Aspirin
- Probenecid
- Vitamin K
- Nitrofurantoin
- Fava beans
- Mothballs

Acetylation is another important instance of genetic variability in drug metabolism. Rapid-metabolizing and slow-metabolizing polymorphic variants of *N*-acetyl-transferase-2 can have therapeutic implications for several drugs, most notably the tuberculosis drug isoniazid. Slow acetylators do not metabolize the drug quickly, and must be given lower doses in order to prevent toxic effects. Rapid acetylators require substantially higher doses, and therapeutic failure rates are more common than with normal or slow acetylators.

DRUG EXCRETION

The other process by which the body eliminates substances is excretion. Unlike metabolism, excretion eliminates substances without further chemical change. The kidney is the primary organ involved, and most substances are excreted in the urine. Polar, water-soluble drugs are usually excreted unchanged; lipophilic drugs are generally excreted as metabolites. There are three components to renal excretion:

1. Glomerular filtration:
   - Blood passes through the capillary network (glomerulus) inside Bowman's capsule.
   - Fenestrated endothelium allows paracellular transport of most solutes (other than macromolecules) into Bowman's capsule.
   - Filtrate (including drug) moves from Bowman's capsule into renal tubules.
   - All nonprotein bound, small-molecule drugs undergo glomerular filtration; the concentration of drug or metabolite in the filtrate will be equal to the concentration of unbound drug in the plasma.

2. Tubular reabsorption:

- Many nutrients and ions are actively reabsorbed into the bloodstream.

- Water is reabsorbed, and filtrate becomes more concentrated as it moves along the tubule.

- No transporters exist for reabsorption of drug; passive diffusion process is dependent on filtrate pH. Acidic (citrus fruits, cranberry juice, aspirin) and basic (milk products, sodium bicarbonate) foods and drugs can alter urine pH enough to affect reabsorption.

  » In alkaline urine: Acidic drugs are ionized → less reabsorbed → more readily excreted

  » In acidic urine: Basic drugs are ionized → less reabsorbed → more readily excreted

  » Pentobarbital (weak acid) overdose: Treated by alkalinizing urine with sodium bicarbonate injection

3. Tubular secretion:

- This occurs simultaneously with tubular reabsorption.

- This removes certain substances from the blood and secretes them back into the filtrate.

- This occurs against concentration gradients and is an energy-requiring process that uses protein transporters.

- Only ionized drug is bound to and secreted by the transporter proteins; drugs that are highly ionized at pH 7.4 will be secreted to a greater extent.

- Plasma protein binding has little effect on this process; transporters can strip drug off of protein.

  » Competitive process; can lead to drug interactions

    - Desirable: Probenecid and penicillin

    - Undesirable: Cimetidine and procainamide

    - Saturable process; at high dose, process plateaus → less drug excreted → higher plasma concentration than expected

The rate of renal excretion of drugs is the net result of the above processes. It depends on blood flow in addition to the physicochemical properties of the drugs in question. More rapid blood flow through the nephron generally leads to an increase in all three processes, with an overall higher drug excretion rate. Glomerular filtration rate (GFR) is normally about 120 mL/min, but may vary widely with the patient's age, size, and disease state. GFR for an individual is determined by calculating the clearance of creatinine, an endogenous substance that is not reabsorbed or secreted. This value gives an indication of kidney function.

Renal clearance is a measure of the efficiency of renal excretion in removing unchanged drug in the urine. It is an indirect measurement expressed by the following equation, where C_U and V_U are concentration of drug in the urine and volume of urine formation per unit time:

$$CL_r = \frac{excretion\ rate\ in\ urine}{plasma\ concentration} = \frac{C_U V_U}{C_p}$$

Nonrenal Excretion

Drugs may also be excreted by the liver into the bile; at this point, one of two things can happen:

- Biliary excretion: Bile (including drug) is emptied into the small intestine, where it is eventually excreted from the body in the feces.
- Enterohepatic recycling: The drug is partially reabsorbed from the intestines (based on pKa and partition coefficient) and re-enters the bloodstream. Drugs undergoing this process may show a secondary peak in plasma concentration; with multiple dosing regimens, the blood-level curve can be altered significantly.

Some drugs are excreted into other fluids, though this is usually not a significant route:

- Saliva: Swallowed, leading to salivary recycling; routine and noninvasive way of monitoring for levels of certain drugs
- Breast milk: Mostly occurs by passive diffusion (primarily of weak bases); can lead to drug transfer to breastfeeding infants
- Sweat: Small volume, so not a significant mode of drug excretion; could become a convenient method for detecting use of illegal or restricted drugs (cocaine, amphetamines, morphine, and ethanol)
- Expired air: Significant route of excretion for volatile drugs (anesthetics, ethanol); drug volatility is more important than polarity for this method of excretion

LEARNING POINTS

- The prime body location for drug absorption is the small intestine, due to the high surface area; the drug must be dissolved in order to be absorbed, however, and factors affecting dissolution in the small intestine (i.e., pH) may prevent this from being the prime absorption location for a particular drug.

- Only drugs that are unbound to plasma protein can pass from the plasma to reach the site of action.

- Enzyme inhibition can often lead to toxicity; enzyme induction can lead to inadequate blood levels of drug.

- Genetic variations in CYP metabolism lead to fast and slow metabolizers of a variety of drugs; dosage adjustments or alternate therapies must be made in some cases.

- Tubular reabsorption decreases drug and metabolite concentration in the urine, while tubular secretion increases the amount. Water-soluble, ionized drugs are more likely to be excreted.

PRACTICE QUESTIONS

1. A single IV dose of a drug is given and the AUC is calculated. After an adequate washout period, a single oral dose of the same drug is given. If the doses are the same size, which of the following results is possible?

    (A) $AUC_{PO} = AUC_{IV}$
    (B) $AUC_{PO} > AUC_{IV}$
    (C) $AUC_{PO} < AUC_{IV}$
    (D) A and B
    (E) A and C

2. The quality-control test required for tablets, intended to reflect the absorption of the drug, is the

    (A) weight variation test.
    (B) content uniformity test.
    (C) dissolution test.
    (D) disintegration test.
    (E) friability test.

3. A 15-year-old patient taking Focalin XR for his ADHD is experiencing inattention later in the day. He admits that after having a cold 2 weeks ago, he started taking 2 g of vitamin C per day to "boost his immune system." What do you think is causing his symptoms?

    (A) He is experiencing vitamin C toxicity.
    (B) The vitamin C is acidifying his urine, causing decreased excretion of Focalin XR.
    (C) The vitamin C is acidifying his urine, causing increased excretion of Focalin XR.
    (D) The vitamin C is inducing CYP2D6, causing increased metabolism of Focalin XR.
    (E) The vitamin C is inhibiting CYP2D6, causing increased metabolism of Focalin XR.

ANSWERS

1. **E**

Because the bioavailability of a drug administered intravenously is 1, by definition, the oral bioavailability of a dosage form containing the same drug may be as high as the IV bioavailability (assuming complete absorption and no first-pass metabolism). It will usually be lower than the IV dose. However, because bioavailability can never be greater than 1, the oral bioavailability may never exceed the IV bioavailability. The AUC_{PO} may, therefore, be less than or equal to the AUC_{IV}, but never greater.

2. **C**

The quality-control test intended to reflect the absorption of the drug is the dissolution test. It is only an approximation; going into solution is the last step before absorption. Weight variation and content uniformity tests assess the distribution of the active ingredients across the tablets and ensure that each dose is approximately the same weight. The disintegration test evaluates how quickly or slowly a tablet disintegrates; disintegration is a necessary step prior to dissolution. The friability test determines how well tablets will hold up to handling.

3. **C**

Focalin (dexmethylphenidate) is a weakly basic drug primarily excreted via the renal route. Acidification of the urine will cause trapping of the ionized form of the drug in the urine, increasing urinary excretion. Although some quantity of Focalin is metabolized by CYP2D6, vitamin C does not induce this enzyme. Symptoms of vitamin C toxicity do not include inattention.

Pharmacokinetics and Graph Interpretation

20

 Suggested Study Time: **2 hours**

Pharmacokinetics is the mathematical study of drug concentration in the body. It is dependent on the absorption, distribution, metabolism, and excretion (ADME) discussed in this book's biopharmaceutics chapter and is the quantitative description of what happens to the drug in the body. Clinical pharmacokinetics applies the concepts directly to individual patients, making individualized drug therapy and therapeutic drug monitoring possible.

Many equations are employed in pharmacokinetics. The more complicated of these are unlikely to be used in calculations on the NAPLEX due to time constraints, but you should be familiar with their concepts because they could form the basis for theoretical questions. Study for this section of the exam should focus primarily on being able to perform calculations related to the basic pharmacokinetic parameters discussed below and being able to properly interpret graphs of blood level data. Calculations involving drugs most likely to be monitored clinically (phenytoin, aminoglycosides) are the most important to focus on.

PLASMA DRUG CONCENTRATION PROFILES

Plasma level-versus-time curve charts are used extensively in pharmacokinetics. A known dose of drug is given to a patient, and blood samples are taken at various time intervals following drug administration. The concentration of drug in plasma is measured and plotted in the figure below. The shape of the curve depends on the relative rates of absorption, distribution, and elimination of the drug.

Figure 20-1: **Blood Level-versus-Time Curves for IV and Oral Drug Administration**

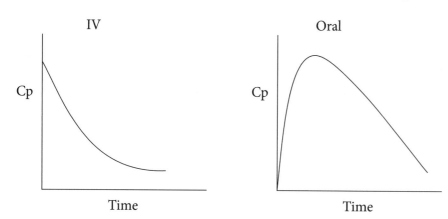

PK MODELING (Compartmental)

From a pharmacokinetic perspective, the body is considered to consist of compartments, inside each of which the drug can be considered evenly distributed. These compartments are interconnected, and the drug moves between them at defined rates. Although compartments are completely theoretical (consisting of groups of tissues with similar blood flow and drug affinity, not actual body regions), they serve a useful purpose in simplifying calculations. Several models exist, but only two are likely to be considered on the NAPLEX:

- One-compartment model:
  - » Body consists of homogenous central compartment.
  - » Drug distributes rapidly and uniformly to this compartment.
  - » This is generally the preferred model.
- Two-compartment model:
  - » Central compartment is still present, and includes highly perfused organs (liver, kidneys).
  - » There is a slow distribution of drug into a peripheral compartment of poorly perfused tissue (muscles, connective tissue).

Multicompartmental models exist (hydromorphone [Dilaudid®] is best described by a three-compartment model), but the calculations become very complex, and it is generally possible to group a few compartments together and still obtain an adequate description of the data.

Figure 20-2: **One-Compartment Versus Multicompartment Models**

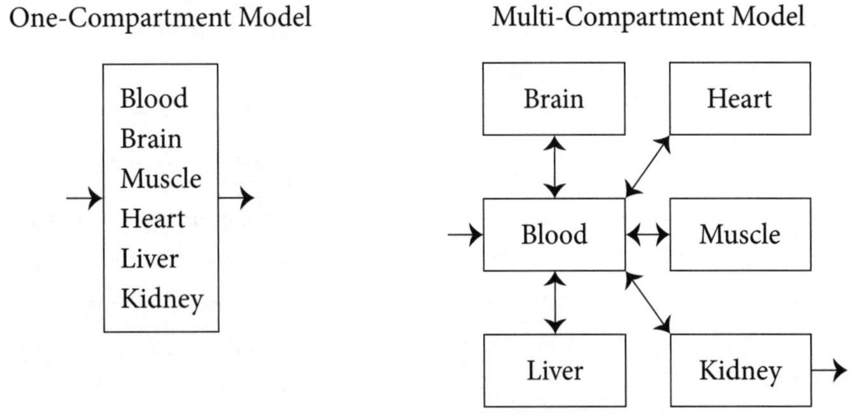

BASIC PHARMACOKINETIC PARAMETERS

Most calculations you are likely to see on the NAPLEX involve the parameters listed below:

Bioavailable Fraction

Bioavailable fraction (F) is the portion of dose administered that reaches the systemic circulation. For IV administration, $F = 1$. Drug given by any other route can have a bioavailable fraction ranging from 0 to 1; the bioavailable fraction will never be greater than 1. Two factors can decrease the bioavailable fraction of a drug:

- Incomplete absorption
- First-pass metabolism

The equation governing bioavailable fraction is given below. *fa* represents the fraction of administered dose absorbed into the bloodstream, and *ffp* represents the fraction of absorbed drug escaping first pass metabolism.

$$F = ffp \cdot fa$$

Hepatic Extraction Ratio

The hepatic extraction ratio (E) is the fraction of drug in the blood that is metabolized during each pass of blood through the liver.

$$(1 - E) = ffp$$

High-*E* drugs are extensively metabolized by liver enzymes. Low-*E* drugs are metabolized by sluggish enzymes with relatively low affinity for the drug. Knowing a drug's *E* value is useful in predicting the effects of first-pass metabolism, disease states, and drug–drug interactions on the metabolism of the drug.

Plasma Level

The plasma level of the drug (*C*) can be determined by a number of equations. The most basic version, for a drug following a one-compartment model, is given below in three formats. You should remember and be able to use at least one of these equations:

$$\log C = \log C_0 - \frac{kt}{2.3}$$
$$\ln C = \ln C_0 - kt$$
$$C = C_0 e^{-kt}$$

When calculating plasma levels following an IV bolus dose, these are the equations you should use.

Elimination Rate Constant

The first-order elimination rate constant, *k*, represents the fraction of drug eliminated per unit time, and thus has units of reciprocal time (i.e., hr^{-1}). It can be obtained graphically (see figure below) or from the drug half-life:

$$k = \frac{\ln 2}{t_{1/2}} = \frac{0.693}{t_{1/2}}$$

Figure 20-3: **Graphical Calculation of Elimination Rate Constant**

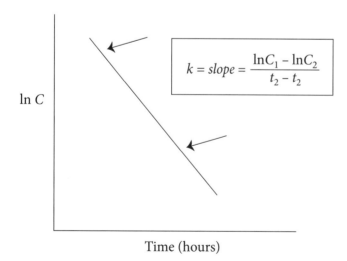

$$k = slope = \frac{\ln C_1 - \ln C_2}{t_2 - t_2}$$

ln *C*

Time (hours)

Half-Life

The elimination half-life of a drug is the time required for its serum concentration to decrease by half. It can be obtained mathematically or graphically:

$$t_{1/2} = \frac{\ln 2}{k} = \frac{0.693}{k}$$

Half-life can also be calculated from clearance and volume of distribution (see sections below). While these parameters do not influence or depend on one another, half-life depends on both of them:

$$t_{1/2} = 0.693 \cdot \left(\frac{Vd}{CL} \right)$$

Clearance

Clearance refers to the efficiency of the body in removing drug from the blood. The liver and kidney are the primary organs involved, and body clearance refers to the sum of the hepatic and renal clearances, plus any clearance from other organs, usually negligible:

$$CL = CL_h + CL_r$$

Some drugs are cleared primarily by one organ (propranolol has a hepatic clearance of 840 mL/min and a total clearance of only 848 mL/min), while others show more mixed clearance (procainamide has a hepatic clearance of 268 mL/min and a renal clearance of 303 mL/min). Knowledge of drug clearance can help determine when dosage adjustments are needed in patients with liver or kidney disease. Using the above examples, patients with kidney disease would need dose adjustments for procainamide but not propranolol. Patients with liver disease would need dose adjustments for both drugs.

If clearance increases, the drug is more efficiently removed from the body and the drug half-life decreases.

Population clearance values are typically based on body weight; clearance corresponds to ideal, not actual, body weight (IBW):

- Tall, lean individuals have larger eliminating organs à higher clearance than a shorter lean person.
- Adipose tissue does not affect the size of eliminating organs à actual body weight should not be used to determine clearance in obese patients (use ideal body weight).

$$IBW(males) = 50kg + [2.3 \cdot (\# \ of \ inches \ of \ height > 60")]$$
$$IBW(females) = 45kg + [2.3 \cdot (\# \ of \ inches \ of \ height > 60")]$$

Volume of Distribution

Apparent volume of distribution (V_d) describes the volume of body fluids required to account for all drugs in the body. As mentioned in the biopharmaceutics chapter, it is not a real volume but a calculated number that helps compare the behavior of different drugs. Several equations can be used to calculate V_d, depending on the information you have available:

$$V_d = \frac{dose}{C_{peak}} = \frac{F \cdot D_0}{AUC \cdot k} = \frac{CL \cdot T_{1/2}}{0.693}$$

Volume of distribution has the following effect on half-life:

- Small V_d:
  - » Drug mostly located in blood
  - » Liver and kidneys can only clear drug in blood
  - » Fewer passes needed to rid body of drug
  - » Shorter half-life
- Large V_d:
  - » Drug extensively distributed into extravascular tissues
  - » More passes required to clear drug from blood
  - » Longer half-life

Area under the Curve

Area under the curve (AUC) is a measure of the extent of drug bioavailability. It is defined as the area under the drug plasma level – time curve from $t = 0$ to infinity. It can be calculated by the trapezoidal rule (unlikely to appear on the NAPLEX, due to time constraints), or by the other listed equations, and has units of concentration/time. S is the salt factor for a given drug formulation and refers to the percentage of administered product that is the active moiety (the acid or base, not the salt). A commonly used example of a drug with a salt factor is aminophylline ($S = 0.8$), as compared to theophylline ($S = 1$).

Trapezoidal rule:

$$AUC = \frac{C_{n-1} + C_n}{2}(tn - t_{n-1})$$

Other equations:

$$AUC = \frac{F \cdot S \cdot D_0}{CL} = \frac{F \cdot D_0}{k \cdot V_D}$$

AUC is often directly proportional to dose, such that increasing the dose of a drug from 500 mg to 1,000 mg will lead to a two-fold increase in *AUC*. This is not always the case, however. If a pathway for drug elimination becomes saturated, as can happen with the enzyme-dependent metabolism of certain drugs (such as phenytoin and salicylates), increasing the dose can lead to a disproportionately large increase in *AUC*.

ORAL DOSING

Most immediate-release oral dosage forms follow a first-order absorption model, as do some nonoral dosage forms such as suppositories and IM injections. When plotting log *C* versus time (see figure below), the following equation of the "y = mx + b" format applies:

$$\log C = \log \frac{F \cdot K_a \cdot D}{V_D(k_a - k)} = \frac{kt}{2.3}$$

Figure 20-4: **First-Order Blood Level-versus-Time Curve**

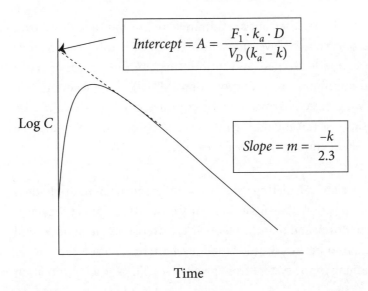

The above equation may also be expressed as:

$$C = \frac{F \cdot K_a \cdot D}{V_D(k_a - k)} = (e^{-kt} - e^{-k_a t}) \quad \text{or} \quad C = Ae^{-kt} - Be^{-k_a t}$$

The absorption rate constant, k_a, cannot be measured directly. It can be calculated by several methods, which are fairly lengthy mathematical processes and are unlikely to be tested on the NAPLEX. General questions about the methods could be asked, however.

- Method of residuals (feathering, peeling)
    - » The difference between the extrapolated line in the above graph and the point directly below it on the absorption portion of the curve (the residual) is plotted versus time.
    - » The slope of this line is equal to $-k_a / 2.3$.
- Wagner-Nelson method
    - » Plots fraction of drug unabsorbed versus time
    - » Can use blood level and/or urinary excretion data
- Loo-Riegelman method
    - » Plots percent of drug unabsorbed versus time
    - » Used for two-compartment model drugs
    - » Must give drug intravenously and orally in order to obtain all necessary information

MULTIPLE DRUG DOSING

Most drugs are not given as single doses but are administered in multiple doses over prolonged periods of time. Since plasma levels must be maintained within certain levels in order to achieve maximum effectiveness and to limit toxicity (minimum effective concentration [MEC] and minimum toxic concentration [MTC]), drug accumulation must be considered. Knowing basic pharmacokinetic parameters for a given drug (k, V_d, and/or CL), as well as the dose (D) and dosing interval (τ), it is possible to predict the plasma level at any time after beginning the dosage regime.

The most common model used in calculating drug levels in the setting of multiple-dosage regimens is that of superposition. It assumes that early doses do not affect the pharmacokinetics of subsequent doses, and that the blood levels after subsequent doses will overlay the previous doses. In other words, the blood level after each dose can simply be added to the level remaining in the system from prior doses. First-order elimination kinetics are assumed.

If the same dose of drug is given at a fixed-dose frequency, eventually the plasma level curve reaches a plateau and a steady-state plasma level is reached (C_{SS}). At this point, the rate of the drug entering the body equals the rate of drug leaving the body. Blood levels are constant from interval to interval provided the patient's pharmacokinetic parameters do not change and the dose and dosing interval stay the same. Ninety percent of the steady-state concentration has been attained after three half-lives; after five half-lives, 97% has been attained. These numbers are very important to remember as they will allow you to estimate some answers on the NAPLEX. Calculation of C_{SS} is discussed below, but two other terms must be accounted for first.

MULTIPLE DOSING FACTOR AND ACCUMULATION FACTOR

The extent of accumulation can be predicted by using the multiple dosing factor (MDF), where N = the number of doses:

$$MDF = \frac{1 \cdot e^{-N \cdot k \cdot t}}{1 - e^{-k \cdot t}}$$

Single-dose equations can be converted to multiple-dose equations simply by multiplying each exponential term that contains time as a variable by the MDF.

At steady state, the MDF simplifies to the following accumulation factor:

$$MDF = \frac{1}{1 - e^{-k \cdot t}}$$

As the equation for AF shows, two things affect how much drug accumulates between the first dose and a dose at steady state:

- Elimination constant or half-life
- Dosing interval

We cannot control the half-life; it is dependent on the drug in question. However, the dosing interval can be adjusted in order to increase or decrease the drug accumulation factor. A simple estimation of this can be described by:

- Dosing interval < drug half-life → C_{SS} will be much higher than the concentration after the first dose.
- Dosing interval = drug half-life → C_{SS} will be twice as high as the concentration after the first dose.
- Dosing interval > drug half-life → C_{SS} will be similar to the concentration after the first dose (because the drug is almost completely washing out before the next dose is given).

Steady-State Equation and Peak-to-Trough Ratio

The steady-state equation is given below. It may be easily rearranged to solve for CL or dose rate (dose/dosing interval):

$$C_{SS,avg} = \frac{F \cdot S \cdot (S/t)}{CL}$$

Another useful equation is the peak-to-trough ratio:

$$P : T = e^{+k(t - T_{max})}$$

Shorter dosing intervals for a particular dose will lead to a decreased $P{:}T$ ratio, meaning that less fluctuation in peak-to-trough is occurring.

The peak-to-trough ratio can be especially useful when predicting the effect of switching a patient from a regular to a sustained-release formulation. T_{max} represents time to peak concentration within the dosing interval; it is smaller for immediate-release formulations than for sustained-release, as the drug is liberated and absorbed more quickly, and so the peak concentration occurs sooner.

Loading Doses

Loading doses are often used to achieve target plasma drug concentrations as quickly as possible. These large initial doses (which may be given as either a single dose or divided doses over a specified period of time) are especially important in life-threatening conditions such as myocardial infarction, status asthmaticus, and status epilepticus. Loading doses should not be used when there is not an urgent need to achieve target blood levels immediately or the patient cannot be supervised for possible toxicity. Loading doses for narrow-therapeutic-index drugs should ideally occur within a clinical setting.

Loading doses that are given slowly can be calculated by the equation given below. If given rapidly (by bolus injection, for example), the volume of the central compartment (V_c) should be used instead of V_d. Lidocaine is an example of a drug that would require a fast loading dose, due to its use in the treatment of life-threatening arrhythmias.

$$LD_{slow} = \frac{(C_{target} - C_{onboard}) \cdot V_d}{F \cdot S}$$

$C_{onboard}$ is included in case the patient is already taking the drug. If this is not the case, that term drops out and the equation simplifies. It is primarily included as a safety factor to avoid overshooting the upper limit of the therapeutic range.

When patients are within 20% of their ideal body weight (IBW), total body weight (TBW) should be used when calculating loading dose. For obese patients, the decision to use IBW versus TBW depends on the drug and its ability to partition into adipose tissue.

- Drug fully partitions into fat: V_d will increase with weight gain à use TBW
  » Example: Lidocaine
- Drug does not partition into fat: V_d does not change with weight gain à use IBW
  » Example: Digoxin
- Drug that partially partitions into fat: an intermediate value should be used
  » Example: Theophylline

Constant IV Infusion

Constant-rate infusions do not generate fluctuations in plasma concentration. Determining the rate for such infusions is relatively simple:

1. Determine the target steady-state plasma concentration.
2. Find the appropriate population CL.
3. Look up S (if drug is a salt).
4. Calculate infusion rate (R).

$$R = \frac{CS \cdot CL}{S}$$

Clearance adjustment factors may be available for some drugs. Some conditions that may have corresponding clearance adjustments include patient age, smoking status, and concurrent use of certain drugs. If available, these factors should be used in order to better predict blood levels in the individual patient.

If a drug is infused at a faster rate, a higher steady-state concentration will result. However, the time to steady-state is based on half-life and will remain the same. In order to achieve and maintain immediate steady-state concentrations:

- Give IV loading dose of R/k.
- Begin IV infusion.

Intermittent IV Infusion

Short IV infusions separated by time for drug elimination are often given to prevent high drug concentration and associated adverse effects. The drug may not reach steady-state in such cases.

$$C = \frac{R}{V_d \cdot k} (1 - e^{-kt})$$

The rate of infusion is equal to the dose/infusion period. After the infusion has stopped, drug concentration at a particular time can be determined by the following equation, given the concentration at the time the infusion was stopped.

$$C = C_{stop} (1 - e^{-kt})$$

Intermittent Oral Dosing

Dose rate in intermittent oral dosing is calculated in a similar fashion to IV infusions. Remember to take F into account with oral dosing, however, since bioavailability may not be equal to IV products. After the dosing rate is determined, dose can be calculated based on the preferred dosing interval.

$$\frac{D}{t} = \frac{C_{SS} \cdot CL}{F \cdot S}$$

NONLINEAR PHARMACOKINETICS

So far, this chapter has referred to general pharmacokinetic principles. These principles are applicable to most drugs without significant modification, and they result in linear mathematical models. Several assumptions are made when different or multiple doses are given:

- Drug clearance remains constant.
- Doubling the dose à doubled C and AUC.

These assumptions are not always accurate. With some drugs, giving a single low dose of the drug leads to the expected linear pharmacokinetics. However, when higher doses are given, or when the medication is taken chronically, the drug no longer fits the linear pharmacokinetic profile.

Figure 20-5: **Pharmacokinetic Relationships: Linear versus Nonlinear**

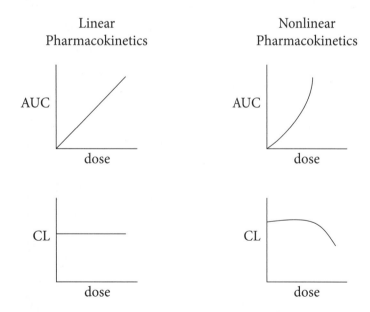

Nonlinear pharmacokinetics generally occur when one or more enzyme- or carrier-mediated systems are saturated. These systems are often referred to as capacity-limited.

- Active drug absorption: Absorption of riboflavin involves saturable gut wall transport
- Drug distribution: Saturable protein binding of salicylates
- Drug metabolism: Saturable metabolism of phenytoin
- Drug excretion: Active secretion of penicillin G

Most elimination processes can be saturated if enough drug is given. Certain drugs (phenytoin in particular) show nonlinear behavior even at normal drug doses.

For drugs exhibiting nonlinear behavior, dose increases lead to half-life increases, and AUC is not proportional to the amount of bioavailable drug. The behavior is described by the Michaelis-Menten equation:

$$\frac{dC}{dt} = \frac{V_{max} - C_{SS}}{K_M + C_{SS}}$$

V_{max} (the maximum elimination rate) and K_M (the Michaelis constant, equal to one-half the concentration at V_{max}) are dependent on both the drug and the enzyme system. Two general situations can apply:

- $C \gg K_m$; rate of change simplifies to V_{max}, a constant $\rightarrow$ zero-order kinetics
- $C \ll K_m$; rate of change is concentration dependent $\rightarrow$ first-order kinetics

In order to determine K_m and V_{max}, steady-state concentrations are measured as the result of two different doses given at different times. Recall that at steady-state, the rate of drug metabolism is assumed to be the same as the rate of drug input. In other words, the change in concentration over time is equal to the dosing rate (DR). As most nonlinear calculations that you will encounter involve phenytoin, remember that the salt factor (S) for phenytoin sodium is 0.92, and the dose must be multiplied by this number when the salt form (capsules and injection) is used.

$$DR = \frac{V_{max} - C_{SS}}{K_M \cdot C_{SS}}$$

K_m may be obtained in two ways:

1. Graph the data and obtain K_m from the slope.
2. Solve simultaneous equations using two dosing rates and respective C_{SS} (algebraic determination; see below).

$$DR_1 = V_{max} - Km \cdot \frac{DR_1}{C_{ss1}}$$

$$-(DR_2 = V_{max} - Km \cdot \frac{DR_2}{C_{ss2}})$$

Subtracting the second equation from the first, V_{max} will drop out and the equation can be solved for K_m.

V_{max} may be obtained in two ways as well:

1. Graph the data, and determine the y-intercept from the graph.
2. Use the dosing rate, C_{ss}, and the newly-calculated K_m to solve mathematically.

Graphical data, if available, is the faster way to obtain K_m and V_{max}.

Figure 20-6: **Graphical Determination of *K*_{*m*} and *V*_{*max*}**

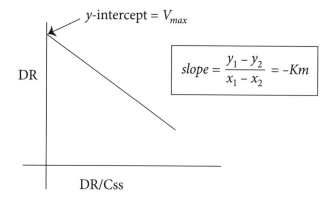

LEARNING POINTS

- Ninety percent of steady-state blood levels have been achieved after three half-lives; 97% after five half-lives.
- Increasing the infusion rate will lead to higher steady-state concentrations, but the drug will not reach steady state more quickly.
- The main parameters you should be able to calculate are half-life, k, CL, V_d, plasma concentration (simple cases), and R.
- When calculating loading doses, the tendency of drug to partition into fat must be considered when determining whether to use TBW or IBW for obese patients (use TBW for drugs that partition heavily into fat).
- Increasing the dose for nonlinear drugs such as phenytoin increases the half-life and can increase AUC above what would be expected for drugs exhibiting linear behavior. Pharmacokinetic monitoring is especially important in such cases.

PRACTICE QUESTIONS

1. A patient is being started on digoxin. What plasma level would you expect after a loading dose of 0.75 mg? Patient weight = 65 kg. V_d = 6 L/kg

   (A) 167 mcg/L
   (B) 2.6 mcg/L
   (C) 125 mcg/L
   (D) 1.95 mcg/L
   (E) 11.5 mcg/L

ANSWERS

1. **D**

Use $C = \dfrac{dose}{V_d} = \dfrac{0.75\ mg}{\dfrac{6L}{kg} \times 65\ kg} = \dfrac{1000\ mcg}{1\ mg} = \dfrac{1.95\ mcg}{L}$

Calculations

 Suggested Study Time: **60 minutes**

This section contains a quick review of the types of calculation questions likely to be covered on the NAPLEX. Practice is the key to this section, and there is only limited space for practice problems within this study guide. However, practice problems are readily available within pharmacy calculation textbooks.

If you do not have a textbook for your review, borrowing older editions from pharmacy libraries will be helpful—the techniques involved have not changed. Two suggestions are *Pharmaceutical Calculations* by Stoklosa and Allen, and *Pharmaceutical Calculations* by Zatz and Teixeria.

PROBLEM-SOLVING TECHNIQUES

Ratio-Proportion and Dimensional Analysis

There are two techniques that can be used to solve most pharmaceutical calculations: Ratio-proportion and dimensional analysis. Either of these techniques is acceptable, and you should use whichever one you fine most comfortable.

Ratio-proportion is a one-step calculation technique that is probably the easiest to use for simple (one- or two-step) calculations. In this process, you set up a likeness between a fraction involving known quantities and one that includes your unknown, and solve the equation by cross-multiplying. An example is given below, illustrating how to convert 3 fluid ounces to milliliters:

$$\frac{29.6\ mL}{1\ fl\ oz} = \frac{x\ mL}{3\ fl\ oz} \quad (29.6\ mL)(3\ fl\ oz) = (x\ mL)(1\ fl\ oz) \quad \frac{(29.6\ mL)(3\ fl\ oz)}{(1\ fl\ oz)} = x\ mL$$

While ratio-proportion is often the most intuitive method, and is something with which you have been familiar since early grades of school, it has no inherent error-checking and it is not ideal for multistep calculations. When using ratio-proportion for multi-step problems, you will have to write down intermediate steps; rounding intermediate answers reduces your accuracy, and writing them down takes time. Both of these can be problems when taking exams, so dimensional analysis might be preferred for these reasons.

Dimensional analysis is a technique, often used in chemistry and other sciences, which allows you to set up long calculations in a single step. Using the short example given above, the problem would be solved:

$$3 \, fl \, oz \, X \, \frac{(29.6 \, mL)}{(1 \, fl \, oz)} = 88.8 \, mL$$

As you can see, the fluid ounces cancel out and leave you with the correct units of milliliters. This serves as an internal error-check and is especially helpful in longer, more complex problems. Also, it saves you from having to write down intermediate steps, and helps prevent "kitchen-sink" syndrome (using every bit of information given, whether it will help solve the problem or not). Finally, it avoids the problem of rounding too early; you round once, when the problem is finished.

When you have completed a calculation, regardless of the method you choose, always ask yourself if the answer makes sense. You won't always be able to determine this, but in many cases you can tell if something has gone wrong in your calculation just by looking at the final answer. For example, it would be impractical to have an IV drip rate of 1,000 mL/min, or a dose rate of 52 tablets per day. If your answer doesn't make sense, check your calculation to find out where you went wrong.

Estimation

Estimation is not always appropriate; when working in pharmacy, you want the most accurate answer possible, especially when working with drugs with narrow therapeutic indices, or for dosing of infants and children. However, for exam purposes you will often be able to eliminate several, if not all, incorrect options by using estimates, particularly of some of the conversion factors listed in the upcoming section. This could allow you more time to focus on other portions of the exam. Use estimation with caution, however, especially if several foils are very similar to each other.

FUNDAMENTALS OF UNITS AND MEASUREMENT

The metric system is the standard system used for science worldwide. It is not, however, the only system used in pharmacy. The avoirdupois, or "common," system is the customary measure in the United States, and most patients will communicate with you in this system. Because of this, you will have to convert between systems of measurement. Unfortunately, cross-system conversions are inherently inexact. Convert from one system of measurement to another only once in a problem, not multiple times, and use the most direct conversion possible. Otherwise, the measurement error will be compounded.

A few key facts about systems of measurement are given below:

- Avoirdupois refers to solid measures only (pounds and ounces).
    » 1 pound = 16 ounces
- Common or household liquid measurements start with the teaspoon:
    » 3 teaspoons (tsp) = 1 tablespoon (T)
    » 2 T = 1 fluid ounce (fl oz) = 1/8 cup
    » 1 cup = 8 fl oz
    » 1 pint = 16 fl oz (or 2 cups)
    » 1 quart = 32 fl oz (or 4 cups)
    » 1 gallon = 128 fl oz (or 16 cups)
- Apothecary measures, the measures pharmacists originally used (drams, grains, and scruples), are no longer used.
    » Some medications (aspirin is one) were traditionally measured in grains, and you may still see strength listed this way; Roman numerals are used instead of Arabic (65 mg = 1 grain [gr]; a gr V aspirin tablet = 325 mg).
    » The apothecary system adopted the common or household liquid measurements of pint, quart, and gallon.
    » Note that the apothecary system has pounds and ounces. These are not the same size as avoirdupois pounds and ounces, and are seldom—if ever—used. The grain, however, is the same size in the avoirdupois and apothecary systems.

Some of the more common conversion factors are given below:

Avoirdupois System	Metric System
1 lb	454 g
2.2 lb	1 kg
1 oz	28.4 g
1 grain	64.8 mg

Apothecary System	Metric System
1 tsp	5 mL
1 T	15 mL
1 fl oz	29.6 mL (30 mL is an acceptable estimate)
1 cup	240 mL
1 pint	473 mL (30 mL/fl oz estimate is no longer exact enough)
1 quart	946 mL
1 gallon	3,785 mL (readjust for accuracy again)

DENSITY, SPECIFIC GRAVITY, AND SPECIFIC VOLUME

Density describes the relationship between the mass of a substance and the volume it occupies. This is a helpful concept in pharmacy, as it allows you to convert between measures of mass and measures of volume. This is most useful with liquid ingredients used in compounded formulations. In compounded recipes, you may see liquid amounts expressed as either weight or volume; and depending on the recipe and the equipment you have available, it might be easier to measure in one form over the other. For instance, viscous liquids might be hard to get out of a graduated cylinder, and if you don't have a dosing syringe in which to measure the liquid, it might be better to weigh the product in a weigh boat.

Density should be treated like a conversion factor, since you are converting between mass and volume. The following example will illustrate:

450 mL of phenol weighs 482.56 g. What is its density? Express your answer in g/mL.

$$\frac{482.56\,g\,phenol}{450\,mL} = 1.07\,g/mL$$

Specific gravity (SG) is a related concept, one that many pharmacy students find confusing. SG is simply the density of a substance relative to a reference substance (usually water). It is a unitless number, because it is equal to density divided by density—the units cancel out. Since water has a density of 1 g/mL, the SG will be numerically identical to the density expressed in g/mL. However, the SG of a substance is the same regardless of what units it was calculated from, so it allows you to compare the relative masses of equal volumes of substances. Also, some sources will list SG instead of density, so you need to be familiar with it to understand these sources. An example is given below:

150 mL of formaldehyde weighs 121.82 g. What is its specific gravity?

$$\frac{\dfrac{121.82\,g\;formaldehyde}{450\;mL}}{\dfrac{1\,g\;water}{1\;mL}} = 0.81$$

REDUCING AND ENLARGING FORMULAS

Most compounding formulas are for stock quantities, and how much the formula makes is rarely the amount you are actually wishing to prepare. However, it is simple to reduce or enlarge the formula to make the amount you need, provided you keep the ingredients in the same proportion with one another. In many ways, this is similar to doubling a recipe when you are cooking for a crowd. Compounding recipes come in two formats:

1. The amount of product produced is specified (formula makes 1,000 mL, for instance).

2. The quantity of each ingredient is specified, either in measured units or in parts. You figure out how much product will be made.

Say you wish to make 50 capsules from the following recipe:

> *Rx* *Ketoprofen 2.5 g*
> *Phenyltoloxamine citrate 6 g*
> *Caffeine 6 g*
> *Lactose 70.5 g*
>
> *M et div caps 200*

First of all, how many doses is this recipe for? "M et div" means "mix and divide," so the recipe is for the entire amount of capsules (200), not for a single capsule. What do you do now? You can either reduce each ingredient by the same proportion (which is easy to figure out but involves lots of writing) or create a single conversion factor and apply it to each ingredient. Since you want 50 capsules and your recipes makes 200, your conversion factor would be 50 capsules/200 capsules = 0.25. Multiplying each ingredient by 0.25 yields:

2.5 g ketoprofen × 0.25	= 0.625 g
6 g phenyltoloxamine citrate × 0.25	= 1.5 g
6 g caffeine × 0.25	= 1.5 g
70.5 g lactose × 0.25	= 17.625 g

This method also works well if you do not have enough of a particular ingredient in stock. Say you have only 4 g of caffeine and want to use the above recipe, which calls for 6 g. You can reduce the recipe to fit the amount of your limiting ingredient. Simply multiply each ingredient by the conversion factor of 4 g/6 g = 0.667.

If you have a recipe that does not have a total amount calculated, you will need to add up the amounts represented by each ingredient to find your total. Remember that you must add like to like, using density if needed in order to make sure that all amounts are specified in the same units (usually either g or mL)

Finally, some recipes are given in parts rather than measurements. If total parts are given (total is listed on the recipe, or one or more ingredients is listed as "qs" or "ad"):

- Set total parts to the amount you want to make
- Solve for the value of one part
- Multiply the size of one part by the number of parts for each ingredient

If total parts are not given:

- Add the number of parts for each ingredient to obtain the total number of parts in the recipe
- Proceed as above

Try this example:

Rx	Bacitracin	105 parts
	Neomycin	35 parts
	Polymyxin B	5 parts
	Petrolatum	qs 10,000 parts

Calculate the quantities of all ingredients to make 30 grams

In this case, 30 g/10,000 parts = 0.003

Multiplying this factor times the other ingredients gives:

105 parts bacitracin × 0.003 = 0.315 g = 315 mg
35 parts neomycin × 0.003 = 0.105 g = 105 mg
5 parts polymyxin B × 0.003 = 0.015 g = 15 mg

The petrolatum needed may be found by subtracting the masses of the other ingredients from the 30 total grams desired:

30 g total − 0.315 g bacitracin − 0.105 g neomycin − 0.015 g polymyxin B = 29.565 g petrolatum

PERCENTAGE AND RATIO STRENGTHS

Since drugs are administered as dosage forms that contain more than just the active ingredient, the amount of the active ingredient needs to be expressed. There are several ways to do this:

- Amount per individual dosage form (capsule, tablet, suppository)
- Concentration per dosing volume (oral liquids, certain topical products)
- Percent
- Ratio strength
- Parts per million or billion

Percent describes the number of parts of active relative to 100 parts of the total. In pharmacy, simply stating % is incomplete; you must attach the appropriate descriptor from the following list:

- % w/w: g of active per 100 g of product
- % w/v: g of active per 100 mL of product
- % v/v: mL of active per 100 mL of product

You may also see concentrations expressed in milligram percent. In this case, the amount in the numerator, usually assumed to be in grams, is expressed in milligrams instead: 0.001% w/w = 1 mg% w/w. This value is the same as mg/dL, a commonly used unit in some blood tests (such as serum glucose).

Ratio strength is another way of expressing concentration, in terms of parts of active related to any number of parts of the whole. Ratio strength is usually expressed in terms of 1 part of active relative to the total number of parts of the product, as opposed to percent, which is any number of parts of active relative to 100 parts of product. For example, 5% means 5 parts per 100, or 5:100, or 1:20. Ratio strength is used for low-concentration solutions, and triturations of high-potency powders (e.g., 1:75 trituration of estradiol).

Express 1 g of epinephrine in 1 L of solution as a percent strength and as a ratio strength:

$$\frac{1\,g\,epinephrine}{1{,}000\,mL} \times \frac{100\,mL\,product}{g\,active} = 0.1\%\ w/v\ \text{or}\ 1{:}1{,}000$$

Using another example:

How much sodium benzoate do you need to preserve 10 L of a solution at a concentration of 1:10,000?

$$\frac{1\,g\,sodium\,benzoate}{10{,}000\,mL} \times \frac{1000\,mL}{1L} \times 10L = 1g$$

Parts per million (ppm) is a special case of ratio strength. Instead of fixing the numerator as 1, in this case you fix the denominator constant as 1,000,000. Parts per billion (ppb) and trillion (ppt) are handled in the analogous fashion. These are used to express very small concentrations; for example, the EPA action level for lead in drinking water is 15 ppb (or 0.015 mg/L).

DOSAGE CALCULATIONS

Pharmacists frequently need to calculate the size of a dose or total amount of medication to dispense, even for noncompounded prescriptions. The following general equation applies:

Number of doses × size of dose = total amount

Example:

How many milliliters of a liquid medicine would provide a patient with 2 teaspoonfuls three times a day for 7 days?

$$2\ tsp \times \frac{3\ doses}{day} \times 7\ days \times \frac{5\ mL}{tsp} = 210mL$$

DILUTION, CONCENTRATION, AND ALLIGATION

In some cases, you may receive a prescription in which you need to either dilute a product you have on hand or make a product more concentrated. These problems can generally be solved by:

1. Using the equation: (quantity) × (concentration) = (quantity) × (concentration)
2. Determining the quantity of active ingredient needed and then calculating the quantity of the available solution (usually a concentrated stock solution), which will provide the needed amount of active

When some ingredients are given as ratio strength, you should convert them to percentage strength before setting up the proportion. Whenever proportional parts enter the calculation, you should reduce them to their lowest terms before beginning (i.e., reduce 75 parts:25 parts to 3 parts:1 part). In both cases, this will simplify your calculations. Example:

If 250 mL of a 15% v/v solution of methyl salicylate in alcohol are diluted to 1,500 mL, what will be the percentage strength?

250 mL × 15% = 1,500 mL × X%   X = 2.5% v/v

Stock Solutions

Stock solutions are strong solutions of known concentration that allow the pharmacist to conveniently prepare weaker solutions. They are generally prepared on a w/v basis and their concentration is expressed as a ratio strength. Example:

How many milliliters of a 1% stock solution of certified red dye should be used in preparing 2,000 mL of an antiseptic that is to contain 1:5,000 of the certified red dye as a coloring agent?

First, how many grams of red dye are needed in the 2,000 mL of antiseptic solution?

$$\frac{1g\ red\ dye}{5000\ mL} \times 2,000\ mL\ antiseptic\ solution = 0.2g$$

Next, how much of the 1% stock solution of red dye contains this amount of dye?

$$0.2g \times \frac{100\ mL}{1g\ red\ dye} = 20\ mL$$

Alligation

Alligation is a method of solving problems that involve mixing multiple products that have different percentage strengths. Two types of alligation exist: Alligation medial and alligation alternate.

Alligation medial

This method allows the calculation of the weighted average percentage strength of a mixture of two or more substances of known quantity and strength. The technique is best shown via illustration:

What is the percentage strength (v/v) of alcohol in a mixture of 3,000 mL of 40% (v/v) alcohol, 1,000 mL of 60% (v/v) alcohol, and 1,000 mL of 70% (v/v) alcohol?

$$40 \times 3,000 = 120,000$$
$$60 \times 1,000 = 60,000$$
$$70 \times 1,000 = 70,000$$
$$\text{Totals: } 5,000 = 250,000$$

$$250,000 / 5,000 = 50\%\ (v/v)$$

Alligation alternate

This method allows calculation of the number of parts of two or more components of a given strength when they are mixed to prepare a mixture of a desired strength. Crosswise subtraction is used to determine the amounts needed of each component. This method can be used regardless of how concentration is expressed (mg/mL, ratio, parts, %). Example:

In what proportion should 20% benzocaine ointment be mixed with an ointment base to produce a 2.5% w/w benzocaine ointment?

Since there is no active drug in the ointment base, its strength can be expressed as 0%.

Strengths to Be Mixed	Desired	Difference in Strength Mixed (crosswise subtraction of absolute values)
20%		2.5 parts (2.5–0) of 20% ointment
	2.5%	
0%		17.5 parts (20 – 2.5) of ointment base

So 2.5 parts of the 20% w/w ointment should be added to 17.5 parts of the ointment base. Remember that the values are subtracted crosswise, but the identities of the substances are read across.

ELECTROLYTE SOLUTIONS

Electrolyte solutions are frequently prescribed for patients who have lost an essential ion through disease, as they play a critical role in maintaining normal body function. Sometimes the necessary amount of the appropriate salt will be stated on the prescription, but often the prescription will ask for a quantity of the needed ion in chemical units, and the pharmacist will need to calculate how much of the salt will contain the desired amount. Milliequivalents are the most common unit used.

Millimoles and Milliequivalents

A review of several chemistry concepts will be useful before beginning milliequivalent calculations.

- Moles (mol): Measurement of the amount of a substance; Avogadro's number of particles (6.023×10^{23})
- Atomic weight: Found on the periodic table; 1 mol of that atom weighs that many grams (also, 1 mmol of that atom weighs that many mg)
- Molecular weight (MW): The sum of all the atomic weights for all of the atoms in the molecule. 1 mol of the molecule weighs MW g; 1 mmol weight MW mg.
- Molar solution: 1 mol of solute in 1 L of solution
  - » Stock solutions often expressed this way
  - » 0.1 M = 0.1 mol of solute/1 L solution

What is the molar concentration of a 5% w/v $MgCl_2$ solution? MW $MgCl_2$ = 95.

$$\frac{1mol\ MgCl_2}{95g\ MgCl_2} \times \frac{5g\ MgCl_2}{100mL} \times \frac{1000mL}{1L} = 0.53mol/L = 0.53M$$

What if you are interested in moles of atoms instead of moles of molecules? In this case, you need to look at the molecular formula. If there is more than one of an atom in a molecule (such as the chloride in the example above), you need to adjust your formula. In that example, you have 1 mol of $MgCl_2$, which contains 1 mol of Mg^{+2} and 2 mol of Cl^-. If you don't have a molecular formula, you can figure one out by balancing charges, provided you know the valencies of the ions involved. In the magnesium chloride example, Mg^{+2} is divalent; it takes two Cl^- to make as much negative charge as one Mg^{+2}. Therefore, the correct formula is $MgCl_2$, not MgCl. NaCl, however, is made up of two monovalent ions, so the charges are equal.

Electrolytes are commonly prescribed in terms of equivalents rather than mass. What does this mean? One mol of hydrogen has 1 mol of positive charge. One equivalent of an ion is the amount required to replace (in positively charged ions) or react with (in negatively charged ions) 1 mol of hydrogen. Monovalent ions (Cl^-, Na^+, K^+, NH_4^+, OH^-) therefore have 1 Eq/mol. Divalent ions like Ca^{+2} are 2 Eq/mol, as it takes 2 mol of hydrogen to replace the charge carried by 1 mol of calcium. Example:

How much potassium citrate powder would we weigh to compound 1 dose of the following prescription?

> Rx   Potassium citrate, 20 mEq of K^+, tid

Recall that potassium has a valence of +1 and citrate has a –3, so the formula must be $K_3(C_6H_5O_7)$ MW = 324.41 mg/mmol.

$$20mEq\ K^+ \times \frac{1mmol\ K^+}{1mEq\ K^+} \times \frac{1mmol\ K_3(C_6H_5O_7)}{3mmol\ K^+} \times \frac{324.41mg\ K^+}{mmol\ K^+} =$$

$$\frac{g}{1000mg} = 2/16g\ K_3(C_6H_5O_7)$$

Be very careful with labeling when performing milliequivalent calculations! Millimoles of ions do not necessarily equal millimoles of molecules.

Osmolarity and Isotonicity

Osmotic pressure is the pressure that exists across a semipermeable membrane due to the free movement of solvent but not solute. Because cell membranes are semipermeable, this concept is important in patients. When administering parenteral drugs, you must balance the osmolarity of your medication with the osmolarity of the body. If not, tissue damage, pain, and possibly death can result due to cells swelling or shrinking with the movement of solvent.

Solutions are considered isotonic when each one has the same osmotic pressure; in pharmacy and medicine, the reference solution is the plasma (280–300 mOsm/L). Hypertonic solutions have higher osmotic pressure than this; hypotonic solutions have lower osmotic pressure. Some other facts you should remember about osmotic pressure are:

- It is a colligative property, based on the number of particles in solution.
- It can be calculated directly, using dissociation constants.
    - » NaCl dissociates 80% in aqueous solution.
    - » For every 100 particles, 80 will have dissociated (making 160 particles) and 20 will not → 180 particles.

$$\frac{180 \ particles \ after \ dissociation}{100 \ particles \ before \ dissociation} = 1.8 = i$$

- It can be calculated by its effect on other colligative properties, including freezing point, boiling point, and vapor pressure.
    - » All colligative properties vary together.
    - » A solution with the same freezing point as a reference solution will have the same osmolarity as that reference solution.

Try this example:

A solute dissociates 50% in aqueous solution. Assuming each molecule of the solute dissociates into two parts, give the dissociation constant (i).

$$\frac{100 \ dissociated \ dissociation + 50 \ undissociated \ particles}{100 \ undissociated \ particles} = 1.5$$

You can use the ratio form of the dissociation constant as a conversion factor. If $i = 1.5$, 1 mol = 1.5 Osm, and 1 mmol = 1.5 mOsm.

Try another example: Calculate the osmolarity of NS in mOsm/L.

NS = normal saline = 0.9% w/v NaCl in water
MW NS = 58.5
$i = 1.8$

$$\frac{0.9g \ NaCl}{100 \ mL} \times \frac{1 \ mol}{58.5g \ NaCl} \times \frac{1000 \ mmol}{mol} \times \frac{1.8 \ mOsm}{mmol} \times \frac{1000 \ mL}{L} = 276.9 \ mOsm/L$$

Because NS is nearly isotonic with plasma, it is useful for comparison. If we know that a product is isotonic to NS, it will be isotonic to body fluids as well. Sodium chloride equivalents are therefore useful, and are for expression of the amount of NaCl it would take to exert the tonic effect of a particular active ingredient. Some baseline assumptions are:

- The tonic effects of solutes are additive and independent.
- The total tonic effect in the solution is the sum of the effect of each solute,.

The following steps can be followed when adjusting tonicity:

1. Determine how much NaCl it would take to exert the tonic effect already seen in the solution.
2. Calculate how much NaCl is required to make the solution isotonic if NaCl is the sole tonicity agent. Compare this to the amount already present (Step 1). Proceed only if the total amount of NaCl equivalent already present is less than the amount needed (i.e., solution is currently hypotonic).
3. Amount needed = Goal amount – Amount you already have
   a. If adjusting tonicity with NaCl, use amount in step 3.
   b. If adjusting tonicity with another substance, figure out how much of your substance is needed to deliver the required tonic effect, using the E value (1 g of substance has the same tonic effect as E g of NaCl).

If one of your ingredients is already isotonic, you can disregard that volume as you calculate your values.

For example, how much boric acid (E = 0.52) should be added to make 15 mL of a 3% w/v pilocarpine HCl (E = 0.24) eyedrop solution isotonic?

Following the steps given above:

1. $\dfrac{3\,g\,pilocarpine}{100\,mL} \times 15\,mL = 0.45\,g\,pilocarpine$

   $0.45\,g\,pilocarpine \times \dfrac{0.24\,g\,NaCl(eq)}{1\,g\,pilocarpine} = 0.108\,g\,NaCl(eq)$

2. $\dfrac{0.9\,g\,NaCl}{100\,mL} \times 15\,mL = 0.135\,g\,NaCl$

3. $0.135\,g - 0.108\,g = 0.027\,g\,NaCl$

   $0.027\,g\,NaCl \times \dfrac{1\,g\,boric\,acid}{0.52\,g\,NaCl(eq)} = 0.05192\,g = 0.52\,g\,boric\,acid$

Another way to describe and calculate osmolarity and isotonicity is freezing-point depression. As mentioned above, this is a colligative property that varies along with other colligative properties of a solution. Some things to remember:

- Plasma freezes at −0.52°C.

- Solutions isotonic to plasma (such as NS) will also freeze at −0.52°C.

- Pure water freezes at 0°C. Therefore, an amount of solute that will make the solution isotonic depresses the freezing point by 0.52°C.

Given the following prescription, how much NaCl must be added to make the solution isotonic? The freezing point of a 1% w/v solution of procaine HCl is −0.122°C.

Rx	Procaine HCl	2% w/v
	NaCl	qs
	Sterile water	qs 30 mL

First, what would be the effect of a 2% w/v solution?

$$\frac{1.22°C}{1\%} \times 2\% = 0.244°C$$

Since the desired freezing point − The depression from the ingredients already in the formulation = The additional depression needed:

$$-0.52°C - (-0.244°C) = -0.276°C$$

So, the required concentration of sodium chloride is:

$$-0.276°C \, \frac{0.9\% \, NaCl}{-0.52°C} = 0.48\% \, NaCl \quad \text{or}$$

$$-30 \, mL \, \frac{0.48 \, g \, NaCl}{100 \, g \, NaCl} = 0.144 \, g \, NaCl$$

COMPOUNDING CALCULATIONS

Use of Prefabricated Dosage Forms in Compounding

When compounding, the source of active ingredient will often be prefabricated dosage forms (tablets, capsules, ointments). When performing such calculations, it is important to remember that if your calculation determines that you need 1.3 tablets as your source drug, you must actually crush 2 tablets and then weigh out a proportional amount of the resultant powder. Remember, a tablet contains far more ingredients than just the drug, so take that into account in your calculations.

> Rx   *Aspirin*   *300 mg*
>   *Lactose*   *qs*
>
> *M.ft. cap DTD #60*

Using 325-mg aspirin tablets (weighing 430 mg each) as the source drug, how many tablets are needed to compound this prescription? How much of the crushed powder should be weighed out?

$$300 \, mg \, ASA \times 60 \, capsules \times \frac{ASA \, tablet}{325 \, mg \, ASA} = 55.38 \, tablets \rightarrow 56 \, tablets$$

$$55.38 \, tablets \times 430 \, mg \, total \, tablet \, weight = 23.813 \, g \, required \, (of \, 24.08 \, g \, produced)$$

Suppository Calculations

The density factor method is often used when preparing suppositories. The density factor expresses the relationship between the mass of an ingredient and the volume of suppository base it displaces. Therefore, a drug will have a different density factor in each suppository base.

$$density \, factor = \frac{weight \, of \, drug}{weight \, of \, base \, displaced}$$

If a pharmacist needs to prepare six 30-mg phenobarbital suppositories in cocoa butter, how many grams each of cocoa butter and phenobarbital should be weighed? Density factor of phenobarbital in cocoa butter is 1.2. Blank suppositories (base only) weigh 2 g.

If one suppository contains 30 mg drug (0.03 g), it will replace:

$$\frac{0.03 \, g \, drug}{1.2 \, g} = 0.025 \, g \, cocoa \, butter$$

2 g – 0.025 g = 1.975 g cocoa butter / suppository × 6 suppositories = 11.85 g cocoa butter

0.025 g × 6 suppositories = 0.15 g phenobarbital

Reconstitution Calculations

Some medications, particularly antibiotics for oral suspension or parenteral use, come as powders for reconstitution. While the container or package will include instructions for reconstitution, including what and how much diluent to use, occasionally the prescriber will need to manipulate the final concentration of the drug. Some simple calculations can help you make these adjustments to provide a more dilute or concentrated product. First, a simple example:

Cefadroxil powder for oral suspension comes in a strength of 250 mg/5 mL. The reconstitution instructions are to add 70 mL of purified water to yield a final solution volume of 100 mL. How many grams of cefadroxil powder are in the bottle?

$$\frac{250 \, mg \, cefadroxil}{5 \, mL \, suspension} \times 100 \, mL = 5000 \, mg = 5 \, g$$

There are a few interesting things to pay attention to here. First, this is an easy example of a question that gives more information than you need to solve the problem (while the 70 mL is necessary for reconstitution, it is not needed to answer this particular question). Be sure to pay attention and use the correct numbers when extra information is given. Second, if you add only 70 mL of water, how do you get 100 mL of total suspension? The powder takes up space in the final product. This volume is called the powder volume: It is a calculated quantity, not corresponding to the physical volume. The powder volume may be greater than, equal to, or less than zero, depending on the drug and the way it was prepared.

When preparing a final concentration that is different from the package directions, you must first calculate the powder volume. The powder volume is equal to the difference between the diluent volume and the final solution volume. Take the following case:

    Rx   *Biaxin 100 mg/5 mL suspension*
            Sig: 1 tsp PO q 12 hr × 10 days

Biaxin comes as a powder for reconstitution with instructions to prepare a final concentration of 125 mg/5 mL by adding 55 mL diluent to make a final volume of 100 mL. The amount of active ingredient in the bottle is 2,500 mg, and the powder volume = total volume – diluent, so 100 mL – 55 mL = 45 mL.

$$2500 \, mg \, Biaxin \, \frac{5 \, mL}{100 \, mg \, Biaxin} = 125 \, mL \, total$$

$$125 \, mL \, total - PV = 125 \, mL - 45 \, mL = 80 \, mL$$

Adding 80 mL of diluent will produce 125 mL of solution with a concentration of 100 mg/5 mL.

Drip Rate Calculations

IV medications are regulated by one of the following methods:

- Drip chambers
    - » Deliver drops of defined volume.
    - » Flow is adjusted by the nurse to a set number of *whole* drops per minute (gH).
    - » Standard sets are 10 gtt/mL or 15 gtt/mL.
    - » Pediatric and critical care drugs may use microdrop infusion sets: 60 gtt/mL.
- Infusion pumps
    - » Deliver a rate of mL/hr.
    - » Round to the nearest 0.1 mL.

17 mL of concentrated vancomycin solution is added to a 100-mL piggyback bag of NS. This solution is to be infused over 1 hour. What is the infusion rate?

$$\frac{17\,mL\;vancomycin + 100\,mL\;NS}{60\;min} = 117\,mL/60\;min = 117\,mL/hr$$

What is the infusion rate in drops/min if the drug is administered using an infusion set that delivers 10 gtt/mL?

$$\frac{117\,mL}{60\;min} \times \frac{10\,gtt}{mL} = 19.5\,gtt/min = 20\,gtt/min$$

Nutrition Calculations

Total parenteral nutrition (TPN) calculations involve many of the calculation techniques described throughout this chapter. Since electrolytes are commonly given via TPN, milliequivalent calculations may be useful. They also supply fluid, calories, essential fatty acids, and vitamins. One example is given below:

Glycerin is sometimes used as an alternative energy source in TPN formulations and produces 4.32 kcal of energy per gram. Given a commercial stock solution of electrolytes, amino acids, and 3% w/v glycerin, how many calories are present in 200 mL of this stock solution?

$$200\,mL \times \frac{3\,g\;glycerin}{100\,ml} \times 4.32\,kcal/g = 26\,kcal$$

LEARNING POINTS

- Always perform a "sanity" check on your answer. Does it make practical sense? If not, recheck your numbers.

- Remember crucial conversion factors (or at least approximations of these): 1 fluid oz = 30 mL, 2.2 lb/kg (*not* the reverse; remember, your weight is always a smaller number when measured in kilograms; if you get an answer to the contrary, you flipped your conversion).

- Valence of a molecule is equal to the total number of negative charges *or* the total number of positive charges, not the two numbers added together.

- When using prefabricated dosage forms as a drug source, fractions of a dosage form must always be rounded up to the next nearest whole.

- Drops must be rounded to the nearest whole drop. You cannot measure partials.

PRACTICE QUESTIONS

1. How many milliliters of water should be mixed with 240 mL of syrup containing 85% w/v sucrose to make a syrup containing 60% w/v sucrose?

   (A) 80 mL
   (B) 100 mL
   (C) 160 mL
   (D) 240 mL
   (E) 340 mL

2. If 10 mL of a solution are to contain 3 mEq of sodium ion, how many 1-g sodium chloride (MW 58.5) tablets would be required to compound 250 mL of solution?

   (A) 2
   (B) 3
   (C) 4
   (D) 5
   (E) 6

3. You have been asked to prepare 500 mL of a benzalkonium chloride solution. The concentration of the solution you prepare must be such that if 20 mL of your solution are diluted to a liter, a 1:1,470 solution is formed. How many milliliters of a 17% benzalkonium chloride solution will you need to compound the solution?

   (A) 17 mL
   (B) 20 mL
   (C) 100 mL
   (D) 147 mL
   (E) 500 mL

4. A pharmacist has 75 grams of 3% w/w zinc oxide paste in stock, to which she adds 5 g of pure zinc oxide. What is the percent concentration of zinc oxide in the final product?

   (A) 2.4% w/w
   (B) 3% w/w
   (C) 7.25% w/w
   (D) 9.06% w/w
   (E) 9.67% w/w

ANSWERS

1. **B**

$$240\,mL \times \frac{85\,g\ sucrose}{100\,mL} = 204\,g\ sucrose$$

$$204\,g\ sucrose \times \frac{100\,mL}{60\,g\ sucrose} = 340\,mL\ total\ volume$$

340 mL total volume – 240 mL 85% w/v sucrose syrup = 100 mL of water to add

2. **D**

$$250\,mL \times \frac{3\,mEq\ Na^+}{10\,mL} \times \frac{1\,mmol\ Na^+}{1\,mEq\ Na^+} \times \frac{1\,mmol\ NaCl}{1\,mmol\ Na^+} \times \frac{58.5\,mg\ NaCl}{1\,mmol\ NaCl} \times$$

$$\frac{1\,g}{1000\,mg} \times \frac{1\,tablet}{1\,g} = 4.4\,tabs = 5\,tabs$$

If you are using a partial tablet, you must always round up. If you use 4.4 tablets, you will actually expend 5 tablets from inventory, use 4.4 for your product, and discard the remainder of the fifth tablet.

3. **C**

Final solution: 1 L of 1:1,470 BC $1000\,mL \times \frac{1\,g\ BC}{1470\,mL} = 0.68\,g\ BC$

This solution was produced by diluting 20 mL of the solution you made. Therefore, the solution you made has 0.68 g of BC in every 20 mL.

$$500\,mL \times \frac{0.68\,g\ BC}{20\,mL} = 17\,g\ of\ BC$$

You need 17 g of benzalkonium chloride. How many milliliters of a 17% w/v stock solution will be required to deliver 17 g?

$$17\,g \times \frac{100\,mL}{17\,g} = 100\,mL\ stock\ solution$$

4. **D**

$$75\,g\ ung \times \frac{3\,g\ ZnO}{100\,g\ ung} = 2.25\,g\ ZnO$$

$$\frac{(2.25 + 5)\,g\ ZnO}{(75 + 5)\,g\ ung} = \frac{7.25\,g\ ZnO}{80\,g\ ung} = \frac{9.0625\,g\ ZnO}{100\,g\ ung} = 9.0626\%\ w/w$$

Biostatistics

 Suggested Study Time: **15 minutes**

Statistics play an important role in the development and interpretation of clinical trials. The following section covers the most important definitions in biostatistics, and discusses various statistical tests, when to use them, and how to interpret them.

GENERAL STATISTICAL DEFINITIONS

The table below lists several general statistical definitions with which you should be familiar.

General Statistical Definitions

Measures of center	Mean	Average value of a sample distribution
	Median	Value that lies closest to the center of a sample distribution
	Mode	Most commonly occurring number in a sample distribution
Estimates of variability	Range	Difference between the smallest and largest values in a sample distribution
	Standard deviation	Average of the distances between each value in a distribution and the mean of the distribution Most widely used estimate of variability
Hypotheses	Hypothesis	Theoretical statement that the study is intended to test
	Null hypothesis	States that there is no difference between the study and control groups
	Alternative hypothesis	States that the null hypothesis is incorrect; there is a difference between the study and control groups

Variables	Independent variable	Known variable(s)
	Dependent variable	Variable with a value dependent upon the value of an independent variable
Error	Type I Error	Rejecting a true null hypothesis: Finding a difference between the study and control groups that does not exist
	Type II Error	Accepting a false null hypothesis: Failing to detect a difference between the study and control groups that does exist
Tests	Parametric	Requires prior knowledge of the nature of the data under examination; data must fall under a normal (Gaussian) distribution and be measured on an interval or a ratio scale
	Non-parametric	Does not require prior knowledge of the distribution of the observations; data need not follow a normal or Gaussian distribution
Miscellaneous definitions	Accuracy	Measure of how close a measured value is to the expected value
	Precision	Measure of how close a particular measured value is to the other values in a set of measurements; does not imply proximity between measured values and the expected value
	Sample	Data set taken under homogenous conditions; a subset of a population
	Population	Entire group from which a sample is taken
	Gaussian (or normal) distribution	A bell-shaped distribution Given a large enough sample size, the Central Limit Theorem states that the distribution of means will follow this type of distribution even if the population is not Gaussian. • 69% of values fall within ± 1 SD of the mean • 95% of values fall within ± 2 SD of the mean • 98% of values fall within ± 3 SD of the mean

Several additional statistical concepts are included below, in slightly greater detail. Many of these concepts apply regardless of the statistical test chosen.

P-value and Statistical Significance

The p-value is the probability that the difference measured between your study group and the control group is the result of random chance rather than a true difference. The p-value is expressed as a value between 0 and 1.

The null hypothesis may be rejected if there is a sufficiently small probability that it is true. A significance level (or α) of 0.05 is most commonly chosen, although it should be chosen based on the relative consequences of making a Type I or Type II error in the particular study setting. When a 0.05 significance level is chosen, if $p \leq 0.05$, a statistically significant difference in treatment effect exists between the control and treatment groups. If $p > 0.05$, the results of the study are considered to be not statistically significant, meaning no difference exists between the treatment and control groups. Choosing a larger significance level, like $p = 0.1$, gives a higher probability of rejecting a true null hypothesis (Type I error, or false positive test).

Confidence Intervals

A confidence interval (CI) is the interval, computed from sample data, such that there is a given probability that the population mean value of the unknown parameter is contained within the interval. Ninety-five percent CI is the most common interval seen, but others may be calculated as well. Wider intervals (such as 99% CI) have a higher probability of containing the population mean; however, they also span more values.

Power

No discussion of statistical significance is complete without a discussion of statistical power. Two factors affect power:

- Sample size
- Amount of variation within the groups (i.e., standard deviation)

Low power may result in Type II errors, where a "not statistically significant" result is obtained even though there truly is a difference between the treatment and control groups. If necessary, the power of a study may be increased by studying more subjects, although there are practical and economic limits on study size. It is not appropriate to conclude that a treatment is ineffective based only on a study with insufficient power.

Correlation

Correlation measures the degree of a linear relationship between two variables. Correlation is often represented by the correlation coefficient (r), which can range in value from –1 to +1. A correlation coefficient of 0 indicates no linear relationship between variables. A coefficient of –1 reflects a perfect inverse relationship between variables, while a value of +1 reflects a perfect direct relationship. A key point to remember is that an observed correlation between two variables does not imply that there is a causal link between the two variables. For example, warm weather causes an increase in both the crime rate and the incidence of sunburn. Crime rate and sunburn incidence will therefore be positively correlated; however, crime does not cause sunburn and sunburn does not cause crime.

Another important point to consider is that correlation coefficient assumes a normal distribution of measured values; if this assumption is incorrect, the coefficient is not relevant.

STATISTICAL TEST SELECTION

The first thing that must be done when determining what statistical test should be employed is to identify the dependent variable and the scale of measurement that will be used for this variable. The scale of measurement may be numeric, ordinal, or nominal.

Tests Appropriate for Numerical Scales of Measurement

Numeric scales (also called interval or ratio scales) of measurement are used when the measured values are numbers. Examples include height, weight, or blood pressure level. When the data follows a Gaussian distribution, parametric statistical tests should be used.

- Two independent groups: T-test
- Two dependent groups: Paired t-test
- Three or more independent groups: Analysis of variance (ANOVA)
- Three or more dependent groups: Repeated measures ANOVA

When the data does not follow a Gaussian distribution, the same tests used for ordinal data should be employed.

Tests Appropriate for Ordinal Scales of Measurement

Ordinal scales of measurement are used when characteristics have an underlying order to their values but the numbers used are arbitrary (such as Likert scales). Various non-parametric tests (such as Mann-Whitney U and Wilcoxon Signed-Rank) are used for analyzing such data.

Tests Appropriate for Nominal Scales of Measurement

Nominal scales are used for characteristics that do not have numerical value (such as gender or race). The Chi-square test and its variants are used to test the null hypothesis that proportions are equal, or that factors or characteristics are not associated with each other.

Finally, Kaplan-Meier is a frequently used statistical test that analyzes patient survival time. Probability of death is recalculated every time a trial subject dies. This method is similar to actuarial analysis in the insurance industry; although, unlike actuarial analysis, Kaplan-Meier gives exact survival proportions because it uses exact survival times instead of group approximations.

LEARNING POINTS

- Smaller p-values associated with a statement reflect a greater likelihood that the statement accurately reflects a difference between groups. Larger p-values mean that the difference detected between groups is more likely to have been due to random chance.

- Power is the ability of a study to detect an actual effect. Power can be increased by increasing the number of patients enrolled in a study. Inadequate power may result in a study failing to detect a difference that actually exists between groups.

- The mean is the numerical average of the entire range of data; the mode is the central point in the data distribution. In a pure Gaussian distribution, the median will be equal or very close to the mode; large variance between median and mode may reflect non-Gaussian distribution or significant outlying data.

- ANOVA and t-tests are appropriate only for numeric data in a Gaussian distribution. Nonparametric tests are appropriate for numeric data in a non-Gaussian distribution, as well as for ordinal data. Chi-square tests should be used for nominal data.

PRACTICE QUESTIONS

1. The median value of a data set is the

    (A) mathematical average of all the values in the data set.
    (B) value equidistant from the extremes of a distribution.
    (C) average of the difference between each value in the set and the mean.
    (D) most commonly occurring value in the data set.
    (E) distance between the smallest and largest values in the data set.

ANSWERS

1. **B**

The median value is the value equidistant from the extremes of the data set. The mathematical average of the values in the data set (A) is the mean. The average of the difference between each value and the mean (C) is the standard deviation. The most commonly occurring value in the data set (D) is the mode. The distance between the smallest and largest values in the data set (E) is the range.

Part Four

Resources and Policy

Drug Information

 23

This chapter provides an overview of common tertiary literature resources that can be used as drug information resources for pharmacists.

Suggested Study Time: **30 minutes**

GENERAL DRUG INFORMATION RESOURCES

American Hospital Formulary Service (AHFS) Drug Information (published by the American Society of Health-System Pharmacists [ASHP])

- Provides FDA-approved and off-label uses
- Each monograph contains general drug information (e.g., pharmacology, pharmacokinetics, side effects, toxicology, drug interactions, dosing, administration, available preparations)

Drug Facts and Comparisons

- Provides information on:
  - » Prescription/over-the-counter (OTC) drugs
  - » Investigational/orphan drugs
- Each monograph contains general drug information
- Also provides helpful comparison tables

United States Pharmacopeia Drug Information (USP DI)

- Volume I: Drug Information for the Healthcare Professional
  - » Provides general drug information
  - » Various appendices (poison control centers, drug-induced side effects, selected therapeutic guidelines, drug identification color inserts)

- Volume II: Advice for the Patient: Drug Information in Lay Language
  - » Provides supplemental information for patient counseling
- Volume III: Approved Drug Products and Legal Requirements
  - » Provides information on therapeutic equivalence (contains FDA Orange Book), labeling/storage/packaging requirements, and pharmacy law

Physicians' Desk Reference (PDR)

- Contains FDA-approved package insert information
- Also contains a colored insert (for drug identification) and manufacturer information

Drug Information Handbook (Lexi-Comp)

- Provides general drug information
- Contains useful charts, tables, and treatment algorithms
- Also available in specialty versions (pediatrics, geriatrics, psychiatric, oncology)

Red Book

- Provides the following information on prescription and OTC drugs:
  - » Cost data (average wholesale price [AWP])
  - » National Drug Code (NDC) numbers
  - » Formulations available (dosage forms, sugar-free/alcohol-free preparations)
  - » Drug identification (colored inserts)
  - » Manufacturer

PHARMACOTHERAPY RESOURCES

Pharmacotherapy: A Pathophysiologic Approach (DiPiro)

- Provides the following information regarding various disease states: Pathophysiology, etiology, clinical presentation, diagnosis, treatment

Applied Therapeutics: The Clinical Use of Drugs (Koda-Kimble)

- Focuses on treatment of disease states
- Case-based format

INTERNAL MEDICINE RESOURCES

Harrison's Principles of Internal Medicine

- Focuses on pathophysiology, etiology, clinical presentation, and diagnosis
- Provides an overview of treatment; does not provide detailed information on drugs or dosing recommendations

Cecil Textbook of Medicine

- Not as comprehensive as Harrison's

Merck Manual of Diagnosis and Therapy

- Provides a quick summary of disease-state information (etiology, pathophysiology, clinical presentation, diagnosis, prognosis, treatment)

DRUG INTERACTION RESOURCES

Hansten and Horn's Drug Interaction Analysis and Management

- Provides the following information on drug interactions: Summary of interaction, proposed mechanism, significance, risk factors, treatment options

Drug Interaction Facts (published by Facts and Comparisons)

- Provides similar information as *Hansten and Horn's*

ADVERSE DRUG REACTION RESOURCES

Meyler's Side Effects of Drugs

- Provides critical review of literature regarding drugs' side effects: Effects on organ systems, interference with lab/diagnostic tests, withdrawal, and overdose

PARENTERAL DRUG COMPATIBILITY/STABILITY RESOURCES

Handbook on Injectable Drugs (published by ASHP)

- Previously known as Trissel's
- Provides information regarding compatibility/stability of parenteral drugs
- Also provides information on commercially available dosages, volumes, and sizes

King Guide to Parenteral Admixtures

- Provides similar information as *Handbook on Injectable Drugs*

PHARMACOLOGY RESOURCES

Goodman & Gilman's: The Pharmacological Basis of Therapeutics

- "Gold standard" pharmacology reference
- Provides very thorough discussion of the pharmacology of drugs; also provides information on the drugs' pharmacokinetics, pharmacodynamics, and toxicology.

COMPOUNDING AND PHARMACEUTICS RESOURCES

Merck Index

- Different from the *Merck Manual*
- Provides chemical and pharmacologic information on drugs (e.g., chemical name, molecular formula, structure, molecular weight, solubility, drug class, toxicity, data, manufacturer)

Remington: The Science and Practice of Pharmacy

- Provides information on numerous issues concerning pharmacy practice (e.g., pharmaceutical calculations, chemistry, radioisotopes, compounding techniques/ingredients)

DRUG IDENTIFICATION RESOURCES

American Drug Index

- Cross-referenced by brand, generic, and chemical names
- Also provides available dosage forms/strengths and manufacturer information
- IDENTIDEX (available through MICROMEDEX)

FOREIGN DRUG INFORMATION RESOURCES

Martindale: The Complete Drug Reference

- Provides information on drugs used throughout the world

Index Nominum: International Drug Directory

- Provides similar information as *Martindale*

PEDIATRIC DRUG INFORMATION RESOURCES

The Harriet Lane Handbook

- Pocket guide that provides brief overview (especially diagnosis and treatment) of common disease states in children

Pediatric Dosage Handbook (Lexi-Comp)

- Provides drug information specific to the pediatric population

PREGNANCY AND LACTATION RESOURCES

Drugs in Pregnancy and Lactation (Briggs)

- "Gold standard"
- Focuses on safety of drugs in pregnancy and lactation

OTC DRUG RESOURCES

Handbook of Nonprescription Drugs: An Interactive Approach to Self-Care (published by the American Pharmacists Association)

- Provides etiology, pathophysiology, clinical presentation, and treatment of disease states that may be amenable to self-care
- Provides comprehensive information on OTC products (e.g., side effects, drug interactions, dosing, dosage forms, patient counseling)

PDR for Nonprescription Drugs, Dietary Supplements, and Herbs

Comparison of Tertiary Drug Information Resources

Reference	Monograph: Basic Info	Approved Uses	Unapproved Uses	Drug Interactions	Language for Patients	Manufacturer Contact Information	Product ID	Cost	Dosage Form Availability	Pathophysiology	Disease State Management	Treatment of Drug Overdoses	Foreign Drug Identification	IV Drug Compatibility	Chemical Properties	Generic Availability	Compounding Information	Lactation Information	Mechanism of Action
American Hospital Formulary Service Drug Information (AHFS)	X	X	X	X					X			X			X	X		X	X
Physicians' Desk Reference (PDR)	X	X		X		X	X		X			X			X			X	X
Drug Information Handbook (Lexi-Comp)	X	X	X	X					X			X				X		X	X
Facts and Comparisons	X	X	X	X					X			X				X		X	X
Martindale: The Complete Drug Reference													X						
USP DI Drug Information for the Healthcare Provider (Vol I)	X	X	X	X			X		X			X						X	X
USP DI Advice for the Patient: Drug Information in Lay Language (Vol II)					X														
USP DI Approved Drug Products and Legal Requirements (Vol III)		X																	
Pharmacotherapy: A Pathophysiologic Approach (DiPiro's)										X	X	X							X
Remington: The Science and Practice of Pharmacy															X		X		
Handbook on Injectable Drugs (Trissel's)									X					X					
King Guide to Parenteral Admixtures														X					

Reference	Monograph: Basic Info	Approved Uses	Unapproved Uses	Drug Interactions	Language for Patients	Manufacturer Contact Information	Product ID	Cost	Dosage Form Availability	Pathophysiology	Disease State Management	Treatment of Drug Overdoses	Foreign Drug Identification	IV Drug Compatibility	Chemical Properties	Generic Availability	Compounding Information	Lactation Information	Mechanism of Action
Goodman and Gilman's: The Pharmacological Basis of Therapeutics																			X
Harrison's Principles of Internal Medicine										X	X	X							
Drug Interactions Analysis and Management (Hansten and Horn's)				X															
Drug Interaction Facts				X															
Harriet Lane Handbook	X	X		X							X							X	
Drugs in Pregnancy and Lactation (Briggs)																		X	
Red Book						X	X	X	X										

LEARNING POINTS

- Learn drug information resources by various categories. Once you know the kind of information that you need, you can select the most appropriate reference.
- Do not memorize the table above; it can be used to assess your general knowledge of tertiary literature sources.
- Remember the differences between primary, secondary, and tertiary literature:
  - Primary literature: Original journal articles (research reports, case reports, editorials); serves as information for development of secondary and tertiary literature resources
  - Secondary literature: Indexing and abstracting services (e.g., MEDLINE, IPA, EMBASE, Cochrane)
  - Tertiary literature: Textbooks and review articles; summarize and interpret primary literature

PRACTICE QUESTIONS

1. A physician calls to ask the pharmacist about the mechanism of action of a new drug that has been approved for hypercholesterolemia. Which of the following references is/are most appropriate for obtaining this information?

    I. AHFS Drug Information
    II. Facts and Comparisons
    III. USP DI Volume III

    (A) I only
    (B) III only
    (C) I and II only
    (D) II and III only
    (E) I, II, and III

2. A patient comes to your pharmacy and gives you a prescription for an ointment that needs to be compounded. Which of the following references would be most appropriate to obtain information regarding the preparation of this ointment?

    (A) *Martindale: The Complete Drug Reference*
    (B) *Pharmacotherapy: A Pathophysiologic Approach*
    (C) *Physicians' Desk Reference*
    (D) *Remington: The Science and Practice of Pharmacy*
    (E) *Harriet Lane Handbook*

ANSWERS

1. **C**

AHFS Drug Information (I) and Facts and Comparisons (II) both contain general drug information in monograph format, so choice (C) is correct. USP DI Volume III (III) contains information on approved drug products (generic availability) and legal requirements.

2. **D**

Remington would be the most appropriate reference to obtain information regarding compounding of an ointment, so choice (D) is correct. *Martindale* (A) provides information on foreign drugs. *Pharmacotherapy: A Pathophysiologic Approach* (B) is a general pharmacotherapy resource. *Physicians' Desk Reference* (C) is a general drug information resource. *Harriet Lane Handbook* (E) is a pediatric drug information resource.

Health Policy

24

This chapter covers three key areas of health policy:

- **HIPAA**
- **FDA regulatory process**
- **JCAHO accreditation process**

 Suggested Study Time: **30 minutes**

HIPAA

What is HIPAA? The Health Insurance Portability and Accountability Act of 1996 (HIPAA) required the U.S. Department of Health and Human Services (HHS) to issue regulations governing healthcare entities that engage in electronic healthcare transactions. HIPAA regulations apply both to the form of electronic healthcare transactions and the privacy of patient information. At the time they were enacted, the regulations were expected to have far-reaching consequences. Compliance with patient privacy regulations was mandated for April 2003.

The purpose of HIPAA is to improve the Medicare program under title XVIII of the Social Security Act, the Medicaid program under title XIX of that act, and the efficiency and effectiveness of the healthcare system, by encouraging the development of a health information system through the establishment of standards and requirements for the electronic transmission of certain health information.

The Office for Civil Rights (OCR) is responsible for enforcing the HIPAA Privacy Rule. One of the ways that OCR carries out this responsibility is to investigate complaints filed with it. OCR may also conduct compliance reviews to determine whether covered entities are in compliance, and OCR performs education and outreach to foster compliance with the requirements of the Privacy Rule.

If OCR accepts a complaint for investigation, OCR will notify the person who filed the complaint and the covered entity named in it. Then the complainant and the covered entity are asked to present information about the incident or problem described in the complaint. OCR may request specific information from each to get an understanding of the facts. Covered entities are required by law to cooperate with complaint investigations.

OCR reviews the information, or evidence, that it gathers in each case. In some cases, it may determine that the covered entity did not violate the requirements of the Privacy Rule. If the evidence indicates that the covered entity was not in compliance, OCR will attempt to resolve the case with the covered entity.

Most Privacy Rule investigations are concluded to the satisfaction of OCR through these types of resolutions. OCR provides written notice of the resolution result to the person who filed the complaint and to the covered entity.

If the covered entity does not take action to resolve the matter in a way that is satisfactory, OCR may decide to impose civil monetary penalties (CMPs) on the covered entity. If CMPs are imposed, the covered entity may request a hearing in which an HHS administrative law judge decides if the penalties are supported by the evidence in the case. Complainants do not receive a portion of CMPs collected from covered entities; the penalties are deposited in the U.S. Treasury.

Every pharmacy, regardless of size, is considered a covered entity under the regulations, and as such, each one is required to comply with the HIPAA regulations. Entities (pharmacies) may be fined for noncompliance (civil fines of up to $25,000 per violation and criminal penalties of up to $250,000 and 10 years imprisonment).

HIPAA protects the information found in your medical record from disclosure (being made available to other persons or organizations) without your authorization. The information protected by HIPAA includes:

- Any information related to your past, present, or future physical or mental health
- The past, present, or future payment for health services you have received
- The specific care that you have received, are receiving, or will receive
- Any information that identifies you as the individual receiving the care
- Any information that another person could reasonably use to identify you as the individual receiving the care

As a covered entity, a pharmacy is required to inform patients of how it may use your protected health information. In providing treatment to patients, a pharmacy should use patients' protected health information only for the purposes of treatment, payment, and healthcare operations.

Other general rules include the requirement that the pharmacy must provide a paper copy of the Notice to patients and the public in general about how the pharmacy will be protecting their privacy.

1. The Pharmacy must make the Notice available upon request to any person, even if that person is not a current pharmacy patient.

2. The Pharmacy must provide the Notice to the patient no later than the date that the Pharmacy first provides service to the patient, including service delivered electronically.

    In emergency treatment situations, the Notice will be provided as soon after the emergency as is reasonably practicable. The Pharmacy may send the Notice to all of its patients at once, give the notice to each patient as s/he comes into the Pharmacy or contacts the Pharmacy electronically, or by any combination of these approaches.

3. The Pharmacy must have the Notice available at the store for individuals who request a copy to take with them.

4. The Pharmacy must post the Notice in a clear and prominent location in the store where patients will be able to read it.

FDA REGULATORY PROCESS

For decades, the regulation and control of new drugs in the United States has been based on the New Drug Application (NDA). Since 1938, every new drug has been the subject of an approval process by the NDA before that drug can be sold commercially in the United States. The NDA application is the vehicle through which drug sponsors formally propose that the FDA approve a new pharmaceutical for sale and marketing in the United States. The data gathered during the animal studies and human clinical trials of an Investigation New Drug (IND) become part of the NDA.

During a new drug's early preclinical development, the sponsor's primary goal is to determine whether the product is reasonably safe for initial use in humans, and if the compound exhibits pharmacological activity that justifies commercial development. When a product is identified as a viable candidate for further development, the sponsor then focuses on collecting the data and information necessary to establish that the product will not expose humans to unreasonable risks when used in limited, early-stage clinical studies.

The FDA's role in the development of a new drug begins when the drug's sponsor (usually the manufacturer or potential marketer), having screened the new molecule for pharmacological activity and acute toxicity potential in animals, wants to test its diagnostic or therapeutic potential in humans. At that point, the molecule changes in legal status under the Federal Food, Drug, and Cosmetic Act and becomes a new drug subject to specific requirements of the drug regulatory system.

There are three IND types:

- Investigator IND is submitted by a physician who both initiates and conducts an investigation, and under whose immediate direction the investigational drug is administered or dispensed. A physician might submit a research IND to propose studying an unapproved drug, or an approved product for a new indication or in a new patient population.

- Emergency Use IND allows the FDA to authorize use of an experimental drug in an emergency situation that does not allow time for submission of an IND in accordance with FDA regulations. It is also used for patients who do not meet the criteria of an existing study protocol, or if an approved study protocol does not exist.

- Treatment IND is submitted for experimental drugs showing promise in clinical testing for serious or immediately life-threatening conditions while the final clinical work is conducted and the FDA review takes place.

There are two IND categories:

- Commercial
- Research (noncommercial)

The IND application must contain information in three broad areas:

- Animal Pharmacology and Toxicology Studies: Preclinical data to permit an assessment as to whether the product is reasonably safe for initial testing in humans. Also included is any previous experience with the drug in humans (often foreign use).

- Manufacturing Information: Information pertaining to the composition, manufacturer, stability, and controls used for manufacturing the drug substance and the drug product. This information is assessed to ensure that the company can adequately produce and supply consistent batches of the drug.

- Clinical Protocols and Investigator Information: Detailed protocols for proposed clinical studies to assess whether the initial-phase trials will expose subjects to unnecessary risks. Also, information on the qualifications of clinical investigators—professionals (generally physicians) who oversee the administration of the experimental compound—to assess whether they are qualified to fulfill their clinical trial duties. Finally, commitments to obtain informed consent from the research subjects, to obtain review of the study by an institutional review board (IRB), and to adhere to the investigational new drug regulations.

Once the IND is submitted, the sponsor must wait 30 calendar days before initiating any clinical trials. During this time, the FDA has an opportunity to review the IND for safety to assure that research subjects will not be subjected to unreasonable risk.

Once the IND data is gathered, the sponsor can then submit an NDA. The goals of the NDA are to provide enough information to permit the FDA reviewer to reach the following key decisions:

- Whether the drug is safe and effective in its proposed use(s), and whether the benefits of the drug outweigh the risks
- Whether the drug's proposed labeling (package insert) is appropriate, and what it should contain
- Whether the methods used in manufacturing the drug and the controls used to maintain the drug's quality are adequate to preserve the drug's identity, strength, quality, and purity

The documentation required in an NDA is supposed to tell the drug's whole story, including what happened during the clinical tests; what the ingredients of the drug are; the results of the animal studies; how the drug behaves in the body; and how it is manufactured, processed, and packaged.

Current Federal law requires that a drug be the subject of an approved marketing application before it is transported or distributed across state lines. Because a sponsor will probably want to ship the investigational drug to clinical investigators in many states, it must seek an exemption from that legal requirement.

Types of Clinical Trials

This section describes the different types of clinical trials used during the IDA and NDA application process following a chemotherapy drug.

Phase 1 (phase I)

These are the earliest trials in the life of a new drug or treatment. They are usually small trials, recruiting anywhere up to about 30 patients, although often a lot less. The trial may be open to people with any type of cancer.

For example, when laboratory testing shows that a new treatment might help treat cancer, phase 1 trials are done to find out:

- The safe dose range
- The side effects
- How the body copes with the drug
- If the treatment shrinks cancer

Patients are recruited very slowly onto phase 1 trials. So although these trials do not recruit many patients, they can take a long time to complete. The first few patients to take part (called a "cohort," or group) will be given a very small dose of the drug. If all goes well, the next group will receive a slightly higher dose. The dose will be gradually increased with each group. The researchers will monitor the effect until they find the best dose to give. This is called a "dose escalation study."

In a phase 1 trial, patients may have many blood tests, as the researchers look at how the drug is affecting the patient and at how the body copes with and gets rid of the drug. Researchers will also record any side effects.

People entering phase 1 trials often have advanced cancer and have usually had all the treatment available to them. This is because they may benefit from the new treatment in the trial, but many will not. The aim of the trial is to study doses and side effects. This work must be done first before the potential new treatment can be tested to see if it works. Phase 1 trials are important because they are the first step in finding new treatments for the future.

Phase 2 (phase II)

Not all treatments tested in a phase 1 trial make it to a phase 2 trial. These trials may include people who all have the same type of cancer, or people who have different types of cancer. Phase 2 trials seek to determine:

- If the new treatment works well enough to test in a larger phase 3 trial
- On which types of cancer the treatment works
- More about side effects and how to manage them
- More about the best dose to use

Although these treatments have been tested at phase 1, patients may still have side effects that the doctors do not yet know about. Drugs can affect people in different ways.

Phase 2 trials are often larger than phase 1; there may be up to 50 or so people taking part. If the results of phase 2 trials show that a new treatment may be as good as (or better than) existing treatment, the drug then moves to phase 3.

Phase 3 (phase III)

Phase 3 trials compare new treatments with the best currently available treatment (the standard treatment). They may compare:

- A completely new treatment with the standard treatment
- Different doses or ways of giving a standard treatment
- A new radiotherapy schedule with the standard one

Phase 3 trials are usually much larger than phases 1 and 2. This is because differences in success rates may be small, so the trial would need to include many patients to show the difference.

For example, six out of 100 (6%) more people get a remission with a new treatment than with standard treatment. If there were 50 people in the new treatment group and 50 people in the standard treatment group, there may be three more people in remission in the new treatment group. The two groups would not look that different. But if each treatment were given to 5,000 people, there could be 300 more remissions in the new treatment group.

Sometimes phase 3 trials involve thousands of patients in many different hospitals, and even in different countries.

Randomization

Phase 3 trials are usually randomized. This means the researchers randomly place the people taking part into two groups. One group receives the new treatment and the other receives the standard treatment.

Overviews

Trial overviews are studies that combine all the results from phase 3 trials of a new treatment. They are sometimes called meta-analyses. The idea is to get a broader picture of how well a treatment works. The more data (information) we have, the more accurate the results are likely to be.

Phase 4 (phase IV)

Phase 4 trials are done after a drug has been shown to work and has been granted a license, so they are looking at drugs that are already available for doctors to prescribe, rather than new drugs that are still being developed.

The main reasons pharmaceutical companies run phase 4 trials are to:

- Find out more about the side effects and safety of the drug
- Identify the long-term risks and benefits
- Determine how well the drug works when it is used more widely than in clinical trials

Orphan Drugs Products

Since its inception in 1982, the Office of Orphan Products Development (OOPD) has been dedicated to promoting the development of products that demonstrate promise for the diagnosis and/or treatment of rare diseases or conditions. OOPD interacts with the medical and research communities, professional organizations, academia, and the pharmaceutical industry, as well as rare-disease groups. The OOPD administers the major provisions of the Orphan Drug Act (ODA), which provide incentives for sponsors to develop products for rare diseases. The ODA has been very successful—more than 200 drugs and biological products for rare diseases have been brought to market since 1983. In contrast, the decade prior to 1983 saw fewer than ten such products come to market. In addition, the OOPD administers the Orphan Product Grants Program, which provides funding for clinical research in rare diseases.

JCAHO ACCREDITATION PROCESS

JCAHO stands for the Joint Commission on Accreditation of Healthcare Organizations. It is a private, nonprofit organization that evaluates medical facility compliance based on a focused set of "requirements" that have long been known as essential to the delivery of good patient care.

The JCAHO sets standards by which healthcare quality is measured. JCAHO accreditation means that healthcare facilities have demonstrated compliance with the standards of performance in meeting the needs of people they serve. To maintain accreditation, healthcare facilities undergo an extensive on-site review by JCAHO professionals. The review evaluates the facilities' performance in all areas that affect patient care. Each facility is evaluated and scored. Accreditation may then be awarded based on how well the facility met JCAHO standards.

LEARNING POINTS

- HIPAA was established due to the advent of electronic healthcare record-keeping and to ensure that patient information remains private.

- All pharmacies, regardless of size, are considered covered entities under the regulations, and as such, they are required to comply with the HIPAA regulations.

- During a new drug's early preclinical development, the sponsor's primary goal is to determine if the product is reasonably safe for initial use in humans, and if the compound exhibits pharmacological activity that justifies commercial development.

- Current Federal law requires that a drug be the subject of an approved marketing application before it is transported or distributed across state lines.

- The OOPD administers the major provisions of the Orphan Drug Act, which provides incentives for sponsors to develop products for rare diseases.

PRACTICE QUESTIONS

1. Which of the following does NOT serve the purpose of HIPAA?

    (A) To improve the Medical program
    (B) To improve the efficiency and effectiveness of the healthcare system
    (C) To encourage the development of health information standards
    (D) To ensure fair prices for procedures
    (E) To ensure safe and private electronic transmission of health information

ANSWERS

1. **D**

HIPAA was not established to ensure fair prices. The purpose of HIPAA is to improve the Medicare program under title XVIII of the Social Security Act, the Medicaid program under title XIX of such Act, and the efficiency and effectiveness of the healthcare system by encouraging the development of a health information system through the establishment of standards and requirements for the electronic transmission of certain health information.

Part Five

Full-Length Practice Test

Full-Length Practice Test

To mimic the realistic conditions of the NAPLEX, allow yourself a total of **four hours and 15 minutes** to complete all 185 questions. Take a ten-minute break at the two-hour time point.

While every test-taker is different, the average candidate takes 2.5 to 3 hours to complete the exam. There are no bonus points for finishing early.

The computer-adaptive format of the exam requires that you **answer all questions in the order in which they are presented**. You cannot skip a question or return to a previous question to review your answer. Again, to make this practice test as realistic as possible, **do not** return to the previous question to change your answer.

ANSWER GRID

1. Ⓐ Ⓑ Ⓒ Ⓓ Ⓔ
2. Ⓐ Ⓑ Ⓒ Ⓓ Ⓔ
3. Ⓐ Ⓑ Ⓒ Ⓓ Ⓔ
4. Ⓐ Ⓑ Ⓒ Ⓓ Ⓔ
5. Ⓐ Ⓑ Ⓒ Ⓓ Ⓔ
6. Ⓐ Ⓑ Ⓒ Ⓓ Ⓔ
7. Ⓐ Ⓑ Ⓒ Ⓓ Ⓔ
8. Ⓐ Ⓑ Ⓒ Ⓓ Ⓔ
9. Ⓐ Ⓑ Ⓒ Ⓓ Ⓔ
10. Ⓐ Ⓑ Ⓒ Ⓓ Ⓔ
11. Ⓐ Ⓑ Ⓒ Ⓓ Ⓔ
12. Ⓐ Ⓑ Ⓒ Ⓓ Ⓔ
13. Ⓐ Ⓑ Ⓒ Ⓓ Ⓔ
14. Ⓐ Ⓑ Ⓒ Ⓓ Ⓔ
15. Ⓐ Ⓑ Ⓒ Ⓓ Ⓔ
16. Ⓐ Ⓑ Ⓒ Ⓓ Ⓔ
17. Ⓐ Ⓑ Ⓒ Ⓓ Ⓔ
18. Ⓐ Ⓑ Ⓒ Ⓓ Ⓔ
19. Ⓐ Ⓑ Ⓒ Ⓓ Ⓔ
20. Ⓐ Ⓑ Ⓒ Ⓓ Ⓔ
21. Ⓐ Ⓑ Ⓒ Ⓓ Ⓔ
22. Ⓐ Ⓑ Ⓒ Ⓓ Ⓔ
23. Ⓐ Ⓑ Ⓒ Ⓓ Ⓔ
24. Ⓐ Ⓑ Ⓒ Ⓓ Ⓔ
25. Ⓐ Ⓑ Ⓒ Ⓓ Ⓔ
26. Ⓐ Ⓑ Ⓒ Ⓓ Ⓔ
27. Ⓐ Ⓑ Ⓒ Ⓓ Ⓔ
28. Ⓐ Ⓑ Ⓒ Ⓓ Ⓔ
29. Ⓐ Ⓑ Ⓒ Ⓓ Ⓔ
30. Ⓐ Ⓑ Ⓒ Ⓓ Ⓔ
31. Ⓐ Ⓑ Ⓒ Ⓓ Ⓔ
32. Ⓐ Ⓑ Ⓒ Ⓓ Ⓔ
33. Ⓐ Ⓑ Ⓒ Ⓓ Ⓔ
34. Ⓐ Ⓑ Ⓒ Ⓓ Ⓔ
35. Ⓐ Ⓑ Ⓒ Ⓓ Ⓔ
36. Ⓐ Ⓑ Ⓒ Ⓓ Ⓔ
37. Ⓐ Ⓑ Ⓒ Ⓓ Ⓔ
38. Ⓐ Ⓑ Ⓒ Ⓓ Ⓔ
39. Ⓐ Ⓑ Ⓒ Ⓓ Ⓔ
40. Ⓐ Ⓑ Ⓒ Ⓓ Ⓔ

41. Ⓐ Ⓑ Ⓒ Ⓓ Ⓔ
42. Ⓐ Ⓑ Ⓒ Ⓓ Ⓔ
43. Ⓐ Ⓑ Ⓒ Ⓓ Ⓔ
44. Ⓐ Ⓑ Ⓒ Ⓓ Ⓔ
45. Ⓐ Ⓑ Ⓒ Ⓓ Ⓔ
46. Ⓐ Ⓑ Ⓒ Ⓓ Ⓔ
47. Ⓐ Ⓑ Ⓒ Ⓓ Ⓔ
48. Ⓐ Ⓑ Ⓒ Ⓓ Ⓔ
49. Ⓐ Ⓑ Ⓒ Ⓓ Ⓔ
50. Ⓐ Ⓑ Ⓒ Ⓓ Ⓔ
51. Ⓐ Ⓑ Ⓒ Ⓓ Ⓔ
52. Ⓐ Ⓑ Ⓒ Ⓓ Ⓔ
53. Ⓐ Ⓑ Ⓒ Ⓓ Ⓔ
54. Ⓐ Ⓑ Ⓒ Ⓓ Ⓔ
55. Ⓐ Ⓑ Ⓒ Ⓓ Ⓔ
56. Ⓐ Ⓑ Ⓒ Ⓓ Ⓔ
57. Ⓐ Ⓑ Ⓒ Ⓓ Ⓔ
58. Ⓐ Ⓑ Ⓒ Ⓓ Ⓔ
59. Ⓐ Ⓑ Ⓒ Ⓓ Ⓔ
60. Ⓐ Ⓑ Ⓒ Ⓓ Ⓔ
61. Ⓐ Ⓑ Ⓒ Ⓓ Ⓔ
62. Ⓐ Ⓑ Ⓒ Ⓓ Ⓔ
63. Ⓐ Ⓑ Ⓒ Ⓓ Ⓔ
64. Ⓐ Ⓑ Ⓒ Ⓓ Ⓔ
65. Ⓐ Ⓑ Ⓒ Ⓓ Ⓔ
66. Ⓐ Ⓑ Ⓒ Ⓓ Ⓔ
67. Ⓐ Ⓑ Ⓒ Ⓓ Ⓔ
68. Ⓐ Ⓑ Ⓒ Ⓓ Ⓔ
69. Ⓐ Ⓑ Ⓒ Ⓓ Ⓔ
70. Ⓐ Ⓑ Ⓒ Ⓓ Ⓔ
71. Ⓐ Ⓑ Ⓒ Ⓓ Ⓔ
72. Ⓐ Ⓑ Ⓒ Ⓓ Ⓔ
73. Ⓐ Ⓑ Ⓒ Ⓓ Ⓔ
74. Ⓐ Ⓑ Ⓒ Ⓓ Ⓔ
75. Ⓐ Ⓑ Ⓒ Ⓓ Ⓔ
76. Ⓐ Ⓑ Ⓒ Ⓓ Ⓔ
77. Ⓐ Ⓑ Ⓒ Ⓓ Ⓔ
78. Ⓐ Ⓑ Ⓒ Ⓓ Ⓔ
79. Ⓐ Ⓑ Ⓒ Ⓓ Ⓔ
80. Ⓐ Ⓑ Ⓒ Ⓓ Ⓔ

81. Ⓐ Ⓑ Ⓒ Ⓓ Ⓔ
82. Ⓐ Ⓑ Ⓒ Ⓓ Ⓔ
83. Ⓐ Ⓑ Ⓒ Ⓓ Ⓔ
84. Ⓐ Ⓑ Ⓒ Ⓓ Ⓔ
85. Ⓐ Ⓑ Ⓒ Ⓓ Ⓔ
86. Ⓐ Ⓑ Ⓒ Ⓓ Ⓔ
87. Ⓐ Ⓑ Ⓒ Ⓓ Ⓔ
88. Ⓐ Ⓑ Ⓒ Ⓓ Ⓔ
89. Ⓐ Ⓑ Ⓒ Ⓓ Ⓔ
90. Ⓐ Ⓑ Ⓒ Ⓓ Ⓔ
91. Ⓐ Ⓑ Ⓒ Ⓓ Ⓔ
92. Ⓐ Ⓑ Ⓒ Ⓓ Ⓔ
93. Ⓐ Ⓑ Ⓒ Ⓓ Ⓔ
94. Ⓐ Ⓑ Ⓒ Ⓓ Ⓔ
95. Ⓐ Ⓑ Ⓒ Ⓓ Ⓔ
96. Ⓐ Ⓑ Ⓒ Ⓓ Ⓔ
97. Ⓐ Ⓑ Ⓒ Ⓓ Ⓔ
98. Ⓐ Ⓑ Ⓒ Ⓓ Ⓔ
99. Ⓐ Ⓑ Ⓒ Ⓓ Ⓔ
100. Ⓐ Ⓑ Ⓒ Ⓓ Ⓔ
101. Ⓐ Ⓑ Ⓒ Ⓓ Ⓔ
102. Ⓐ Ⓑ Ⓒ Ⓓ Ⓔ
103. Ⓐ Ⓑ Ⓒ Ⓓ Ⓔ
104. Ⓐ Ⓑ Ⓒ Ⓓ Ⓔ
105. Ⓐ Ⓑ Ⓒ Ⓓ Ⓔ
106. Ⓐ Ⓑ Ⓒ Ⓓ Ⓔ
107. Ⓐ Ⓑ Ⓒ Ⓓ Ⓔ
108. Ⓐ Ⓑ Ⓒ Ⓓ Ⓔ
109. Ⓐ Ⓑ Ⓒ Ⓓ Ⓔ
110. Ⓐ Ⓑ Ⓒ Ⓓ Ⓔ
111. Ⓐ Ⓑ Ⓒ Ⓓ Ⓔ
112. Ⓐ Ⓑ Ⓒ Ⓓ Ⓔ
113. Ⓐ Ⓑ Ⓒ Ⓓ Ⓔ
114. Ⓐ Ⓑ Ⓒ Ⓓ Ⓔ
115. Ⓐ Ⓑ Ⓒ Ⓓ Ⓔ
116. Ⓐ Ⓑ Ⓒ Ⓓ Ⓔ
117. Ⓐ Ⓑ Ⓒ Ⓓ Ⓔ
118. Ⓐ Ⓑ Ⓒ Ⓓ Ⓔ
119. Ⓐ Ⓑ Ⓒ Ⓓ Ⓔ
120. Ⓐ Ⓑ Ⓒ Ⓓ Ⓔ

ANSWER GRID

121. Ⓐ Ⓑ Ⓒ Ⓓ Ⓔ
122. Ⓐ Ⓑ Ⓒ Ⓓ Ⓔ
123. Ⓐ Ⓑ Ⓒ Ⓓ Ⓔ
124. Ⓐ Ⓑ Ⓒ Ⓓ Ⓔ
125. Ⓐ Ⓑ Ⓒ Ⓓ Ⓔ
126. Ⓐ Ⓑ Ⓒ Ⓓ Ⓔ
127. Ⓐ Ⓑ Ⓒ Ⓓ Ⓔ
128. Ⓐ Ⓑ Ⓒ Ⓓ Ⓔ
129. Ⓐ Ⓑ Ⓒ Ⓓ Ⓔ
130. Ⓐ Ⓑ Ⓒ Ⓓ Ⓔ
131. Ⓐ Ⓑ Ⓒ Ⓓ Ⓔ
132. Ⓐ Ⓑ Ⓒ Ⓓ Ⓔ
133. Ⓐ Ⓑ Ⓒ Ⓓ Ⓔ
134. Ⓐ Ⓑ Ⓒ Ⓓ Ⓔ
135. Ⓐ Ⓑ Ⓒ Ⓓ Ⓔ
136. Ⓐ Ⓑ Ⓒ Ⓓ Ⓔ
137. Ⓐ Ⓑ Ⓒ Ⓓ Ⓔ
138. Ⓐ Ⓑ Ⓒ Ⓓ Ⓔ
139. Ⓐ Ⓑ Ⓒ Ⓓ Ⓔ
140. Ⓐ Ⓑ Ⓒ Ⓓ Ⓔ
141. Ⓐ Ⓑ Ⓒ Ⓓ Ⓔ
142. Ⓐ Ⓑ Ⓒ Ⓓ Ⓔ
143. Ⓐ Ⓑ Ⓒ Ⓓ Ⓔ
144. Ⓐ Ⓑ Ⓒ Ⓓ Ⓔ
145. Ⓐ Ⓑ Ⓒ Ⓓ Ⓔ

146. Ⓐ Ⓑ Ⓒ Ⓓ Ⓔ
147. Ⓐ Ⓑ Ⓒ Ⓓ Ⓔ
148. Ⓐ Ⓑ Ⓒ Ⓓ Ⓔ
149. Ⓐ Ⓑ Ⓒ Ⓓ Ⓔ
150. Ⓐ Ⓑ Ⓒ Ⓓ Ⓔ
151. Ⓐ Ⓑ Ⓒ Ⓓ Ⓔ
152. Ⓐ Ⓑ Ⓒ Ⓓ Ⓔ
153. Ⓐ Ⓑ Ⓒ Ⓓ Ⓔ
154. Ⓐ Ⓑ Ⓒ Ⓓ Ⓔ
155. Ⓐ Ⓑ Ⓒ Ⓓ Ⓔ
156. Ⓐ Ⓑ Ⓒ Ⓓ Ⓔ
157. Ⓐ Ⓑ Ⓒ Ⓓ Ⓔ
158. Ⓐ Ⓑ Ⓒ Ⓓ Ⓔ
159. Ⓐ Ⓑ Ⓒ Ⓓ Ⓔ
160. Ⓐ Ⓑ Ⓒ Ⓓ Ⓔ
161. Ⓐ Ⓑ Ⓒ Ⓓ Ⓔ
162. Ⓐ Ⓑ Ⓒ Ⓓ Ⓔ
163. Ⓐ Ⓑ Ⓒ Ⓓ Ⓔ
164. Ⓐ Ⓑ Ⓒ Ⓓ Ⓔ
165. Ⓐ Ⓑ Ⓒ Ⓓ Ⓔ
166. Ⓐ Ⓑ Ⓒ Ⓓ Ⓔ
167. Ⓐ Ⓑ Ⓒ Ⓓ Ⓔ
168. Ⓐ Ⓑ Ⓒ Ⓓ Ⓔ
169. Ⓐ Ⓑ Ⓒ Ⓓ Ⓔ
170. Ⓐ Ⓑ Ⓒ Ⓓ Ⓔ

171. Ⓐ Ⓑ Ⓒ Ⓓ Ⓔ
172. Ⓐ Ⓑ Ⓒ Ⓓ Ⓔ
173. Ⓐ Ⓑ Ⓒ Ⓓ Ⓔ
174. Ⓐ Ⓑ Ⓒ Ⓓ Ⓔ
175. Ⓐ Ⓑ Ⓒ Ⓓ Ⓔ
176. Ⓐ Ⓑ Ⓒ Ⓓ Ⓔ
177. Ⓐ Ⓑ Ⓒ Ⓓ Ⓔ
178. Ⓐ Ⓑ Ⓒ Ⓓ Ⓔ
179. Ⓐ Ⓑ Ⓒ Ⓓ Ⓔ
180. Ⓐ Ⓑ Ⓒ Ⓓ Ⓔ
181. Ⓐ Ⓑ Ⓒ Ⓓ Ⓔ
182. Ⓐ Ⓑ Ⓒ Ⓓ Ⓔ
183. Ⓐ Ⓑ Ⓒ Ⓓ Ⓔ
184. Ⓐ Ⓑ Ⓒ Ⓓ Ⓔ
185. Ⓐ Ⓑ Ⓒ Ⓓ Ⓔ

Directions: Complete each of the following questions with the best possible answer.

1. Which of the following is/are possible side effects of probenecid?

    I.   GI upset
    II. Rash
    III. Stone formation

    (A) I only
    (B) III only
    (C) I and II only
    (D) II and III only
    (E) I, II, and III

2. Which of the following is NOT true regarding A1c?

    (A) It is used to evaluate glycemic control in patients with diabetes.
    (B) It represents a time frame of approximately 30–45 days.
    (C) It can be inaccurate in cases of severe anemia.
    (D) The most commonly used normal reference range is 4–6%.
    (E) An A1c of 10% would indicate average blood sugar over 200 mg/dL.

3. Which of the following atypical antipsychotics requires rigorous monitoring of WBC and ANC?

    (A) Olanzapine
    (B) Risperidone
    (C) Quetiapine
    (D) Ziprasidone
    (E) Clozapine

4. What information should the doctor know prior to initiating Mirapex in a patient with Parkinson's disease?

    I.   Decrease the levodopa dose by 20–30% when initiating Mirapex
    II. Patient must wear patch for 24 hours for efficacy
    III. Monitor for serious cardiac side effects

    (A) I only
    (B) III only
    (C) I and II only
    (D) II and III only
    (E) I, II, and III

5. A patient has been diagnosed with depression and will begin antidepressant therapy today. Which of the following is MOST appropriate, assuming the patient has no other health conditions?

    (A) Venlafaxine 37.5 mg PO BID
    (B) Lexapro 10 mg PO BID
    (C) Fluvoxamine 80 mg PO weekly
    (D) Nortriptyline 300 mg PO daily
    (E) Mirtazapine 10 mg PO Q a.m.

6. Which of the following counseling points is TRUE?

    I. NuvaRing should be inserted once every month.
    II. Ortho-evra should be applied once every week for three weeks/month.
    III. Seasonale should result in menses approximately every three months.

(A) I only
(B) III only
(C) I and II only
(D) II and III only
(E) I, II, and III

7. Which of the following key monitoring parameters is NOT correctly matched to its corresponding medication?

(A) Blood Glucose – prednisone
(B) CBC – methotrexate
(C) Ocular exam – hydroxychloroquine
(D) Tuberculin skin test (PPD) before initiation – Enbrel
(E) Hepatic enzymes – leflunomide

8. Which of the following statements regarding serum creatinine is TRUE?

(A) Serum creatinine is most commonly used to assess hepatic disease.
(B) Serum creatinine is dependent upon the amount of iron consumed in the diet.
(C) Serum creatinine is a more accurate measure in the very elderly than in young adults.
(D) Serum creatinine is used in the Cockroft-Gault equation.
(E) Serum creatinine is synonymous with microalbumin.

9. Which of the following is TRUE of Natalizumab in multiple sclerosis?

    I. Patients must enroll in TOUCH prior to receiving
    II. Reserved for those unresponsive to other medications
    III. Added to other disease-modifying drugs (DMDs) when relapsing occurs

(A) I only
(B) III only
(C) I and II only
(D) II and III only
(E) I, II, and III

10. Allopurinol is indicated for which of the following gout presentations?

   (A) Prophylaxis in patients with slightly elevated uric acid levels
   (B) Prophylaxis in patients with moderately elevated uric acid and uric acid overproduction
   (C) Prophylaxis in patients with uric acid excretion indicative of underexcretion
   (D) Treatment of acute gout
   (E) Treatment of asymptomatic hyperuricemia

11. Which medication(s) require monitoring of serum drug concentrations?

   I. Lamotrigine
   II. Valproic acid
   III. Lithium

   (A) I only
   (B) III only
   (C) I and II only
   (D) II and III only
   (E) I, II, and III

12. Which of the following trade names is NOT correctly matched with its generic name?

   (A) Zyprexa – Olanzapine
   (B) Risperdal – Risperidone
   (C) Geodon – Ziprasidone
   (D) Abilify – Aripiprazole
   (E) Haldol – Clozapine

13. Migraine prophylaxis could be achieved with which of the following medication classes?

   (A) ACE-inhibitors
   (B) Acetaminophen
   (C) Antidepressants
   (D) Calcium channel blockers
   (E) Anticholinergics

14. What is the MOST appropriate recommendation for a patient with osteoarthritis and stomach ulcers?

   (A) Aspirin 325 mg PO every 4–6 hours
   (B) Tramadol 25 mg PO every 4–6 hours
   (C) Diclofenac 50 mg PO BID
   (D) Daypro 600 mg PO daily
   (E) Mobic 7.5 mg PO daily

Questions 15–19 refer to the following patient profile.

Patient Name: Tamara Yates

Age: 40   **Height:** 5'2"
Sex: F   **Weight:** 90 lb

Allergies: Geodon

Diagnosis

    <u>Primary:</u>
        Hypertension
        Depression
        Schizophrenia

    <u>Chief Complaint:</u> tardive dyskinesia, dystonia

Lab/Diagnostic Tests

Date	Test/Result	
03/02	Sodium	133 mEq/L
(last week)	Potassium	3.5 mEq/L
	Serum creatinine	1.0 mg/dL
	Blood pressure	166/98 mmHg
	Heart rate	80 bpm

Medications

Date	Name and Strength	Route	Directions
02/20	HCTZ 25 mg	PO	1 tablet in the morning
	Citalopram 20 mg	PO	1 tablet daily
	Haloperidol 2 mg	PO	1 tablet twice daily

Additional Information

Date	Comment
03/02	Patient has been suspected of bulimia by her primary physician and dentist.

---

15. Which of the following is likely causing Ms. Yates' chief complaint?

    (A) HCTZ
    (B) Citalopram
    (C) Haloperidol
    (D) Low sodium
    (E) Uncontrolled blood pressure

16. What additional monitoring is needed to assess the haloperidol?

    (A) Serum drug levels
    (B) A1c
    (C) Ejection fraction
    (D) Bone mineral density
    (E) CBC

17. Which of the following is/are appropriate recommendations to address Ms. Yates' chief complaint?

    I. Switch to the liquid formulation of haloperidol
    II. Switch the haloperidol to ziprasidone
    III. Switch the haloperidol to Risperdal

    (A) I only
    (B) III only
    (C) I and II
    (D) II and III
    (E) I, II, and III

18. What education should be provided to Ms. Yates concerning her antipsychotic medications?

    (A) Medications for schizophrenia are absorbed better in an acidic environment and should be taken with orange juice or vitamin C.
    (B) Medications for schizophrenia work quickly and should start to take effect within two to three doses.
    (C) If side effects are bothersome, stop taking the medication.
    (D) Alcohol should be avoided.
    (E) If side effects are bothersome, cut the dose in half.

19. Ms. Yates was told by a friend that her citalopram is bad for her. Although you have tried to talk with her about it, she wants another antidepressant. Which of the following is the MOST appropriate recommendation?

    (A) Bupropion 100 mg PO BID
    (B) Alprazolam 1 mg PO TID
    (C) Lexapro 10 mg PO daily
    (D) Venlafaxine 37.5 mg PO BID
    (E) Propranolol 80 mg PO daily

20. What is the purpose of adding carbidopa to levodopa in the treatment of Parkinson's disease?

    I. Prevents the peripheral degradation of levodopa
    II. Allows for extended dosing intervals
    III. Carbidopa prevents some of the side effects of levodopa from occurring

    (A) I only
    (B) III only
    (C) I and II only
    (D) II and III only
    (E) I, II, and III

21. Which of the following is first-line treatment for acute gout?

    (A) Acetaminophen 1,000 mg PRN up to QID
    (B) Colchicine 2 mg PRN
    (C) Indomethacin 25 mg TID
    (D) Allopurinol 100 mg daily
    (E) Probenecid 250 mg BID

22. Which of the following agents is/are correctly matched with common side effects?

    I. Mirtazapine – somnolence
    II. Paroxetine – disorder of ejaculation/impotence
    III. Amitriptyline – weight gain

    (A) I only
    (B) III only
    (C) I and II only
    (D) II and III only
    (E) I, II, and III

23. Phenytoin is available in which supplied dosage forms?

    I. Chewable tablets
    II. Oral suspension
    III. Parenteral solution

(A) I only
(B) III only
(C) I and II only
(D) II and III only
(E) I, II, and III

24. What is the role of NSAIDs in rheumatoid arthritis?

(A) NSAIDs function as a disease-modifying antirheumatic drug (DMARD).
(B) NSAIDs are used for PRN symptomatic relief of symptoms.
(C) NSAIDs are used as adjunctive therapy in patients with refractory symptoms.
(D) NSAIDs can prevent the flushing associated with biological injections.
(E) NSAIDs must be given in combination with infliximab.

25. What recommendation(s) for abortive therapy would be BEST for a patient who experiences severe nausea and vomiting every time a migraine occurs?

    I. Amerge oral tablets
    II. Relpax oral tablets
    III. Maxalt MLT

(A) I only
(B) III only
(C) I and II only
(D) II and III only
(E) I, II, and III

26. Which of the following statements is TRUE?

(A) Oxcarbazepine and lamotrigine both have a possibility of causing Stevens-Johnson rash.
(B) Oxcarbazepine is generic for Tegretol.
(C) Lithium has a significant drug interaction with beta-blockers.
(D) Valproic acid is contraindicated in renal disease.
(E) Lithium works by increasing gamma-aminobutyric acid (GABA) in the brain.

27. Which of the following is a contraindication bupropion?

    I. Current smoker
    II. Bulimia
    III. Seizure disorder

(A) I only
(B) III only
(C) I and II only
(D) II and III only
(E) I, II, and III

28. Which of the following is NOT true of methotrexate?

    (A) It may cause folate deficiency.
    (B) It should be taken with food.
    (C) It is the first-line disease-modifying antirheumatic drug (DMARD) for treatment of rheumatoid arthritis.
    (D) The usual dose is 7.5 mg once weekly.
    (E) It requires ophthalmic exams every three months.

29. Which of the following is/are TRUE regarding oxybutynin?

    I.   It is available in oral and transdermal patch formulations.
    II. It is an anticholinergic medication.
    III. Common side effects include dry mouth and dry eyes.

    (A) I only
    (B) III only
    (C) I and II only
    (D) II and III only
    (E) I, II, and III

30. Which of the following can be used for both treatment and prevention of gout?

    I.   NSAIDs
    II. Corticosteroids
    III. Colchicine

    (A) I only
    (B) III only
    (C) I and II only
    (D) II and III only
    (E) I, II, and III

Questions 31–35 apply to the following case.

Patient Name: Janelle Brown

Age: 21   **Height: 5'2"**
Sex: F   **Weight: 120 lb**

Allergies: Pollen

Diagnosis

Primary:
1. Acne vulgaris
2. Migraine headaches

Chief Complaint: Acne lesions and frequent migraine headaches

Lab/Diagnostic Tests

Date	Test/Result	
03/02	Sodium	134 mEq/L
(last week)	Potassium	3.5 mEq/L
	Serum creatinine	1.0 mg/dL
	Blood pressure	116/82 mmHg
	Heart rate	78 bpm

Medications

Date	Name and Strength	Route	Directions
02/20	Ovcon-50	PO	1 tablet daily utd
	Maxalt MLT 10 mg	PO	Take PRN

---

31. Which of the following side effects is MOST common with Ms. Brown's oral contraceptive?

    (A) Hot flushes
    (B) Decreased libido
    (C) Breast tenderness
    (D) Spotting
    (E) Dyspareunia

32. After talking with Ms. Brown, it seems she may be experiencing some side effects from her Ovcon-50. You call her physician, who provides you with a new prescription for Seasonale. Which of the following is/are the MOST appropriate counseling for this medication?

    I. Take one tablet by mouth daily.
    II. Smoking while on this medication will increase your risk of serious side effects.
    III. Apply one patch each week.

    (A) I only
    (B) III only
    (C) I and II only
    (D) II and III only
    (E) I, II, and III

33. Ms. Brown is prescribed amoxicillin 500 mg PO TID for one week. Which of the following is the MOST appropriate counseling for her?

   (A) There is no drug interaction present. Take the antibiotic three times daily as prescribed.

   (B) There is a drug interaction between the antibiotic and oral contraceptive which renders the oral antibiotic less effective. Hold the contraceptive until the antibiotic regimen is complete.

   (C) There is a drug interaction between the antibiotic and oral contraceptive which renders the oral contraceptive less effective. Do not take the antibiotics.

   (D) There is a drug interaction between the antibiotic and oral contraceptive which renders the oral contraceptive less effective. Take two Ovcon-50 tablets daily of during the week of antibiotic therapy.

   (E) There is a drug interaction between the antibiotic and oral contraceptive, which renders the contraceptive less effective. Take both medications as prescribed and use a backup method of contraception for at least seven days after finishing the antibiotic therapy.

34. Ms. Brown has several noninflammatory comedones on her face. She states that she has never tried therapy for her acne and requests a recommendation for a medication. Which of the following would be the MOST appropriate initial recommendation?

   (A) Tetracycline 500 mg PO QID
   (B) Isotretinoin 20 mg PO daily
   (C) Benzoyl peroxide 5% topical cream daily
   (D) Benzoyl peroxide 5% topical cream and tretinoin 0.1% gel applied daily
   (E) Isotretinoin 20 mg PO daily and tretinoin 0.1% gel applied daily

35. Ms. Brown asks for information about prophylactic migraine medications. She states that she is currently experiencing about four migraine headaches per week. Which of the following would be the MOST appropriate recommendation for migraine prophylaxis?

   (A) Not a good candidate for migraine prophylaxis because she does not have headaches frequently enough
   (B) Imitrex
   (C) Topiramate
   (D) Propranolol
   (E) Hydrocodone

36. Which of the following has no known drug interaction with oral contraceptives?

   (A) Neurontin
   (B) Carbamazepine
   (C) Valproic acid
   (D) Phenytoin
   (E) Topiramate

37. Which of the following trade/generic combinations is correctly matched?

    (A) Detrol – Oxybutinin
    (B) Vesicare – Tolterodine
    (C) Enablex – Darifenacin
    (D) Ditropan – Imipramine
    (E) Tofranil – Solifenacin

38. When should biologics be initiated in rheumatoid arthritis?

    I.   Within three months of a diagnosis
    II. For PRN symptom relief
    III. DMARDs have been ineffective

    (A) I only
    (B) III only
    (C) I and II only
    (D) II and III only
    (E) I, II, and III

39. Which of the following is/are TRUE of tricyclic antidepressants?

    I.   They may exhibit anticholinergic side effects.
    II. They are very dangerous and often fatal in overdosage.
    III. They have a significant drug–food interaction with aged cheese.

    (A) I only
    (B) III only
    (C) I and II only
    (D) II and III only
    (E) I, II, and III

40. A patient was started on a selegiline patch three days ago for major depression. The family states that it is not working. The best recommendation is to

    (A) add fluoxetine if it is still not working in two weeks.
    (B) add duloxetine if it is not better in 6–8 weeks.
    (C) have the patient start a high caffeine intake so that the drug will be absorbed better.
    (D) inform the family that the medication has not had time to work yet and may take 1–2 months.
    (E) switch the patient to the oral formulation for better efficacy.

41. Which of the following products contains aspirin with butalbital and caffeine?

    (A) Fiorinal
    (B) Fioricet
    (C) Excedrin Migraine
    (D) Midrin
    (E) Migranal

42. A 15-year-old female patient is given a new prescription for Retin-A. Which of the following would be an appropriate counseling point?

    (A) This medication works best if combined with an astringent or abrasive soap.
    (B) This medication should result in rapid improvement within 1–2 days.
    (C) This medication should be used only as a "spot treatment" for blemishes.
    (D) It is important to use sunblock prior to sun exposure due to the risk of photosensitivity.
    (E) It is important to apply this product to wet skin immediately after washing the face.

43. Which of the following is/are alternative treatment for osteoporosis in patients who are unable to tolerate bisphosphonates?

      I. Zoledronic acid
     II. Calcium 600 mg + Vitamin D 200 mg TID
    III. Raloxifene

   (A) I only
   (B) III only
   (C) I and II only
   (D) II and III only
   (E) I, II, and III

44. The medication used to treat anxiety, which takes 2–3 weeks to reach maximal efficacy, is

   (A) Xanax.
   (B) Librium.
   (C) Buspar.
   (D) Valium.
   (E) Vistaril.

45. Common side effects of isotretinoin include which of the following?

      I. Cheilitis
     II. Pruritus
    III. Hypertrichosis

   (A) I only
   (B) III only
   (C) I and II only
   (D) II and III only
   (E) I, II, and III

46. Which of the following is NOT a treatment option for psoriasis?

   (A) Methotrexate
   (B) Prednisone
   (C) Coal tar
   (D) Benzoyl peroxide
   (E) Anthralin

47. In the TNM classification of cancer staging, N represents

   (A) the size of the tumor in centimeters.
   (B) the number of tumors.
   (C) the number of involved lymph nodes.
   (D) the number of involved organs.
   (E) the presence of distant metastases.

48. Which of the following is/are TRUE regarding neoadjuvant chemotherapy?

      I. It is given prior to surgery.
     II. The goal is to reduce tumor burden.
    III. It is given to relieve symptoms and has no effect on survival.

   (A) I only
   (B) I and II
   (C) II and III
   (D) I and III
   (E) I, II, and III

49. Leucovorin should be given as rescue therapy to patients receiving _____, but will increase both the toxicity and the chemotherapeutic activity of _____ _____.

   (A) fluorouracil; methotrexate
   (B) doxorubicin; fluorouracil
   (C) fluorouracil; cytarabine
   (D) methotrexate; fluorouracil
   (E) methotrexate; doxorubicin

50. Which of the following is/are TRUE regarding cytarabine?

    I. Its main mechanism of action is inhibition of DNA polymerase.
    II. Patients should be monitored for neurotoxicity at each office visit.
    III. Pre- and post-treatment corticosteroid eyedrops should be given to prevent conjunctivitis.

(A) I only
(B) I and II
(C) II and III
(D) I and III
(E) I, II, and III

51. The most significant adverse drug effect of anthracyclines is

(A) ototoxicity.
(B) infusion-related reactions.
(C) folate deficiency.
(D) cardiotoxicity.
(E) hand-and-foot syndrome.

52. The brand name for bevacizumab is

(A) Gleevec.
(B) Herceptin.
(C) Avastin.
(D) Tarceva.
(E) Platinol.

Questions 53–56 refer to the following patient profile.

Patient Name: Mary Jefferson

Age: 42   **Height:** 5'6"
Sex: F   **Weight:** 125 lb

Allergies: None known

Diagnosis
  Primary:
    1. Adenocarcinoma
    2. Asthma

Lab/Diagnostic Tests
  WBC 1×10^3 50% segs 10% bands
    30% lymphs 10% monos
  Hgb: 14.5 mg/dL
  Blood pressure: 134/85 mmHg
  Heart rate: 75 bpm

---

53. Calculate Ms. Jefferson's absolute neutrophil count using the lab values above.

(A) 3,000
(B) 750
(C) 600
(D) 300
(E) 50

54. Ms. Jefferson's neutropenia would be considered

(A) transient.
(B) mild.
(C) moderate.
(D) severe.
(E) This patient is not neutropenic, the ANC is within normal range.

55. _____ will put neutropenic patients at risk for developing infection.

    (A) Severe neutropenia (ANC <100/mm³)
    (B) Rapid fall in ANC
    (C) Invasive procedures such as enemas, catheter placement, or dental procedures
    (D) Neutropenia lasting more than seven days
    (E) All of the above increase the risk of infection.

56. On the basis of her lab values, which of the following drugs would be appropriate for the Ms. Jefferson?

    (A) Neupogen®
    (B) Epogen®
    (C) Procrit®
    (D) Aranesp®
    (E) None of the above

57. Which of the following scales of measurement would be appropriate to use when the measured values in a study are gender or race?

    (A) Numeric scale
    (B) Nominal scale
    (C) Kaplan-Meier
    (D) Ordinal scale
    (E) ANOVA

58. To increase the power of a study, the researchers could

    (A) decrease the sample size.
    (B) lengthen the duration of the study.
    (C) decrease the duration of the study.
    (D) increase the number of dependent variables being studied.
    (E) increase the sample size.

59. Which of the following is NOT true regarding Type II errors?

    (A) A Type II error occurs when a study fails to detect a difference between study groups but in fact a difference does exist.
    (B) Not achieving power in a study may increase the likelihood of Type II errors.
    (C) A Type II error means that a false null hypothesis was accepted.
    (D) A Type II error occurs when researchers find a difference between study groups when no difference actually exists.
    (E) All of the above are true regarding Type II errors.

60. When a clinical trial is studying three or more independent groups and using numeric scales, the preferred statistical test is

    (A) t-test
    (B) Paired t-test
    (C) Chi-square test
    (D) ANOVA
    (E) Mann-Whitney

61. You need to make 30 g of 0.4% w/w hydrocortisone ointment. You have 2.5% w/w hydrocortisone ointment in stock. How much of the 2.5% ointment must you mix with white petrolatum to make the appropriate quantity of 0.4% ointment?

    (A) 2.4 g
    (B) 2.5 g
    (C) 4.8 g
    (D) 9.6 g
    (E) 30 g

62. The formula for hydrophilic petrolatum USP is given below. How much white wax do you need to weigh out to compound 70 g of hydrophilic petrolatum?

Hydrophilic petrolatum:
3% w/w cholesterol
3% w/w stearyl alcohol
8% w/w white wax
86% w/w white petrolatum

(A) 2.1 g
(B) 8 g
(C) 5.6 g
(D) 60.2 g
(E) 70 g

63. How many 4-mg tablets of chlorpheniramine maleate would be required to compound 4 fluid ounces of a syrup containing 2 mg of chlorpheniramine maleate in every tablespoonful dose?

(A) 1
(B) 2
(C) 4
(D) 8
(E) 12

64. A 60-kg patient is to receive a constant infusion of dobutamine at a rate of 5 mcg/kg/min. The available solution has a concentration of 0.5 mg/mL. For what rate should the infusion pump be set?

(A) 0.6 mL/hr
(B) 36 mL/hr
(C) 18 mL/hr
(D) 600 mL/hr
(E) 3.6 mL/hr

65. A patient is given an IV bolus dose of 1 g of Drug A. The plasma level is measured shortly after administration and is found to be 0.2 mg/mL. The same patient is later given an IV bolus dose of Drug B. The plasma level of Drug B shortly after administration is 83 mcg/mL. On the basis of this data, which of the following statements can you make?

    I. Drug A has a smaller volume of distribution than Drug B.
    II. Drug A is better absorbed than Drug B.
    III. Drug A induced the metabolism of Drug B.

(A) I only
(B) II only
(C) III only
(D) I and III
(E) I, II, and III

66. To treat preeclampsia, a patient receives an infusion of 40 mL of a 10% w/v solution of magnesium sulfate for injection. How many mEq of magnesium did she receive?
(MW $MgSO_4 \cdot (H_2O)_7$ = 246.36)

(A) 8.63 mEq Mg^{2+}
(B) 16.25 mEq Mg^{2+}
(C) 32.5 mEq Mg^{2+}
(D) 65 mEq Mg^{2+}
(E) 130 mEq Mg^{2+}

67. You receive a prescription for 240 mL of a potassium citrate solution with a concentration of 15 mEq/15 mL. How much potassium citrate must you weigh out to compound this prescription? (MW $C_6H_5K_3O_7 = 306$)

    (A) 8.16 g
    (B) 24.48 g
    (C) 2.72 g
    (D) 367.2 g
    (E) 73.44 g

68. You are considering adding HgbA1c monitoring services to your clinical pharmacy offerings and are evaluating an HgbA1c monitor to decide if it sufficiently precise and accurate to be used in your clinic. Using a test solution that produces a value of 7.5% on standardized laboratory tests, you perform ten sample tests on the monitor. The values you obtain are:

    7.9
    8.1
    7.9
    8.0
    7.9
    7.9
    8.0
    8.1
    7.9
    8.0

    You would say that the monitor being evaluated produces readings that are

    (A) accurate but not precise.
    (B) precise but not accurate.
    (C) both precise and accurate.
    (D) neither precise nor accurate.
    (E) You do not have enough information to answer this question.

69. How much sodium chloride must be added to the prescription to make the solution isotonic?

    Rx: Tetracaine hydrochloride   0.5% w/v
           (E = 0.18)
         NaCl   qs
         Sterile water   add 30 mL

    M et ft isotonic eyedrops

    (A) 0.027 g NaCl
    (B) 0.243 g NaCl
    (C) 0.27 g NaCl
    (D) 0.83 g NaCl
    (E) 0.9 g NaCl

70. Given the capsule recipe provided below, how much diphenhydramine must you weigh out to compound 60 capsules?

    Diphenhydramine hydrochloride: 0.5 g
    Acetaminophen: 6.5 g
    Lactose qs: M et div caps #10

    (A) 30 g
    (B) 3 g
    (C) 0.5 g
    (D) 7 g
    (E) 42 g

**Questions 71–74 refer to
the following patient information:**

AJ is a 70-kg male with a creatinine clearance of 100 mL/min. You have the following information about the behavior of a particular drug in this patient:

CL = 400 mL/min;
    CLr = 25 mL/min

Vd = 140 L

95% bound to plasma proteins

71. What is the filtration clearance of this drug?

(A)   0 mL/min
(B)   1.25 mL/min
(C)   5 mL/min
(D)   20 mL/min
(E)   95 mL/min

72. You can conclude that this drug is

(A)   only filtered.
(B)   both filtered and reabsorbed.
(C)   both filtered and secreted.
(D)   secreted and reabsorbed but not filtered.
(E)   You do not have enough information to answer this question.

73. The half-life of this drug in this patient is

(A)   4 hours.
(B)   12 hours.
(C)   24 hours.
(D)   48 hours.
(E)   60 hours.

74. What blood level would you expect after a single IV bolus dose of 250 mg of this drug?

(A)   0.1 mg/dL
(B)   0.13 mg/dL
(C)   0.15 mg/dL
(D)   0.18 mg/dL
(E)   0.2 mg/dL

75. MT is being treated for a serious infection with *Pseudomonas aeruginosa*. After obtaining culture and sensitivity data, her physician starts her on tobramycin 70 mg IV TID. During her hospital stay, MT's serum creatinine was found to increase from 0.8 to 1.6 mg/dL. What kinetic parameters have been affected and what modification should be made to MT's tobramycin therapy?

(A)   The bioavailability for tobramycin is increased, resulting in kidney impairment, so tobramycin should be discontinued.
(B)   The clearance for tobramycin has decreased, resulting in a longer half-life. MT may experience drug accumulation, so the tobramycin dose should be decreased.
(C)   The clearance for tobramycin has increased, resulting in a shorter half-life. MT may experience subtherapeutic drug concentrations, so the tobramycin dose should be increased.
(D)   The clearance for tobramycin has decreased, resulting in a longer half-life. MT may experience subtherapeutic drug concentrations, so the tobramycin dose should be increased.
(E)   The Vd of tobramycin has increased, resulting in a longer half-life. MT may experience drug accumulation, so the tobramycin dose should be decreased.

76. Penicillin is a weakly acidic drug that is secreted by the kidney. Probenecid, also a weakly acidic drug, competes for the carrier system that is responsible for the secretion of penicillin. When penicillin and probenecid are administered together, what do you expect will happen to penicillin's CL and steady-state plasma concentrations?

    (A) CL decreases and steady-state concentrations increase.
    (B) CL increases and steady-state concentrations increase.
    (C) CL increases and steady-state concentrations decrease.
    (D) CL decreases and steady-state concentrations decrease.
    (E) CL and steady-state concentrations are nearly unchanged.

77. Which of the following modifications to a drug will increase its aqueous solubility?

    (A) Convert anhydrous to trihydrate form.
    (B) Convert crystalline to amorphous form.
    (C) Add a lipophilic group.
    (D) Remove a hydroxyl group.
    (E) All of the above will increase aqueous solubility.

78. The pKa of a weak base is 8.4. What form will the drug be in at an intestinal pH of 7.4?

    (A) 75% un-ionized
    (B) Greater than 90% un-ionized
    (C) 75% ionized
    (D) Greater than 90% ionized
    (E) Approximately equal amounts ionized / un-ionized

79. Which dosage form would be the best option for a drug that is prone to first-pass metabolism?

    (A) Tablet
    (B) Syrup
    (C) Capsule
    (D) Rapid-dissolve strip
    (E) Transdermal patch

80. Structured vehicles form suspensions by what means?

    (A) Promoting loose aggregation of suspended particles
    (B) Increasing viscosity, thereby slowing sedimentation
    (C) Maximizing sedimentation volume
    (D) Reducing repulsive forces between particles
    (E) All of the above

81. Phenytoin is formulated in a co-solvent system. Intravenous administration of this drug should occur slowly because

    (A) the onset of drug action will be faster.
    (B) slow injection will prevent precipitation of the drug from solution.
    (C) rapid infusion will lead to hemolysis.
    (D) it will prevent the drug from being metabolized too quickly.
    (E) the cosolvent system is too viscous for rapid administration.

82. Which of the following ophthalmic products must contain a preservative?

    I. Saline in a multiple-dose container
    II. Saline in a single-dose container
    III. Single-use rinse solution used in eye surgery

(A) I only
(B) I and II
(C) II and III
(D) I and III
(E) I, II, and III

83. Drug(s) may be administered rectally to provide local treatment for

(A) nausea.
(B) chronic pain.
(C) ulcerative colitis.
(D) hormone replacement.
(E) migraine headache.

84. Metronidazole leads to a disulfiram reaction when taken with alcohol. Which of the following liquid dosage forms would be the MOST appropriate way of delivering metronidazole?

(A) Spirit
(B) Elixir USP
(C) Tincture
(D) Suspension
(E) Fluid extract

85. A bottle of drug solution was left open in a dark room. After one day, the solution had changed from colorless to pink. An identical bottle, left capped, remained unchanged. The solution has undergone what type of degradation?

(A) Hydrolysis
(B) Photolysis
(C) Oxidation
(D) Sedimentation
(E) Polymorphism

86. Calamine lotion remains thick when sitting on the shelf, yet pours easily when shaken. What type of flow is calamine lotion exhibiting?

(A) Dilatant
(B) Newtonian
(C) Plastic
(D) Pseudoplastic
(E) Thixotropic

87. How many 50-mg phenytoin tablets should a 5-year-old child receive per day, given the following information?

$$V_{max} = 300 \text{ mg/day}$$
$$K_m = 6.5 \text{ mg/L}$$
$$C_{ss} \text{ (desired)} = 14 \text{ mg/L}$$

Salt factor for phenytoin tablets = 1

(A) 1 tablet
(B) 4 tablets
(C) 5 tablets
(D) 6 tablets
(E) 7 tablets

88. Which of the following tablet excipients would be most expected to decrease product bioavailability?

    (A) Starch
    (B) Microcrystalline cellulose
    (C) Lactose
    (D) Magnesium stearate
    (E) Mannitol

89. Poor metabolizers of CYP 2D6 are most likely to receive therapeutic benefit from which of the following opioids?

    (A) Codeine
    (B) Morphine
    (C) Hydrocodone
    (D) Oxycodone
    (E) Dextromethorphan

90. Patients taking protease inhibitors should avoid drinking grapefruit juice because it

    (A) inhibits CYP 3A, leading to toxic levels of the drug.
    (B) inhibits CYP 3A, leading to subtherapeutic levels of the drug.
    (C) induces CYP 3A, leading to toxic levels of the drug.
    (D) induces CYP 3A, leading to subtherapeutic levels of the drug.
    (E) binds to the drug, preventing absorption.

91. You receive an order for 10 mL of epinephrine 1:10,000 solution. What is another way to express this concentration?

    (A) 10% w/v
    (B) 1% w/v
    (C) 0.1% w/v
    (D) 0.01% w/v
    (E) 0.001% w/v

92. You need to measure out 100 g of methyl salicylate to use in a compound. The specific gravity of methyl salicylate is 1.18. How much methyl salicylate should you measure, by volume, to deliver the appropriate amount?

    (A) 69.5 mL
    (B) 84.75 mL
    (C) 100 mL
    (D) 115.25 mL
    (E) 130.5 mL

Questions 93–97 refer to the following patient profile.

Patient Name: John Marx

Age: 70   **Height:** 5'10"
Sex: M   **Weight:** 198 lb
Race: Black

Allergies: None known

Diagnosis

Primary:

1. Hypertension
2. Dyslipidemia
3. Heart failure

Secondary:

1. MI (5 years ago)

Chief Complaint: Swelling in legs

Medications

Date	Name and Strength	Route	Directions
10/25	Aspirin 81 mg	PO	1 daily
	Digoxin 0.125 mg	PO	1 daily
	Furosemide 20 mg	PO	1 in the morning
	Lisinopril 20 mg	PO	1 daily
	Toprol XL 25 mg	PO	1 daily
	Vytorin 40/10 mg	PO	1 at bedtime

Lab/Diagnostic Tests

Date	Test/Result	
11/10	Sodium	145 mEq/L
	Potassium	3.9 mEq/L
	Serum creatinine	1.1 mg/dL
	Digoxin	0.8 ng/mL
	Blood pressure	122/80 mmHg
	Heart rate	70 bpm
	LVEF	35%

Additional Information

Date	Comment
11/10	Patient has gained 3 lb in the past week.

93. Vytorin is the brand name for which of the following combinations?

   (A) Atorvastatin and amlodipine
   (B) Atorvastatin and ezetimibe
   (C) Lovastatin and niacin
   (D) Simvastatin and ezetimibe
   (E) Simvastatin and lisinopril

94. Which of the following is/are appropriate nonpharmacological recommendations for Mr. Marx?

     I. Restrict fluid intake.
     II. Restrict sodium intake.
     III. Restrict vitamin K intake.

   (A) I only
   (B) III only
   (C) I and II only
   (D) II and III only
   (E) I, II, and III

95. Which of the following signs/symptoms is/are associated with digoxin toxicity?

     I. Anorexia
     II. Arrhythmias
     III. Visual disturbances

   (A) I only
   (B) III only
   (C) I and II only
   (D) II and III only
   (E) I, II, and III

96. Which of the following medications is contraindicated in Mr. Marx?

   (A) Aldactone
   (B) BiDil
   (C) Diovan
   (D) Calan SR
   (E) Inspra

97. Mr. Marx's furosemide is increased to 40 mg PO BID. The pharmacist should counsel the patient on which of the following?

   (A) He should separate both doses of furosemide from other medications by two hours.
   (B) He should take the second dose of furosemide before 5 P.M. each day.
   (C) He should take both doses of furosemide with food or milk.
   (D) He should take the second dose of furosemide at bedtime.
   (E) He should take both doses of furosemide on an empty stomach.

Questions 98–101 refer to the following patient profile.

Patient Name: Susan Brown

Age: 42   **Height:** 5'4"
Sex: F   **Weight:** 162 lb

Allergies: None known

Diagnosis

Primary:
1. UTI
2. DVT (secondary to oral contraceptive use)
3. Hypertension

Chief Complaint: Pain with urination

Medications

Date	Name and Strength	Route	Directions
3/3	Depo-Provera 150 mg	IM	Every 3 months
5/5	Coumadin 5 mg	PO	1 daily
	HCTZ 25 mg	PO	1 daily
	Lisinopril 10 mg	PO	1 daily

Lab/Diagnostic Tests

Date	Test/Result	
5/22	Urinalysis:	pyuria, nitrite (+)
	Sodium	145 mEq/L
	Potassium	3.9 mEq/L
	Serum creatinine	0.9 mg/dL
	INR	2.3
	Blood pressure	125/72 mmHg
	Heart rate	71 bpm

Additional Information

Date	Comment
5/5	Patient contemplating smoking cessation
5/22	Patient prescribed Bactrim DS 1 tablet PO BID × 3 days, #6

---

98. Bactrim DS is probably being used to treat which of the following microorganisms?

    (A) *Chlamydia pneumoniae*
    (B) *Clostridium difficile*
    (C) *Enterococcus faecalis*
    (D) *Escherichia coli*
    (E) *Pseudomonas aeruginosa*

99. Which of the following lab alterations would you expect to see in Ms. Brown as a result of starting the Bactrim DS?

    (A) Increased INR
    (B) Decreased INR
    (C) Increased potassium
    (D) Decreased potassium
    (E) Increased sodium

100. Bactrim DS is the brand name for which of the following medications?

    (A) Amoxicillin and clavulanic acid
    (B) Ciprofloxacin and doxycycline
    (C) Imipenem and cilastatin
    (D) Isoniazid and rifampin
    (E) Trimethoprim and sulfamethoxazole

101. Lisinopril belongs to which of the following classes of drugs?

    (A) Angiotensin-converting enzyme inhibitor
    (B) Angiotensin II receptor blocker
    (C) Aldosterone receptor antagonist
    (D) Calcium channel blocker
    (E) Potassium-sparing diuretic

102. A patient recently moved to the United States from England. She brings in her prescription bottle and asks the pharmacist if he carries the antibiotic that she has been taking for a UTI. Which of the following references could be used by the pharmacist to determine if there is an equivalent antibiotic available in the United States?

    (A) Facts and Comparisons
    (B) Martindale
    (C) Merck Index
    (D) PDR
    (E) Red Book

103. A patient presents with a prescription for Xalatan. Xalatan is probably being used to treat which of the following disease states?

    (A) Anxiety
    (B) Asthma
    (C) Depression
    (D) Glaucoma
    (E) Sepsis

104. Which of the following drugs is/are classified as macrolide(s)?

    I. Keflex
    II. Keppra
    III. Ketek

    (A) I only
    (B) III only
    (C) I and II only
    (D) II and III only
    (E) I, II, and III

105. Patients taking sulfasalazine for inflammatory bowel disease should be counseled on which of the following?

    I. Take on an empty stomach.
    II. It may cause orange bodily fluids.
    III. Wear sunscreen and protective clothing.

(A) I only
(B) III only
(C) I and II only
(D) II and III only
(E) I, II, and III

106. During a hospital stay for pneumonia, David Jones developed *Clostridium difficile*. Which of the following antibiotics would be the BEST treatment for Mr. Jones?

(A) Amoxicillin
(B) Azithromycin
(C) Levofloxacin
(D) Metronidazole
(E) Tobramycin

107. A 22-year-old woman comes to the pharmacy to pick up her new prescription for oral contraceptives. Which of the following references would be the MOST appropriate source of important counseling advice for this patient?

(A) Harriet Lane Handbook
(B) Index Nominum
(C) Merck Index
(D) USP-DI Volume I
(E) USP-DI Volume II

108. Cytotec is the brand name of which of the following medications?

(A) Cimetidine
(B) Metoclopramide
(C) Misoprostol
(D) Olsalazine
(E) Sucralfate

109. Which of the following drugs would be an appropriate treatment for genital herpes?

(A) Acyclovir
(B) Indinavir
(C) Lamivudine
(D) Oseltamivir
(E) Valganciclovir

110. Which of the following references is the BEST source for obtaining the cost information of drugs?

(A) Facts and Comparisons
(B) The Harriet Lane Handbook
(C) PDR
(D) Red Book
(E) USP-DI Volume I

111. Which of the following is/are potential side effects of niacin?

    I. Flushing
    II. Hyperglycemia
    III. Hyperuricemia

(A) I only
(B) III only
(C) I and II only
(D) II and III only
(E) I, II, and III

112. Cosopt is the brand name for which of the following c ombinations?

    (A) Timolol and brimonidine
    (B) Timolol and dorzolamide
    (C) Latanoprost and carbachol
    (D) Pilocarpine and brinzolamide
    (E) Pilocarpine and carbachol

113. Which of the following medications could be used intravenously to treat an invasive *Aspergillus* infection?

    I. Caspofungin
    II. Linezolid
    III. Miconazole

    (A) I only
    (B) III only
    (C) I and II only
    (D) II and III only
    (E) I, II, and III

114. Which of the following is/are appropriate nonpharmacological recommendations for a patient with gastroesophageal reflux disease?

    I. Avoid chocolate
    II. Stop smoking
    III. Lose weight

    (A) I only
    (B) III only
    (C) I and II only
    (D) II and III only
    (E) I, II, and III

115. Which of the following intravenous medications should be protected from light?

    (A) Enalaprilat
    (B) Esmolol
    (C) Fenoldopam
    (D) Nitroglycerin
    (E) Nitroprusside

116. A patient presents to the pharmacy with prescriptions for Biaxin, Amoxil, and Nexium. The patient is probably being treated for which of the following infections?

    (A) *Helico*bacter pylori
    (B) Haemophilus influenzae
    (C) Klebsiella pneumoniae
    (D) Morax*ella catarrhalis*
    (E) *Neisseria meningitidis*

117. Trusopt belongs to which of the following classes of drugs?

    (A) Antihistamine
    (B) Beta-blocker
    (C) Carbonic anhydrase inhibitor
    (D) Cholinergic agonist
    (E) Prostaglandin analog

118. The Commission E Monographs provide information on which of the following?

    (A) Dietary supplements
    (B) Foreign drugs
    (C) Herbal products
    (D) Homeopathic products
    (E) Nonprescription drugs

119. Clotrimazole is available in which of the following dosage forms?

    I. Troche
    II. Capsule
    III. Powder

    (A) I only
    (B) III only
    (C) I and II only
    (D) II and III only
    (E) I, II, and III

120. Which of the following is/are the most appropriate monitoring recommendations for a patient receiving amiodarone?

    I. Chest x-ray should be performed every six months.
    II. Thyroid function tests should be performed annually.
    III. Liver function tests should be performed every six months.

(A) I only
(B) III only
(C) I and II only
(D) II and III only
(E) I, II, and III

121. A patient using ophthalmic preparations should be counseled that

(A) the preparations can be used safely with contact lenses.
(B) the dropper tip should be placed on the edge of the lower eyelid.
(C) the upper eyelid should be pulled outward to form a pocket in which the medication can be placed.
(D) the eyes should be rubbed after the eyedrops are administered.
(E) the administration of different medications should be separated by intervals of at least ten minutes.

122. Information on intravenous medication compatibility can be found in which of the following references?

    I. Facts and Comparisons
    II. Physician's Desk Reference
    III. Trissel's Handbook on Injectable Drugs

(A) I only
(B) III only
(C) I and II only
(D) II and III only
(E) I, II, and III

123. Tagamet belongs to which of the following classes of drugs?

(A) Aminosalicylate
(B) H2 receptor antagonist
(C) Immunosuppressant
(D) Prostaglandin analog
(E) Proton pump inhibitor

124. A patient brings in a prescription for methotrexate for the treatment of Crohn's disease. Which of the following tests should be monitored in this patient?

    I. Electrocardiogram
    II. Complete blood count
    III. Liver function tests

(A) I only
(B) III only
(C) I and II only
(D) II and III only
(E) I, II, and III

125. Which of the following medications may result in hyperkalemia?

    I. Candesartan
    II. Eplerenone
    III. Triamterene

(A) I only
(B) III only
(C) I and II only
(D) II and III only
(E) I, II, and III

126. Which of the following medications can be administered via a nasogastric tube?

    I. Esomeprazole
    II. Lansoprazole
    III. Pantoprazole

(A) I only
(B) III only
(C) I and II only
(D) II and III only
(E) I, II, and III

127. A patient is prescribed felodipine for her hypertension. She should be counseled to do which of the following?

(A) Avoid drinking grapefruit juice.
(B) Avoid foods with tyramine.
(C) Take the felodipine with folic acid.
(D) Take the felodipine on an empty stomach.
(E) Take the felodipine two hours before taking other medications.

128. An otherwise healthy patient develops community-acquired pneumonia. Which of the following antibiotics would be the best empiric treatment option for this patient?

(A) Azithromycin
(B) Metronidazole
(C) Penicillin
(D) Rifampin
(E) Vancomycin

129. Amoxicillin is available in which of the following dosage forms?

    I. Intravenous injection
    II. Oral suspension
    III. Capsule

(A) I only
(B) III only
(C) I and II only
(D) II and III only
(E) I, II, and III

130. Which of the following drugs would be most appropriate to use for the treatment of hypertension in a pregnant patient?

(A) Doxazosin
(B) Lisinopril
(C) Methyldopa
(D) Metolazone
(E) Valsartan

131. A patient is prescribed Prevacid for his peptic ulcer disease. He should be counseled to take it

(A) 15 to 30 minutes before breakfast.
(B) 30 minutes after breakfast.
(C) two hours before taking other medications.
(D) with the first bite of a meal.
(E) with a high-fat meal.

132. Sporanox is the brand name for which of the following medications?

    (A) Aripiprazole
    (B) Fluconazole
    (C) Itraconazole
    (D) Lansoprazole
    (E) Rabeprazole

133. A patient presents to the pharmacy with a prescription for simvastatin 40 mg PO at bedtime and gemfibrozil 600 mg PO BID. Which of the following adverse reactions is this patient likely to experience?

    (A) Dyspnea
    (B) Edema
    (C) Headache
    (D) Insomnia
    (E) Myopathy

134. A patient presents with a new prescription for Synthroid. Which of the following medications might have contributed to her recent diagnosis of hypothyroidism?

    (A) Amiodarone
    (B) Bisoprolol
    (C) Dofetilide
    (D) Hydralazine
    (E) Propafenone

135. Levaquin belongs to which of the following classes of drugs?

    (A) Aminoglycosides
    (B) Cephalosporins
    (C) Fluoroquinolones
    (D) Macrolides
    (E) Tetracyclines

136. Which of the following statements regarding amiodarone is/are CORRECT?

    I. It is only effective for the treatment of atrial arrhythmias.
    II. It does not undergo cytochrome P450 metabolism by the liver.
    III. If pulmonary fibrosis develops, the amiodarone should be discontinued.

    (A) I only
    (B) III only
    (C) I and II only
    (D) II and III only
    (E) I, II, and III

137. Which of the following drug classes is/are used in the treatment of inflammatory bowel disease?

    I. Aminosalicylates
    II. Corticosteroids
    III. Immunosuppressants

    (A) I only
    (B) III only
    (C) I and II
    (D) II and III
    (E) I, II, and III

138. Which of the following drugs can be used in an appropriate combination regimen to treat *H. pylori*?

    I. Amoxicillin
    II. Lansoprazole
    III. Clarithromycin

    (A) I only
    (B) III only
    (C) I and II
    (D) II and III
    (E) I, II, and III

Questions 139–143 refer to the following patient profile.

Patient Name: William Boyd

Age: 56   **Height:** 5'8"
Sex: M   **Weight:** 148 lb

Allergies: Codeine, PCN, Sulfa

Diagnosis

Primary

1. Hypertension
2. Hypothyroidism
3. Type 2 diabetes × 5 years

Secondary

1. Heartburn

Chief Complaint: Fatigue, tiredness, cold fingers, feeling down

Medications

Date	Name and Strength	Route	Directions
7/10	Prilosec OTC 10 mg	PO	3 daily
	Synthroid 100 mcg	PO	1 daily
	Metformin 1,000 mg	PO	1 three times day
	Lantus	SC	Inject 20 units HS
	Lisinopril 10 mg	PO	1 daily
	Ferrous sulfate 325 mg	PO	1 daily

Lab/Diagnostic Tests

Date	Test/Result	
7/9	Sodium	141 mEq/L
	Potassium	3.5 mEq/L
	Serum creatinine	0.9 mg/dL
	TSH	28 uU/mL
	T4	4 ug/dL
	A1c	5.5%
	Blood pressure	139/80 mmHg
	Heart rate	90 bpm
	GDS	4

Additional Information

Date	Comment
7/10	Patient complains of fatigue and lack of energy.
3/9	Pharmacist advised patient to start taking Prilosec OTC.
3/9	Pharmacist counseled patient to check blood sugars.

---

139. With respect to the metformin, the pharmacist should

    (A) recommend that it be discontinued due to the A1c level.
    (B) call the doctor to discuss.
    (C) do nothing.
    (D) The metformin is not indicated in this patient.
    (E) inform the doctor that it interacts with lisinopril.

140. Which of the following is/are appropriate recommendations for Mr. Boyd?

    I. Continue taking all medications as prescribed.
    II. Start taking a multivitamin for energy.
    III. Call the doctor regarding the patient's heartburn.

    (A) I only
    (B) III only
    (C) I and II only
    (D) II and III only
    (E) I, II, and III

141. Which of the following is/are most likely associated with Mr. Boyd's chief complaints?

    I. Undertreated hypothyroidism
    II. Hypoglycemia
    III. Untreated depression

    (A) I only
    (B) III only
    (C) I and II only
    (D) II and III only
    (E) I, II, and III

142. Lisinopril helps to do which of the following for this patient?

    (A) Improve blood sugars by inhibiting ACE
    (B) Block angiotensin to lower blood pressure
    (C) Inhibit ACE, which blocks the ACE receptor
    (D) Block angiotensin-converting enzyme to vasodilate
    (E) Protect his kidneys by lowering bradykinin

143. Mr. Boyd's Synthroid was increased to 125 mcg by the medical resident. The pharmacist should counsel Mr. Boyd to

    (A) watch for symptoms of tachycardia.
    (B) avoid taking the Synthroid with ferrous sulfate.
    (C) take the Synthroid only in the evening.
    (D) take the Synthroid with metformin.
    (E) do nothing.

144. Nevirapine is the generic name of which brand drug, and to which drug class does it belong?

    (A) Viramune; non-nucleoside reverse transcriptase inhibitors
    (B) Rescriptor; non-nucleoside reverse transcriptase inhibitors
    (C) Kaletra; protease inhibitors
    (D) Videx; nucleoside reverse transcriptase inhibitors
    (E) Fuzeon; fusion inhibitors

145. When should antiviral therapy for HIV be initiated?

    I. At the time diagnosis is confirmed by Western blot
    II. Viral load greater than 100,000 copies and/or CD4 less than 350 cells/mm3
    III. Signs of opportunistic infections

(A) I only
(B) III only
(C) I and II only
(D) II and III only
(E) I, II, and III

146. Which of the following drugs is/are inhaled corticosteroids?

    I. Pulmicort Respules
    II. Tilade
    III. Zyflo

(A) I only
(B) III only
(C) I and II only
(D) II and III only
(E) I, II, and III

Questions 147–151 refer to the following patient profile.

Patient Name: Mary Christensen

Age: 75   **Height:** 5'4"

Sex: F   **Weight:** 183 lb

Allergies: NKDA

Diagnosis

   Primary

      1. Asthma

      2. Hypertension

      3. Osteoarthritis

   Chief Complaint: Thrush, dizziness, SOB, tachycardia, nausea, and vomiting

Lab/Diagnostic Tests

Date	Test/Result	
7/9	Sodium	140 mEq/L
	Potassium	3.5 mEq/L
	Serum creatine	0.9 mg/dL
	Personal best	325 L/sec
	FEV1	300 L/sec
	Blood pressure	90/70 mmHg
	Heart rate	60 bpm
	Theophylline level	23 mcg/mL

Medications

Date	Name and Strength	Route	Directions
7/20	Advair	PO	1 puff BID
	Theophylline 500 mg	PO	1 TID
	Albuterol MDI	PO	1–2 puffs TID PRN
	Metoprolol 50 mg	PO	1 BID
	Aspirin 325 mg	PO	1 QD
	Omega fish oils 1,000 mg	PO	1 QD
	Hydrocodone/ APAP 5/500	PO	1–2 Q 6 hours for pain
	Tylenol Arthritis 650 mg	PO	1 TID

Additional Orders

Date	Comment
5/10	Pharmacist counseled on swish and spit after Advair usage
6/15	Pharmacist counseled on use of peak flow meter
7/2	Patient stated she got a new cat

147. The patient's chief complaint is likely caused by which of the following?

    I. Theophylline toxicity
    II. Lack of swishing and spitting
    III. Excessive metoprolol dose

(A) I only
(B) III only
(C) I and II only
(D) II and III only
(E) I, II, and III

148. Which of the following medications would you recommend discontinuing?

(A) Advair because of thrush
(B) Metoprolol because of bronchoconstriction
(C) Albuterol due to excessive usage
(D) Theophylline because of generic substitution
(E) Hydrocodone

149. What is the generic ingredient of Advair?

(A) Fluticasone
(B) Salmeterol
(C) Fluticasone and salmeterol
(D) Flunisolide
(E) Flunisolide and salmeterol

150. What is the likely reason that this patient is taking omega fish oils?

(A) To reduce total cholesterol
(B) To reduce LDL cholesterol
(C) To increase HDL cholesterol
(D) To reduce HDL cholesterol
(E) To reduce triglycerides

151. This patient is potentially taking excessive doses of acetaminophen. Your best recommendation to the patient is to

(A) call her doctor.
(B) discuss how much acetaminophen is appropriate per day.
(C) discontinue the hydrocodone/APAP.
(D) discontinue the Tylenol Arthritis.
(E) consider switching the Tylenol Arthritis to an ibuprofen-containing product.

152. What are the major differences between Spiriva and Atrovent?

    I. Atrovent has fewer side effects.
    II. Spiriva is taken once daily.
    III. Spiriva is a dry powder inhaler.

(A) I only
(B) III only
(C) I and II only
(D) II and III only
(E) I, II, and III

153. Zyban's active ingredient is bupropion. What is its mechanism of action?

(A) It inhibits reuptake of serotonin.
(B) It inhibits reuptake of norepinephrine.
(C) It inhibits reuptake of dopamine.
(D) It inhibits reuptake of dopamine and norepinephrine.
(E) It inhibits reuptake of serotonin, norepinephrine, and dopamine.

154. Which of the following drugs is NOT commonly used in the treatment of nonresistant tuberculosis?

    (A) Isoniazid
    (B) Rifampin
    (C) Pyrazinamide
    (D) Ethambutol
    (E) Streptomycin

155. What are the current recommendations for use of ipecac syrup in the home for acute poisoning?

    (A) Use ipecac syrup liberally due to few contraindications.
    (B) Store at home and call poison center for guidance with administration.
    (C) Do not store at home and do call poison center for guidance.
    (D) Use only if you are unable to contact the poison center.
    (E) Consider activated charcoal instead of ipecac syrup.

156. Flumazenil is used to treat which of the following overdosages?

    (A) Benzodiazepines
    (B) Opioids
    (C) Ethanol
    (D) Methotrexate
    (E) Cisplatin

157. Cytomel is the brand name for which active ingredient?

    (A) Liothyronine
    (B) Levothyroxine
    (C) Dessicated thyroid
    (D) T4
    (E) T3 and T4

158. Which of the following drugs is/are considered category X for pregnancy?

    I. Finasteride
    II. Isotretinoin
    III. ACE inhibitor

    (A) I only
    (B) III only
    (C) I and II only
    (D) II and III only
    (E) I, II, and III

159. When counseling a patient about medroxyprogesterone, which of the following is/are important factors to discuss?

    I. Weight gain
    II. Osteoporosis
    III. Risk of pulmonary embolism

    (A) I only
    (B) III only
    (C) I and II only
    (D) II and III only
    (E) I, II, and III

160. How long does it take for the fentanyl patch to begin working?

    (A) 12 hours
    (B) 24 hours
    (C) 48 hours
    (D) 72 hours
    (E) 84 hours

161. Which of the following is/are important points to discuss with a patient taking morphine for chronic pain?

    I. The need for a stimulant laxative
    II. The importance of not driving a vehicle
    III. Compliance

(A) I only
(B) III only
(C) I and II only
(D) II and III only
(E) I, II, and III

162. A woman comes into the pharmacy and requests an OTC medication for pain in her knee, though she can't remember what her physician told her to purchase. She informs you that she has kidney problems. Which of the following medications is acceptable?

(A) Ibuprofen
(B) Ketoprofen
(C) Naprosyn
(D) Acetaminophen
(E) Aspirin

163. A PPD should be performed on which of the following individuals?

    I. Healthcare worker
    II. HIV-infected patient
    III. Immigrant

(A) I only
(B) III only
(C) I and II only
(D) II and III only
(E) I, II, and III

164. Which of the following pain medications must be renally adjusted?

    I. Morphine
    II. Codeine
    III. Oxycodone

(A) I only
(B) III only
(C) I and II only
(D) II and III only
(E) I, II, and III

165. Which NSAID has a maximum dose of 1,250 mg per day?

(A) Naproxen
(B) Ibuprofen
(C) Relafen
(D) Ketoprofen
(E) Daypro

166. Which of the following is NOT a warning sign of stroke?

(A) Numbness or weakness of the face, arm, or leg
(B) Sudden confusion, trouble speaking or understanding
(C) Sudden trouble seeing in one or both eyes
(D) Sudden seizure for no known reason
(E) Sudden trouble walking, dizziness, loss of balance

167. Folic acid is important in which of the following conditions?

    I. Methotrexate treatment
    II. Neural tube defects
    III. Iron deficiency anemia

(A) I only
(B) III only
(C) I and II only
(D) II and III only
(E) I, II, and III

168. Which of the following is/are the most common side effects of long-term treatment with ferrous sulfate?

     I. Constipation
     II. Dark stools
     III. Discoloration of urine

     (A) I only
     (B) III only
     (C) I and II only
     (D) II and III only
     (E) I, II, and III

169. A patient with osteomalacia would best be given a nutritional supplement high in

     (A) pyridoxine.
     (B) ascorbic acid.
     (C) beta-carotene.
     (D) nicotinic acid.
     (E) cholecalciferol.

170. Iron deficiency anemia requires a minimum of how many months of treatment?

     (A) 1 month
     (B) 3 months
     (C) 6 months
     (D) 9 months
     (E) 12 months

171. What is the mechanism of epoetin-alpha?

     (A) It induces reticulocytes to create more iron stores.
     (B) It induces erythropoiesis and the release of reticulocytes.
     (C) It stimulates granulocyte colony-stimulating factor to generate more reticulocytes.
     (D) It is a thrombopoietic growth factor, which stimulates iron absorption in the gut.
     (E) It stimulates colony-stimulating factor to generate more iron absorption.

172. A patient taking chronic doses of isoniazid should be supplemented with which of the following?

     (A) Beta-carotene
     (B) Ascorbic acid
     (C) Cyanocobalamin
     (D) Thiamine
     (E) Pyridoxine

173. The organization responsible for the enforcement of control substances is the

     (A) Federal Drug Association.
     (B) Food and Drug Administration.
     (C) Drug Enforcement Administration.
     (D) National Provider Indicators.
     (E) State Patrol.

174. Lifestyle modifications are an important aspect of disease management. Pharmacists play a vital role in ensuring that patients understand this message. Which lifestyle modification is NOT correct?

    (A) Smoking cessation for more than a year can lead to an improvement in lung function.
    (B) Avoidance of asthma triggers such as mold, pollen, dust, cockroaches, grass, and smoke can replace the need for a short-acting B2 bronchodilator.
    (C) NCEP guidelines recommend six months of lifestyle modifications prior to starting medical therapy in most cases.
    (D) Patients with heartburn may raise the head of the bed by 2–3 inches to relieve symptoms during sleeping hours.
    (E) Patients with hypertension should limit their salt intake to less than 2.4 g/day.

175. Which of the following statements is false regarding the Dietary Supplement Health and Education Act of 1994?

    (A) Manufacturers are not required to demonstrate safety, purity, or efficacy of supplements.
    (B) Labeling must include the FDA statement: "This drug [medication?] not evaluated by FDA, and not intended to diagnose, treat, cure, or prevent disease."
    (C) Products cannot have specific claims on their labels or use phrases such as "helps boost/support/ enhance."
    (D) The FDA requires certain standards for manufacturing practices.
    (E) Manufacturers are not required to demonstrate safety.

176. Which of the following herbal products does NOT have the potential to interact with anticoagulant/antiplatelet agents?

    (A) Ginkgo biloba
    (B) Ginseng
    (C) Garlic
    (D) Saw palmetto
    (E) Feverfew

177. The best therapeutic substitution for Robitussin AC is

    (A) Robitussin.
    (B) Robitussin CF.
    (C) Robitussin DAC.
    (D) Robitussin DM.
    (E) Robitussin PE.

178. Which of the following is NOT a setting within an insulin pump?

    (A) Basal insulin rate
    (B) Insulin to carbohydrate ratio
    (C) Insulin sensitivity factor
    (D) Rule of 1,800
    (E) Goal blood sugar

179. Doses of Vitamin E over 400 IU are known to increase

    (A) cardiovascular events.
    (B) Alzheimer's disease.
    (C) hepatotoxicity.
    (D) kidney dysfunction.
    (E) gastrointestinal discomfort.

180. Compilations of information concerning parenteral drug solutions are found in

    (A) Goodman and Gilman.
    (B) Martindale.
    (C) Merck Index™.
    (D) Remington.
    (E) Trissel's Handbook on Injectable Drugs.

181. Solubility data for potassium gluconate will be found in which of the following?

    I. Merck Index™
    II. USP-NF
    III. Remington

    (A) I only
    (B) III only
    (C) I and II only
    (D) II and III only
    (E) I, II, and III

182. _____ are currently available on the market.

    (A) Metformin 1,250-mg tablets
    (B) Ferrous sulfate 5-grain tablets
    (C) Synthroid 212-mcg tablets
    (D) Boniva 3.5-mg tablets
    (E) Lisinopril 80-mg tablets

183. Which statin is equivalent to Lipitor 10 mg?

    (A) Rosuvastatin 10 mg
    (B) Simvastatin 20 mg
    (C) Pravastatin 20 mg
    (D) Simvastatin 80 mg
    (E) None of the above

184. St. John's wort interacts with which of the following medications?

    I. Pravachol
    II. Sertraline
    III. Warfarin

    (A) I only
    (B) III only
    (C) I and II only
    (D) II and III only
    (E) I, II, and III

185. A patient who is experiencing a runny nose, sneezing, headache, and watery eyes should be counseled to take which of the following OTC agents?

    I. Diphenhydramine
    II. Acetaminophen
    III. Pseudoephedrine

    (A) I only
    (B) III only
    (C) I and II only
    (D) II and III only
    (E) I, II, and III

Full-Length Practice Test
Answers & Explanations

1. E

Probenecid has the potential to cause stone formation (III). Patients taking probenecid should be advised to drink six to eight 8-oz glasses of water to avoid formation of kidney stones. Probenecid may also cause GI upset and a rash (I and II). I, II, and III are correct, so the answer is (E).

2. B

A1c is the gold standard for monitoring glycemic control in patients with diabetes. Because A1c measures glycosylated hemoglobin, the timeframe it represents correlates with the lifespan of a red blood cell (90–120 days). Similarly, in patients with severe anemia, low hgb values can make the A1c value inaccurate. The most common normal reference range is 4-6% while an A1c of 10% correlates with blood sugar values averaging in excess of 200 mg/dL.

3. E

Clozapine requires rigorous monitoring with a minimum of monthly WBC and ANC. This is due to the possibility of clozapine-induced agranulocytosis or severe granulocytopenia. Due to these frequent monitoring requirements, clozapine is used less than other atypical antipsychotics and is often used for refractory cases. Answer choices (B), (C), (D), and (E) all have similar monitoring parameters involving markers of metabolic syndrome, cardiovascular effects, and unwanted side effects.

4. A

When initiating a dopamine agonist such as Mirapex, the levodopa dose should be decreased by 20–30%. II is incorrect because Mirapex does not come in a patch, which eliminates answer choices (C), (D), and (E). Rotigotine is a dopamine agonist that is available in a patch. The ergot-derivative bromocriptine must be monitored for the cardiac side effects (III), which is why the nonergot derivatives such as Mirapex are much more commonly used.

5. A

Venlafaxine is appropriate medication and dosage. (B) Lexapro is dosed once daily. (C) Fluvoxamine should be dosed once daily; fluoxetine is the SSRI that can be dosed weekly. (D) The maximum dose of Nortriptyline is 150 mg/day. (E) Mirtazapine does not come in a 10-mg formulation and should be dosed at bedtime due to somnolence.

6. E

NuvaRing should be inserted once per month; ortho-evra is applied once each week for three consecutive weeks followed by one patch-free week per month; and Seasonale is a continuous oral contraceptive that is taken as 84 active pills followed by seven inactive pills, resulting in menses approximately once every three months.

7. D

Corticosteroids such as prednisone may increase blood glucose (A) and blood pressure. Methotrexate may cause a folate deficiency; therefore, a CBC must be monitored (B). Hydroxychloroquine may cause macular damage, corneal deposits, or retinopathy, so ocular exams must be performed every three months (C). The tuberculin skin test (PPD) must be done before the initiation of Humira, not Enbrel, because untreated latent TB is a contraindication to the use of Humira. (D). Leflunomide is contraindicated in hepatic disease and may elevate liver enzymes so ALT must be monitored monthly for six months, then periodically (E).

8. D

Serum creatinine is most commonly used to assess renal function, not hepatic function. Serum creatinine is not dependent upon the amount of iron in the diet and is sometimes an inaccurate representation of renal function in the very elderly. Serum creatinine is commonly used in the Cockroft-Gault equation to calculate creatinine clearance. Microalbumin, a microscopic protein, is measured in the urine and is not synonymous with serum creatinine.

9. C

Natalizumab is reserved for patients that have not responded to other disease-modifying drugs (DMDs) (II). Natalizumab is available only through a restrictive prescribing program called TOUCH, in which both prescribers and patients must enroll (I), eliminating choices (A) and (D). Natalizumab should be used only as monotherapy and not in combination with other DMDs (III), eliminating choices (B), (D), and (E). Using Natalizumab with DMDs increases the risk of progressive multifocal leukoencephalopathy.

10. B

Allopurinol is indicated for prophylaxis of gout exacerbations in patients with moderately elevated serum uric acid levels and a history of nephrolithiasis, tophi, serum creatinine >2 g/dL, or urinary uric acid excretion indicative of overproduction (B). If the serum uric acid levels are only slightly elevated, colchicine is used for prophylaxis (A). In patients that have urinary uric acid excretion levels indicative of underexcretion, uricosuric drugs are used for prophylaxis (C). Acute gout is never treated with allopurinol and can actually worsen the symptoms (D). Asymptomatic hyperuricemia does not require therapy (E).

11. D

Lamotrigine (I) does not require monitoring of serum drug concentrations. Valproic acid (II) should be monitored to achieve serum drug concentrations of 50–100 mcg/mL. Lithium (III) should maintain serum drug concentration levels of 0.6–1.5mEq/L. Therefore, II and III are both correct and require close monitoring of serum drug concentrations, efficacy, and side effects.

12. E

All of the trade/generic names are correctly matched except that Haldol is the trade name for haloperidol and clozapine is generic for Clozaril.

13. **C**

Available prophylactic agents include beta-blockers such as propranolol, atenolol, and metoprolol, not ACE-inhibitors (A) or calcium channel blockers (D). Antidepressants such as amitriptyline, paroxetine, fluoxetine, and sertraline can be used as prophylaxis, as well as anticonvulsant medications such as valproic acid, gabapentin, tiagabine, and topiramate (C). Acetaminophen (B) is considered abortive treatment and is not taken for prophylaxis. Anticholinergics (E) have no role in prevention of migraines.

14. **B**

Tramadol is an oral analgesic that does not cause GI upset or bleeding (B). Aspirin (A) is an NSAID that may cause GI bleeding. Diclofenac is an acetic acid (C) and Daypro is a propionic acid (D), both of which may cause GI upset and bleeding. Although Mobic (E) is an oxicam and more COX-2–selective than traditional NSAIDs, it still possess the potential to cause GI upset and stomach bleeding.

15. **C**

Haloperidol is a first-generation antipsychotic. First-generation antipsychotics are known for the potential to cause extrapyramidal symptoms (EPS) such as tardive dyskinesia and dystonia. (A) is a common antihypertensive that does not cause EPS; nor does citalopram (B), a common antidepressant. Although low sodium (D) can be dangerous, it does not cause EPS. Uncontrolled blood pressure (E) may lead to organ damage but does not cause EPS.

16. **E**

Haloperidol requires periodic monitoring of a CBC because of its potential to cause agranulocytosis. (A) Serum drug levels are not mea-

sured with haloperidol. Although a baseline EKG is recommended upon haloperidol initiation, monitoring of ejection fraction (C) is not necessary. (B) HbgA1c could be monitored in atypical antipsychotics due to their likelihood of causing metabolic syndrome. (D) A bone mineral density is not routine monitoring in any antipsychotic.

17. **B**

Switching between formulations (I) would not provide any benefit with extrapyramidal side effects. Changing the patient to an atypical antipsychotic would be the best option since atypicals have fewer extrapyramidal side effects. This patient is allergic to Geodon (ziprasidone) so (II) would not be appropriate. This leaves the atypical Risperdal, which would be appropriate.

18. **D**

(D) Alcohol should be avoided in combination with antipsychotics due to the excessive CNS depression it may cause. (A) Acidic environment is not required and patients may take most of the medications with food if GI upset occurs. Medications for schizophrenia may take 2–4 weeks to work, so (B) is not correct. It is also important that these medications not be abruptly stopped (C) or self-adjusted (E). If bothersome side effects occur, physicians should be contacted to make adjustments and changes in the medications.

19. **C**

(B) Alprazolam is not used for depression but may be used in anxiety disorders. (E) Propranolol is a beta-blocker which may actually worsen depression; however, it can be used for situational anxiety. Although not contraindicated, venlafaxine (D) may not be the best option for this patient considering her uncontrolled blood pressure. Venlafaxine can increase blood pressure and should be monitored closely. Bupropion (A) is contraindicated if the patient actually has an eating disorder. Since this woman is suspected of having an eating disorder, this is not the most appropriate recommendation. Lexapro (C) is an SSRI similar to her current citalopram and would be an appropriate substitution.

20.　A

Carbidopa is a dopa-decarboxylase inhibitor, which must be combined with levodopa to prevent the peripheral degradation of levodopa (I). If the levodopa is degraded in the periphery, it does not enter into the blood-brain barrier for site of action. The carbidopa does not extend the dosing interval (II), nor does it prevent side effects from occurring (III), therefore eliminating answer choices (B)–(E).

21.　C

NSAIDs such as indomethacin are the first-line treatment for acute gout. If the patient is unable to take NSAIDs, the time course of the event must be evaluated. If the symptoms have been present for less than 48 hours, colchicine (B) is recommended. If the symptoms have been present for >48 hours, a corticosteroid is recommended. Allopurinol (D) should never be used in the treatment of acute gout and can worsen the symptoms. Probenecid (E) is not useful in acute exacerbation and should be avoided as it may precipitate attacks. Acetaminophen (A) plays no role in the treatment of acute gout.

22.　E

All of the medications are correctly matched with their common side effects. Mirtazapine is typically dosed at bedtime because of the somnolence it causes. All of the SSRIs (paroxetine) have the potential to cause ejaculation disorders or impotence. The TCAs (amitriptyline) have the potential to cause weight gain along with anticholinergic side effects.

23.　E

Phenytoin is available in many supplied dosage forms: Chewable tablets (I), capsules, and extended-release capsules. It is also available as an oral suspension (II). Phenytoin can also be given IM or IV, as it comes in a parenteral solution (III); therefore, (E) is the correct answer.

24.　B

NSAIDs are used for symptomatic relief during the onset of disease-modifying antirheumatic drug (DMARD) therapy and PRN symptomatic relief (B). NSAIDs do not alter the disease progression of rheumatoid arthritis therefore are not DMARDs. (A). Although NSAIDs can be given along with DMARDs for symptoms, they are not considered adjunctive therapy for patients with refractory symptoms (C); that is the role of corticosteroids. The biologics are not known to cause flushing with the injections (D), although NSAIDs could be used for PRN symptom relief with the biologics. Methotrexate must be given in combination with infliximab, not NSAIDs (E).

25.　B

If the patient is experiencing severe nausea and vomiting whenever a migraine occurs, most likely she will not receive maximum benefit from a regular oral tablet (I and II) due to the emesis. Many other dosage forms are available just within the Triptan class of abortive therapies. Maxalt MLT (III) is a rapidly disintegrating tablet that is one possible option for treatment in these patients. Other Triptan options include Imitrex injection or nasal spray and Zomig ODT.

Choice (C) is incorrect because caffeine should be avoided in combination with MAOIs as well as many other foods and medications. Choice (E) is not correct because although there is an oral formulation, it is not indicated for depression and the efficacy would not increase.

41. A

Fiorinal contains aspirin with butalbital and caffeine. Fioricet (B) contains acetaminophen with butalbital and caffeine. Midrin (D) contains isometheptene/dichloral-phenazone/acetaminophen. (E) Migranal is a dihydroergotamine nasal spray.

42. D

Photosensitivity is a common side effect with Retin-A, and the use of sunblock prior to sun exposure is very important. Retinoids such as Retin-A should not be used with astringents or abrasive soaps due to the increased risk of excessive drying of the skin (A). Topical retinoids take significantly longer than 1–2 days to result in a benefit (B). Topical retinoids are not used as spot treatment (C) and should be applied sparingly over the face after the face has been allowed to dry fully (E) after cleansing.

43. B

Although calcium and vitamin D are prerequisites to pharmacological therapy, they are not a treatment option for osteoporosis (II). Zoledronic acid (I) is an annual infusion for the treatment of osteoporosis but is a bisphosphonate, so it is not an alternative to bisphosphonate therapy (I). Raloxifene is a selective estrogen receptor modulator (SERM) that is recommended as an alternative choice for the treatment of osteoporosis (III), so (B) is the correct answer.

44. C

The benzodiazepines including Xanax (alprazolam), Librium (chlordiazepoxide), and Valium (diazepam) vary in their peak activity and duration of action, but all have an onset of effect of minutes to hours. Vistaril or hydroxyzine also works within minutes to hours, while BuSpar takes up to two to three weeks to reach maximal efficacy.

45. C

Cheilitis (chapped lips) is the most common side effect of isotretinoin therapy. Pruritus (itching) related to dry skin is also a very common side effect of isotretinoin therapy. Hypertrichosis, or excessive hair growth, is not a known side effect of this medication.

46. D

Topical agents such as coal tar and anthralin are commonly used in the treatment of psoriasis. Systemic agents such as antimetabolites (methotrexate) and corticosteroids (prednisone) are often used in combination with topical agents in the treatment of psoriasis. Benzoyl peroxide is not an effective treatment option.

47. C

In the TNM classification, T represents the severity of the primary tumor, N represents the severity of lymph node involvement, and M represents the severity of distant metastases. Generally, N0 and M0 mean no nodal involvement and no metastases, respectively. The only choice that includes information about nodal involvement is (C).

48. B

Adjuvant chemotherapy is chemotherapy given after surgical treatment to provide further reduction in tumor burden. Neoadjuvant chemotherapy is given prior to surgical treatment, to provide an initial decrease in tumor burden. Both adjuvant and neoadjuvant chemotherapy are expected to increase survival. Palliative chemotherapy is given to relieve symptoms without expectation of survival benefit. The answer, therefore, is (B).

49. D

Methotrexate inhibits dihydrofolate reductase; when administered at the appropriate time in a chemotherapy cycle, leucovorin permits healthy cells to continue DNA replication and RNA transcription by providing a folic acid source that is not dependent on the action of dihydrofolate reductase. 5-Fluorouracil inhibits thymidylate synthase, as does leucovorin. The two agents therefore have a synergistic effect. Doxorubicin is an anthracycline antibiotic that works as an intercalating agent, interrupting DNA synthesis. Cytarabine inhibits DNA polymerase. Leucovorin does not interact with the mechanism of action of either of these medications. Thus, the answer is (D).

50. E

The primary mechanism of action of cytarabine is inhibition of DNA polymerase. Common side effects of cytarabine treatment include conjunctivitis and neurotoxicity. Therefore, choice (E) is correct.

51. D

The most clinically important side effect of anthracyclines is cardiac damage, including acute arrhythmias and cardiomyopathy following prolonged exposure. The risk of cardiotoxicity increases with cumulative lifetime dose. Hand-and-foot syndrome, or palmarplantar erythrodysesthesia, is more common with 5-fluorouracil. Ototoxicity is rarely seen

in anthracyclines, and is more commonly a side effect of platinum compounds and nitrogen mustards. Methotrexate can cause symptoms of folate deficiency. Infusion reactions are more common with etoposide, platinum compounds, and mustard compounds.

52. C

Avastin is the brand name for bevacizumab (C). Gleevec is imatinib, Herceptin is trastuzumab, Tarceva is erlotinib, and Platinol is cisplatin.

53. C

ANC = white blood cell × (% neutrophils/sig/bands)/100; therefore, the answer is (C), 600.

54. B

The range for mild neutropenia is 500–1,000/mm^3, so the answer is (B). Moderate ANC is 100–500/mm^3, severe is less than 100/mm^3, and normal is 3,000–7,000/mm^3.

55. E

Severe or prolonged neutropenia or a sudden drop in ANC are all risk factors for infection. Invasive procedures, including dental procedures, catheter placement, and enemas, also increase the risk of infection. Thus, choice (E) is the answer.

56. E

None of the erythropoietin derivatives (Epogen, Procrit, and Aranesp) are indicated in this patient, as her hemoglobin level is normal at 14.5 mg/dL. She is suffering mild neutropenia, which does not warrant treatment with a colony-stimulating factor. Therefore, none of the listed drugs are appropriate and choice (E) is correct.

57. B

The nominal (or categorical) scale is used for measurements that have no numerical value, such as gender and race. Therefore, the answer is choice (B). A numeric scale is used for data that already consists of numbers, like weight or blood pressure. An ordinal scale is used when the data are ordered but not inherently numbered; satisfaction surveys and pain scales are examples of ordinal data. Kaplan-Meier is a statistical measure of patient survival, not a measurement scale. ANOVA is an analysis of variance, conducted on three or more independent sets of data that are distributed in a Gaussian fashion.

58. E

Power depends on sample size and variation within groups. The easiest way to increase power is to increase the sample size of a study. Altering the duration of the study or decreasing the sample size will not increase power. Increasing the number of dependent variables being studied will also not increase the power of the study.

59. D

Type II errors occur when a real difference between study and control groups is not found. The null hypothesis is the hypothesis that there is no difference between study groups; not detecting a true difference between groups will lead to a type II error. Insufficient study power may mean that a difference between groups will not be discovered or will not be found to be statistically significant. Therefore, choices (A), (B), and (C) are all true statements about type II errors. Type I errors occur when a difference between groups is detected that does not actually exist. Because the question is asking for

which statement regarding type II errors is false, the answer is (D).

60. D

ANOVA is the only test listed that is appropriate for such data (D). T-tests and paired t-tests are appropriate only when studying two groups; Mann-Whitney is a nonparametric test appropriate for ordinal data, and Chi-square tests are used on nominal data.

61. C

$$0.12\,g \times \frac{100\,g\,ung}{2.5\,g\,HC} = 4.8\,g\,ung$$

$$30\,g\,ung \times \frac{0.4\,g\,HC}{100\,g\,ung} = 0.12\,g\,HC\,required$$

4.8 g of the 2.5% ointment is required to deliver the correct amount of hydrocortisone.

62. C

$$70\,g\,HPet \times \frac{8\,g\,WW}{100\,g\,HPet} = 5.6\,g\,WW$$

63. C

$$4\,fl\,oz \times \frac{30\,mL}{1\,fl\,oz} \times \frac{1\,tbsp}{15\,mL} \times \frac{2\,mg}{1\,tbsp} \times \frac{1\,tab}{4\,mg} = tabs$$

64. B

$$60\,kg \times \frac{5\,mcg}{kg \times min} \times \frac{1\,mg}{1000\,mcg} \times$$

$$\frac{1\,mL}{0.5\,mg} \times \frac{60\,min}{1\,hr} = 36\frac{mL}{hr}$$

65. A

The initial concentration (C0) will be obtained by drawing blood very soon after administration. Using the equation $V_d = \frac{dose}{C_0}$, we can see that for equal doses, Vd will vary inversely with C0. Drug A has a higher C0 than Drug B (0.2

mg/mL > 83 mcg/mL); therefore, Drug A has a smaller volume of distribution.

66. C

$$40\,mL\,so\ln \times \frac{10\,g\,MgSO_4}{100\,mL\,so\ln} \times \frac{1000\,mg}{1\,g} \times$$

$$\frac{1\,mmol\,MgSO_4}{246.36\,mg\,MgSO_4} \times \frac{1\,mmol\,Mg^{2+}}{1\,mmol\,MgSO_4} \times$$

$$\frac{2\,mEq\,Mg^{2+}}{1\,mmol\,Mg^{2+}} = 32.5\,mEq\,Mg^{2+}$$

67. B

$$240\,mL \times \frac{15\,mEq}{15\,mL} \times \frac{1\,mmol\,K^+}{1\,mEq\,K^+} \times$$

$$\frac{1\,mmol\,C_6H_5K_3O_7}{3\,mmol\,K^+} \times \frac{1\,mol}{1000\,mmol} \times$$

$$\frac{306\,g\,C_6H_5K_3O_7}{1\,mol\,C_6H_5K_3O_7} = 24.48\,g\,C_6H_5K_3O_7$$

68. B

Accuracy refers to how closely test values approach the true value. Precision refers to how closely test values approach each other. Because the test values given are tightly grouped (8.0 ± 0.1) but differ significantly from the true value given (7.5), it can be said the values are precise but not accurate.

69. B

$$\frac{0.9\,g\,NaCl}{100\,mL} \times 30\,mL = 0.27\,g\,NaCl$$

needed to make volume isotonic

$$30\,mL \times \frac{0.5\,g\,TetHCl}{100\,mL} \times \frac{0.18\,g\,NaCl(Eq)}{1\,g\,TetHCl} = 0.027\,g$$

NaCl equivalent present

0.27 g – 0.027 g = 0.243 g NaCl needed to make the solution isotonic

70. B

The recipe makes 10 capsules (M et div caps #10). Therefore each capsule contains (0.5/10) or 0.05 g diphenhydramine. Then, 0.05 × 60 = 3 g.

71. C

fup = 1 – (fraction bound to proteins) = 0.05

Filtration clearance = fup × CLcr =
    0.05 × 100 mL/min = 5 mL/min

72. C

CLr = amount filtered + amount secreted – amount reabsorbed

All molecules small enough to pass through the glomerular membrane, which includes most nonprotein-bound small molecule drugs, are filtered.

If CLr > filtration clearance, some drug must be secreted. (Some reabsorption may also occur, but less is reabsorbed than secreted.)

If CLr < filtration clearance, some drug must be reabsorbed. (Some secretion may also occur, but less is secreted than is reabsorbed.)

Because CLr = 25 mL/min, while filtration clearance is only 5 mL/min, the drug must be secreted as well as filtered.

73. A

$$k = \frac{CL}{V_d} = \frac{400\,mL/min}{140\,L} \times \frac{1\,L}{1000\,mL} \times$$

$$\frac{60\,min}{hr} = 0.171\,hr^{-1}$$

$$t_{1/2} = \frac{0.693}{k} = \frac{0.693}{0.171\,hr^{-1}} = 4.04\,hr$$

74. D

$$C_{peak} = \frac{dose}{V_d} = \frac{250\,mg}{140\,L} = 1.79\,mg/L = 0.179\,mg/dL$$

75. B

Tobramycin is predominantly cleared by the kidney. The increase in serum creatinine concentration indicates a decrease in creatinine clearance, which in turn implies a decrease in tobramycin clearance. Therefore, choices (C) and (E) are wrong. The bioavailability of any drug given IV is 1; therefore, choice (A) is wrong. When clearance decreases, the half-life and serum concentration will increase, leading to drug accumulation. Therefore, choice (D) is wrong and (B) is correct.

76. A

Because penicillin and probenecid compete for the same saturable excretion pathway, administration of probenecid will decrease the secretion and therefore the overall clearance of penicillin. Choices (B), (C), and (E) are incorrect. When CL decreases, the steady-state plasma concentration of the drug will increase, so choice (D) is incorrect and (A) is the right answer.

77. B

Amorphous compounds are more soluble in water than their crystalline counterparts, so the answer is choice (B). Hydrates are less soluble in water than anhydrous drugs, and adding lipophilic groups and removing hydroxyl groups will also decrease water solubility.

78. D

For weak bases, when pH < pKa the drug will be mostly ionized. Therefore the answer is choice (D).

79. E

All medication given by mouth is subject to first-pass metabolism. Only medications given by routes that bypass the gastrointestinal tract can escape first-pass metabolism. Syrups, tab-lets, and capsules are all swallowed, and their contents undergo first-pass metabolism. The rapid-dissolve strip is also an oral product: The strip dissolves in the mouth, and the resultant solution is swallowed. Do not confuse a rapid-dissolve strip with a sublingual or buccal tab-let—in these latter two dosage forms, the drug is absorbed across the oral mucosa, escaping the first-pass effect. Of the choices listed, only the patch is given by a nonoral route. Therefore (E) is the only choice that is not subject to first-pass metabolism.

80. B

Maximizing sediment volume and promoting loose aggregation of suspended particles are functions of controlled flocculation, not structured vehicles. Reducing repulsion between particles will lead to increased sediment density, causing caking. Only slowing sedimentation by increasing viscosity is a behavior of structured vehicles, so (B) is correct.

81. B

The cosolvent system for phenytoin injection contains water, propylene glycol, and alcohol. The cosolvent system is necessary to keep phenytoin in solution, as phenytoin has only limited aqueous solubility. Rapid infusion would dilute the cosolvents, creating a super-saturated concentration of drug in a primarily aqueous environment, leading to precipitation. Onset of action will not be faster as a result of slow injection. Rapid injection is unlikely to lead to hemolysis; this is a complication of hypertonic solutions. The viscosity of the solution is not high enough to prevent rapid injection. Therefore, choice (B) is the correct answer.

82. A

Ophthalmic products must contain preservative if they are in multiple-use containers to limit the possibility of severe eye infections. They do not require preservative when packaged in single-dose containers (II), and must not contain preservative when being used as rinse solutions in eye surgery or trauma (III).

83. C

Ulcerative colitis is a local condition of the intestinal tract; medications administered rectally are providing treatment at the site of action. Nausea, chronic pain, hormone deficiency, and migraine headaches may be treated with medications administered rectally; however, these drugs are absorbed into the systemic circulation to act at distant sites of action.

84. D

The disulfiram reaction results from the inhibition of acetaldehyde dehydrogenase. Ethanol consumption leads to the buildup of acetaldehyde, causing nausea, vomiting, and severe discomfort. Tinctures, spirits, fluid extracts, and Elixir USP all contain ethanol, and will trigger this reaction if taken in combination with metronidazole. Suspensions do not customarily contain ethanol and would be an appropriate way to deliver metronidazole.

85. C

Hydrolysis (A) results when the drug reacts with water in the dosage form. Because the reaction occurred in only one of the two bottles, this is unlikely. Photolysis (B) is chemical breakdown caused by light exposure; however, the drug was stored in a dark room. Sedimentation (D) and polymorphism (E) are physical changes, rather than chemical changes, and there was no difference in conditions between the capped and uncapped bottles that would explain a difference in the occurrence of these changes. Because only the open bottle was affected, while the capped bottle did not change color, the oxygen in the atmosphere likely caused the degradation.

86. E

Dilatant substances (A) become more viscous on agitation, and thin at rest. Newtonian substances (B) do not change viscosity when stirred or agitated. Plastic flow (C) occurs when a substance is thick at rest and remains thick until it receives sufficiently vigorous agitation, after which it behaves in a Newtonian manner. Pseudoplastic flow (D) is similar to plastic flow, but the material continues to thin if agitated more vigorously. Thixotropy is the property where a suspension remains thick until agitated, and then becomes easily pourable.

87. B

$$DR = \frac{V\max Css}{Km + Css} = \frac{(300)(14)}{6.5 + 14} =$$
$$205mg / day = 4\ tablets$$

88. D

Magnesium stearate is a lubricant, and at high concentration has a tendency to waterproof particles, preventing them from dissolving. Starch, microcrystalline cellulose, lactose, and mannitol would not be expected to affect bioavailability.

89. B

Morphine is the only one of these products not metabolized by CYP 2D6. All of the others require metabolism by CYP 2D6 in order to be activated to a therapeutically useful form.

90. A

Grapefruit juice inhibits CYP 3A, the enzyme that metabolizes protease inhibitors. Therefore, choices (C), (D), and (E) can be eliminated. Inhibition of CYP 3A will decrease clearance of drugs metabolized by that enzyme, leading to increased serum concentrations. Increased serum concentration will lead to toxic, rather than subtherapeutic (B), levels.

91. D

$$1:10,000 = \frac{1\,g}{10,000\,mL} = \frac{0.01\,g}{100\,mL} = 0.01\%\,w/v$$

92. B

$$SG = \frac{density_{substance}}{density_{water}}$$

$$SG \times density_{water} = density_{substance}$$

$$1.18 \times 1\,g/mL = 1.18\,g/mL$$

$$100\,g \times \frac{1\,mL}{1.18\,g} = 84.75\,mL$$

93. D

Simvastatin and ezetimibe combined are called Vytorin, so choice (D) is correct. The combination of atorvastatin and amlodipine (A), is called Caduet; and the combination of lovastatin and niacin (C) is called Advicor. There are no combinations of atorvastatin and ezetimibe (B), or simvastatin and lisinopril (E).

94. C

Nonpharmacological therapies that can be recommended to patients with heart failure include restricting sodium intake (≤3 g/day) and restricting fluid intake (<2 L/day), so choice (C) is correct. There is no specific reason why a patient with heart failure needs to restrict vitamin K in the diet.

95. E

Anorexia, arrhythmias, and visual disturbances are all associated with digoxin toxicity, so choice (E) is correct.

96. D

Calan SR (verapamil) is a nondihydropyridine calcium channel blocker, which is contraindicated in systolic heart failure (LVEF ≤40%), so choice (D) is correct. Aldactone (spironolactone) (A) and Inspra (eplerenone) (E), which are both aldosterone receptor antagonists, as well as the angiotensin receptor blocker, Diovan (valsartan) (C), would be safe to use in a patient with heart failure. In addition, BiDil (B), the combination of hydralazine and isosorbide dinitrate, would also be appropriate to use in a heart failure patient.

97. B

The second dose of furosemide should be taken before 5 P.M. to minimize nocturia, so choice (B) is correct. Furosemide does not need to be separated from other medications, does not need to be taken with food or milk, and does not need to be taken on an empty stomach, so choices (A), (C), and (E), respectively, are incorrect. The second dose should not be taken at bedtime, as this will likely result in increased nocturia, so choice (D) is also incorrect.

98. D

Bactrim DS is most likely being used to treat Escherichia coli, a common cause of UTIs. Bactrim DS does not cover the other bacteria listed, so choice (D) is correct.

99. A

The combination of Bactrim DS and Coumadin (warfarin) may lead to a significant drug interaction that would result in an increase in

Ms. Brown's INR, so choice (A) is the correct answer.

100. **E**

The combination of trimethoprim and sulfamethoxazole is called Bactrim DS, so choice (E) is correct. The combination of amoxicillin and clavulanic acid (A) is called Augmentin, and the combination of imipenem and cilastatin (C) is called Primaxin. There are no combinations of ciprofloxacin and doxycycline (B), or of isoniazid and rifampin (D).

101. **A**

Lisinopril is an angiotensin-converting enzyme inhibitor, so choice (B) is correct.

102. **B**

Martindale is the only reference that contains foreign drug information, so choice (B) is correct.

103. **D**

Xalatan (latanoprost) is an ophthalmic prostaglandin analog used to treat glaucoma, so choice (D) is correct.

104. **B**

Ketek (telithromycin) is a macrolide antibiotic, so choice (B) is the correct answer. Keflex (cephalexin) is a cephalosporin antibiotic, and Keppra (levetiracetam) is an anticonvulsant.

105. **D**

Sulfasalazine may cause bodily fluids (e.g., urine, tears) to turn orange and may cause photosensitivity. Sulfasalazine should be taken with food rather than on an empty stomach. Therefore, choice (D) is the correct answer.

106. **D**

Metronidazole is the only option listed that can be used to treat Clostridium difficile, so choice (D) is correct.

107. **E**

USP-DI Volume II contains information for the patient in lay language; therefore, choice (E) is the correct answer. The other choices are all references for the healthcare professional.

108. **C**

Cytotec is the brand name for misoprostol, so choice (C) is correct. Cimetidine (A) is Tagamet. Metoclopramide (B) is Reglan. Olsalazine (D) is Dipentum. Sucralfate (E) is Carafate.

109. **A**

Acyclovir is an appropriate treatment for genital herpes, so choice (A) is correct. Indinavir (B) and lamivudine (C) are used to treat HIV. Oseltamivir (D) is used to treat influenza. Valganciclovir (E) is used to treat cytomegalovirus.

110. **D**

The Red Book is the only choice listed that contains cost information, so choice (D) is correct.

111. **E**

Potential side effects of niacin include flushing, hyperglycemia, and hyperuricemia, so choice (E) is correct.

112. **B**

The combination of timolol and dorzolamide is called Cosopt, so choice (B) is correct. The combination of timolol and brimonidine (A), is called Combigan. There are no combinations of latanoprost and carbachol (C), pilocarpine and brinzolamide (D), or pilocarpine and carbachol (E).

113. **A**

Caspofungin is an intravenous antifungal that could be used to treat an invasive Aspergillus infection, so choice (A) is correct. While miconazole is also an antifungal drug, it is available only in topical formulations and is used to treat superficial fungal infections. Linezolid is used to treat gram-positive bacterial infections, such as methicillin-resistant Staphylococcus aureus or vancomycin-resistant Enterococcus faecium.

114. **E**

Avoiding chocolate, smoking cessation, and weight loss are all nonpharmacological recommendations for a patient with GERD, so choice (E) is correct.

115. **E**

Nitroprusside should be protected from light, so choice (E), is correct. None of the other IV medications listed need to be protected from light.

116. **A**

The three-drug combination regimen of Biaxin (clarithromycin), Amoxil (amoxicillin), and Nexium (esomeprazole) would be used to treat a Helicobacter pylori infection, so choice (A) is correct.

117. **C**

Trusopt (dorzolamide) is an ophthalmic carbonic anhydrase inhibitor used in treating glaucoma, so choice (C) is correct.

118. **C**

The Commission E monographs provide information on herbal products, so choice (C) is correct.

119. **A**

Clotrimazole is available as a troche, topical cream, vaginal cream, topical solution, and vaginal tablet. However, it is not available as a capsule or powder. Therefore, choice (A) is the correct answer.

120. **B**

In patients receiving amiodarone, liver function tests should be performed every six months to monitor for potential hepatotoxicity, so choice (B) is correct. A chest x-ray should be performed every 12 months to monitor for pulmonary toxicity. Thyroid function tests should be performed every six months to monitor for hyper- or hypothyroidism.

121. **E**

Patients should separate the administration of different ophthalmic preparations by intervals of at least 10 minutes, so choice (E) is correct. Contact lenses should be removed before using ophthalmic products, so choice (A) is incorrect. Patients should not touch the tip of the dropper to any part of the eye, so choice (B) is incorrect. Patients should pull out the lower eyelid (not the upper eyelid) to form a pocket for the medication to be placed, so choice (C) is incorrect. Patients should not rub their eyes after administration of ophthalmic preparations, so choice (D) is incorrect.

122. **B**

Trissels contains information on intravenous drug compatibility, so choice (B) is correct. Facts and Comparisons and the Physician's Drug Reference contain general drug information and do not contain intravenous drug compatibility information.

123. **B**

Tagamet (cimetidine) is an H2 receptor antagonist, so choice (B) is correct..

124. **D**

Patients taking methotrexate should have their complete blood count monitored for potential bone marrow suppression, and their liver function tests monitored for potential hepatotoxicity. It is not necessary to have an electrocardiogram while taking this medication, so choice (D) is correct.

125. **E**

Candesartan (angiotensin II receptor antagonist), eplerenone (aldosterone receptor antagonist), and triamterene (potassium-sparing diuretic) may all result in hyperkalemia, so choice (E) is the correct answer.

126. **C**

Esomeprazole and lansoprazole can be administered via a nasogastric tube, whereas pantoprazole cannot. Therefore, choice (C) is correct.

127. **A**

A patient who is taking felodipine should avoid drinking grapefruit juice because grapefruit juice inhibits CYP3A4, which would result in increased concentrations of felodipine. Therefore, choice (A) is correct. Tyramine-containing foods (B) should be avoided in patients taking monoamine oxidase inhibitors. Felodipine does not cause folate deficiency, and therefore does not to be administered with folic acid (C). Felodipine does not need to be taken on an empty stomach (D), and does not need to be separated from other medications (E).

128. **A**

Azithromycin is the best option, as it will cover the most likely bacteria that would cause community-acquired pneumonia in this patient (Streptococcus pneumoniae, Mycoplasma pneumoniae, Haemophilus influenzae). Therefore, choice (A) is correct. The other choices would not cover the appropriate bacteria.

129. **D**

Amoxicillin is available as a suspension or a capsule, but not as intravenous injection, so choice (D) is correct. A related antibiotic, ampicillin, can be administered intravenously.

130. **C**

Antihypertensives that can be used safely in pregnancy are methyldopa, a calciumchannel blocker, and labetalol, so choice (C) is correct. Angiotensin-converting enzyme inhibitors (such as lisinopril; B) and angiotensin II receptor blockers (such as valsartan; E) are contraindicated in pregnancy. Diuretics (such as metolazone; D) and α1-receptor antagonists (such as doxazosin; A) are not recommended in pregnant patients.

131. **A**

Proton pump inhibitors should be taken 15–30 minutes before breakfast, so choice (A) is correct.

132. **C**

Sporanox is the brand name for itraconazole, so choice (C) is correct. Abilify is the brand name of aripiprazole (A). Diflucan is the brand name of fluconazole (B). Prevacid is the brand name of lansoprazole (D). Aciphex is the brand name of rabeprazole (E).

133. E

Simvastatin plus gemfibrozil is likely to result in myopathy (and possibly rhabdomyolysis), so choice (E) is correct. In fact, if a fibric acid derivative must be used with a statin, gemfibrozil should be avoided and fenofibrate should be used alternatively.

134. A

Amiodarone contains iodine and may potentially cause hyper- or hypothyroidism, so choice (A) is correct.

135. C

Levaquin (levofloxacin) is a fluoroquinolone, so choice (C) is correct.

136. B

Amiodarone-induced pulmonary fibrosis is a potentially life-threatening condition. Therefore, if this adverse effects occurs in a patient taking amiodarone, this antiarrhythmic must be discontinued, so choice (B) is correct. Amiodarone undergoes significant P450 metabolism and is a substrate of the CYP3A4 isozyme. It is also an inhibitor of the CYP1A2, CYP2C9, CYP2D6, and CYP3A4 isozymes. Amiodarone is effective for the treatment of both ventricular and atrial arrhythmias.

137. E

Aminosalicylates, corticosteroids, and immunosuppressants can all be used to treat IBD, so choice (E) is correct. Other drug therapy includes biological agents, such as infliximab.

138. E

All three of the drugs listed can be used in a 3-drug combination regimen to treat H. pylori, so choice (E) is correct. A 3-drug combination regimen for H. pylori consists of 2 antibiotics and a proton pump inhibitor.

139. B

The maximum daily dose of metformin is 2,550 mg/day, so the doctor should be contacted. Choice (A) is incorrect because this patient has controlled blood sugars based on A1c less than 7%. Choice (D) is incorrect because metformin is indicated by the ADA as the drug of choice in newly diagnosed patients and this patient has no contraindications such as heart failure, renal disease, or age greater than 80 years. Lisinopril does not interact with metformin, so choice (E) is incorrect. There truly are no major drug interactions with metformin.

140. B

Choice (B) is the most correct answer because this patient is taking more than the recommended daily dose of Prilosec OTC: 20 mg 1QD × 14 days, which can be repeated in four months. Mr. Boyd has continued the treatment longer than the recommended 14 days for Prilosec OTC. A multivitamin (II) is not a bad option for any patient in any circumstances; however, Mr. Boyd's complaint of fatigue that he is experiencing is likely due to the symptoms of hypothyroidism.

141. A

Hypothyroidism is the most correct answer because Mr. Boyd's TSH is well out of the normal range (4.5–12.5 mcg/dL). His symptoms are very consistent with hypothyroidism: Weakness, fatigue, depression, cold feeling, weight gain. Hypoglycemia (II) is incorrect because he is taking metformin only, which does not cause hypoglycemia in monotherapy. Depression (III) is incorrect because his general depression score

(GDS) was not greater than 7 and the hypothyroidism must be ruled out first.

142. D

Choice (A) is incorrect because current literature does not support ACE-I lowering blood sugars. We are beginning to see published data supporting the idea that ACE-1 may prevent diabetes, but this is still being researched. Choice (D) is the most correct answer because ACE-Is block the conversion of angiotensin II to angiotensin III, which is the most potent vasoconstriction hormone in the body. Choices (B), (C), and (E) are all incorrect because ARBs block the receptor and bradykinin is produced but does not protect the kidneys.

143. B

The most correct choice is (B); Mr. Boyd should avoid taking the Synthroid with ferrous sulfate. Ferrous sulfate will bind to the levothyroxine and prevent it from absorbing. Tachycardia (A) could be a concern because the patient is presenting with hypothyroidism and that increase could increase his chances; however, this is a very small increase so tachycardia is unlikely. Choice (C), taking Synthroid only in the evening, is possible but the patient must be informed not to take it with the ferrous sulfate so (B) is still the best option. There is no drug interaction with the metformin, so Mr. Boyd could take the Synthroid at the same time as the metformin; however, ferrous sulfate is more correct.

144. ~~B~~ A

The best way to learn the HIV medications is to memorize the generic and brand names and the drug classes. Remember: There are only three drugs in the non-nucleoside reverse transcriptase inhibitors. Never Eat Sushi at Dela Restaurant is a great acronym to remember this. (Nev = Nevirapine [Viramune]; E = Efavirenz [Sustiva]; Dela = Delavirdine [Rescriptor]). Nearly all the proteases inhibitors end in –vir, which leaves the remaining drugs to be nucleoside reverse transcriptase inhibitors. Kaletra (lopinavir/ritonavir) are protease inhibitors. Videx (didanosine) is a nucleoside reverse transcriptase inhibitor. Fuzeon (enfuvirtide) is the only drug in the fusion protein inhibitors.

145. D

Patients diagnosed with HIV will need to have a Western blot performed; however, starting highly active antiviral therapy is not recommended because of the long-term side effects and because some patients' viral load and CD4 rise and drop differently. However, when the viral load reaches greater than 100,000 copies and the CD4 drops to less than 350, it is recommend to start therapy. In addition, if patients show signs of opportunistic infections regardless of their viral or CD4, antiviral therapy should be initiated as well as treatment for the opportunistic infection.

146. A

The correct choice is (A) because Pulmicort Respules (budesonide) is the only nebulized inhaled corticosteroid available on the market. Tilade (nedocromil) is a mass cell stabilizer and Zyflo (zileuton) is a 5-lipoxygenase inhibitor, eliminating the other answer choices.

147. E

Thrush is a common side effect of inhaled corticosteroids. The classic toxicity symptoms for theophylline include tachycardia and nausea and vomiting along with an elevated theophylline level outside of 5-15 mcg/mL. Shortness of breath is likely due to metoprolol causing bronchoconstriction by blocking beta-2 receptors in the lungs. Although metoprolol is a selective beta-2 agonist, at higher dosages it loses its selectivity.

148. B

Metoprolol could very likely be causing bronchoconstriction (as discussed in the previous question) and should be discontinued; therefore, it is the answer. Thrush must be treated with Nystatin and the patient must be counseled to swish and spit after each use of Advair. Choice (C) states that the albuterol is excessive, but there is not enough information to assess this; more frequent than 1 albuterol MDI per month would determine excessiveness. Theophylline should be discontinued due to toxicity symptoms, not because of a generic substitution problem, so theophylline (D) should not be discontinued.

149. C

Fluticasone and salmeterol combined are called Advair, so (C) is correct. Fluticasone alone (A) is called Flovent or Flonase; and salmeterol alone (B) is called Serevent and is available only as a dry powder inhaler (DPI). (D) Flunisolide alone (D) is the ingredient of AeroBid, AeroBid-M (mint), and Nasarel. There are no combinations of flunisolide and salmeterol (E).

150. E

Omega fish oils target triglyceride reduction. They are available over-the-counter and as a prescription called Lovaza. Lovaza is concentrated fish oil made through a distilling process. Omega fish oils are thought to inhibit acylCA:1,2 diacylglycerol acyltransferase and to increase hepatic beta-oxidation, causing a reduction in the hepatic synthesis of triglycerides or an increase in plasma lipoprotein lipase activity. Fish oils have only modest effects on the other lipid profiles, so choices (A), (B), (C), and (D) are incorrect.

151. B

The maximum daily dose of acetaminophen is 4,000 mg per day. Ms. Christensen could potentially take 5,950 mg/day by taking two hydrocodone/APAP every six hours and the Tylenol 650 mg TID. Choice (B) is the best option because the pharmacist can easily educate the patient on the 4,000-mg guideline and help develop a plan of administration. There is no need to call the doctor (A); and the patient can have the flexibility to decide if she needs OTC acetaminophen or the combination product with hydrocodone for more severe pain, so choices (C) and (D) are also incorrect. Ibuprofen is not a good option because it may aggravate her asthma symptoms, so choice (E) is incorrect.

152. D

Spiriva (tiotropium) and Atrovent (ipratropium) both block the action of acetylcholine at parasympathetic sites at the M3-receptor located on bronchial smooth muscle, causing bronchodilation. Ipratropium is a metered-dose inhaler used 4 times per day and tiotropium is a dry powder inhaler (DPI) administered with the HandiHaler device once daily. DPIs are breath-actuated, lessening the need for hand and breath coordination and allowing for better lung deposition. Tiotropium is longer-acting due to structural differences from ipratropium allowing for higher affinity to the M3 receptor. Ipratropium and tiotropium have virtually the same side effect profile, so (I) is incorrect.

153. C D

Bupropion is indicated both as an antidepressant and smoking-cessation agent. It is not a serotonergic inhibitor, ruling out choice (A).

As a result, bupropion does not cause sexual dysfunction like most serotonin antidepressants. Bupropion inhibits both norepinephrine and dopamine, so choice (C) is correct. Effexor (venlafaxine) inhibits serotonin, norepinephrine, and dopamine, ruling out choice (E).

154. E

Choice (E) is the correct answer because streptomycin is used only as a substitute for ethambutol and for drug-resistant MTB. It does not penetrate the CNS and cannot be used for TB meningitis. The other choices are commonly used in combination for treatment.

155. C

Due to a recent study, it is no longer recommended that ipecac be used liberally in the home because benefit remains to be proven, so (C) is correct. Choices (B) and (D) are incorrect because there was no difference in adverse outcome rates between the poison centers that more commonly recommended ipecac compared with those centers that did not. Choice (A) is incorrect because there are several contraindications including lack of a gag reflex, lethargy, and/or seizures. After the ingestion of caustic agents, corrosive agents, ammonia, or bleach, chronic misuse of ipecac may lead to cardiomyopathy. Although activated charcoal (E) could be considered, calling the poison control center before administration is highly recommended.

156. A

Choice (A) is correct because flumazenil is the antidote for benzodiazepines. Choice (B) is incorrect because there are several antidotes for opioids, including naloxone, nalmefene, and naltrexone. With ethanol (C), the antidote is Fomepizole. The antidote to overdose of metho-

trexate (D) is leucovorin; and to cisplatin (E) is amifostine.

157. A

Liothyronine is called Cytomel, so choice (A) is correct. Levothyroxine (B) has multiple brand name products: Levothyroid, Levoxyl, Synthroid, Tirosint, Unithroid. Choice (C) is the natural animal thyroid which is desiccated from pig or cow and is called Armour Thyroid. Choices (D) and (E) are the abbreviated names for levothyroxine and liothyronine.

158. C

ACE inhibitors decrease placental blood flow, lower birth weight, cause fetal hypotension, and cause preterm delivery but as a class are not category X drugs. They are category C for the first trimester and category D for the second and third trimesters, so option III is not correct. Finasteride (I) causes abnormalities of external male genitalia; and isotretinoin (II) causes major fetal abnormalities, both internal and external, making (C) the correct answer.

159. E

Weight gain, osteoporosis, and pulmonary embolism are all side effects of medroxyprogesterone administration and should be discussed with the patient.

160. B

During the initial application, the absorption of transdermal fentanyl requires 12 to 24 hours to reach plateau. The transdermal fentanyl, then, is inappropriate for management of acute pain, so choice (B) is correct and (E) is not. Choice (D) is misleading, as the patch needs to be changed every 72 hours.

161. **E**

For a patient who is taking morphine, it is highly recommended that a stimulant laxative be started for the risk of constipation. Due to possible sedation, it is not recommended that antihistamines or other pain medication be used, as these can add to morphine's sedative effects. Likewise, it is not recommended that the patient drive a motorized vehicle. Compliance is important within the treatment of chronic pain so the patient is able to prevent and stay ahead of the pain.

162. **D**

This question is designed to assess whether you know that choices (A), (B), (C), and (E) are all forms of NSAIDs. NSAIDs inhibit prostaglandins, which help to keep the afferent arterioles of the kidneys open. As a result, a recommendation other than acetaminophen (D) could compromise the patient's kidney function.

163. **E**

A PPD is a tuberculin test for tuberculosis. Tuberculosis results in individuals becoming sensitized to certain antigenic components of the M. tuberculosis organism. Healthcare workers (I) are at risk for being exposed to patients with TB. HIV-infected patients (II) are immunocompromised, which allows for easier inoculation and growth of the organism. Immigrant workers (III) have a higher rate of infection and lack of access to health care. Considering all this, choice (E) is the correct answer.

164. **C**

Morphine and codeine should be renally adjusted to 75% with the CrCl between 10 and 50 mL/min. When the CrCl is less than 10 mL/min, only 50% of the dose should be administered. Morphine has a metabolite, morphine-6-glucuronide, which can become toxic in renal insufficiency. Oxycodone should be hepatically adjusted but does not require renal adjustment, so choice (C) is correct.

165. **A**

Naproxen's maximum daily dose is 1,250 mg/day. Other maximum daily doses are: Ibuprofen (B), 3,200 mg/day; Relafen (nabumetone) (C), 2,000 mg/day; and ketoprofen (D), 300 mg/day. Daypro (oxaprozin) (E) maximum daily dose is 1,200 mg/day in patients who weigh less than 50 kg and 1,800 mg/day in patients who weigh more than 50 kg.

166. **D**

There are four warning signs for stroke. Of the five answer choices, only sudden seizure for no reason (D) is not considered common with stroke. Regardless, a patient should be rushed to the emergency room for care if a seizure occurred. The four warning signs for stroke (choices A, B, C, and E) are important in helping patients and clinicians to reach and begin treatment as soon as possible.

167. **C**

Folic acid is used with methotrexate treatment because methotrexate is a folate antimetabolite that inhibits DNA synthesis. Methotrexate irreversibly binds to dihydrofolate reductase and inhibits the formation of reduced folates. Use of folate acid is important in preparation for pregnancy to not affect fetal growth and to prevent neural tube defects. Iron deficiency anemia (III) is a deficiency of iron. Folate deficiency is found in megablastic and macrocytic anemias, so (C) is correct.

168. E

All three of these side effects are common with ferrous sulfate. It is important to recommend a stool softener and to counsel patients regarding the dark stools and discoloration of urine.

169. E

Choice (E) is correct because cholecalciferol is dietary supplement of vitamin D for the treatment of vitamin D deficiency. Pyridoxine (A) is used for vitamin B6 deficiency, acute toxicity from isoniazid, cycloserine, or hydrazine overdose. Ascorbic acid (B) is used for prevention and treatment of scurvy and to acidify the urine. Beta-carotene (C) is used for prophylaxis and treatment of polymorphous light eruption, and for erythropoietic protoporphyria. Nicotinic acid (D) is used for dyslipidemias to lower the risk of recurrent MI and slow the progression of coronary artery disease.

170. C

One of the problems with treating iron deficiency anemia (IDA) is the side effects associated with treatment. Patients are often unable to tolerate the side effects, which limits the length of therapy. The minimum length of therapy with the lowest rates of relapsing IDA is six months.

171. B

The mechanism of action of epoetin-alpha is inducing erythropoisis and releasing reticulocytes, which are immature red blood cells. Choices (A), (C), (D), and (E) are all combinations of other drug mechanisms of actions.

172. E

Choice (E) is correct. The other options are not used with isoniazid treatment.

173. C

The Drug Enforcement Administration is the organization that is ultimately responsible for controlling and regulating controlled substances. The Federal Drug Association (A) is not a known association. The Food and Drug Administration (B) is in charge of approving medication for market. The National Provider Indicators (D) is a group that assigns a national provider number to all healthcare professionals. The State Patrol (E) is often called on to arrest or investigate persons involved in drug diversion.

174. C

Choices (A), (B), (D), and (E) are all correct lifestyle modifications for their respective diseases. Choice (C) is incorrect (and thus the correct answer) because the most recent NCEP guidelines recommend only three months of lifestyle modifications. This is updated from the previous recommendation of six months before starting pharmacological therapy.

175. D

Choices (A), (B), and (C) are all correct statements within the Dietary Supplement Health and Education Act of 1994. Choice (D) is not written into that act and has created much debate and controversy; the FDA is considering making a change but to date, has not.

176. D

Saw palmetto has very few drug interactions. This is important because its prescription counterparts finasteride and dutasteride do interact with warfarin. Choices (A), (B), (C), and (E) all interact with warfarin by increasing INR levels by inhibiting CYP 450 enzymes 1A2, 2D6, and 3A4.

177. D

Robistussin DM contains dextromethorphan and guaifenesin for cough and mucus; this is the most correct answer as it does not involve treating any other symptoms. Robitussin AC contains guaifenesin to enhance mucus thinning and codeine as a cough suppressant. The active ingredient in Robitussin (A) is guaifenesin for mucus. In Robitussin CF (B), the active ingredients are guaifenesin, dextromethorphan, and phenylephrine for cough, mucus, and cough, respectively. Robitussin DAC (C) contains guaifenesin, pseudoephedrine, and codeine for mucus, congestion, and cough, respectively. (D) Robitussin PE (E) contains guaifenesin and pseudoephedrine for mucus and cough.

178. D

The most modern insulin pumps have basal insulin rates that typically run for 24 hours per day, providing a small amount of continuous insulin. Insulin-to-carbohydrate ratio settings are used for bolus injections during carbohydrate intake, and insulin sensitivity factor settings are used for elevated blood sugars that are not related to food intake. The goal blood-sugar setting is used to determine how tightly controlled the patient should be. The rule of 1,800 is used to determine the insulin sensitivity factor but is not within the insulin pump, so choice (D) is an incorrect statement and is thus the correct answer.

179. A

It has been suggested that vitamin E has several benefits, including antioxidants, prevention of Alzheimer's disease and hemolytic anemia, and treatment of tardive dyskinesia. However, a recent meta-analysis suggests that doses greater than 400 IU can increase the risk for cardiovascular events, so choice (A) is correct.

180. E

Trissel's is the only book that provides a single compilation of all currently available stability information on drugs in compounded oral, enteral, topical, and ophthalmic formulations. Goodman and Gilman (A) focuses on medical pharmacology. Martindale (B) is a comprehensive drug list in which the first volume contains the preface and the drug monographs, and the second volume holds all proprietary preparations as well as manufacturer's contact information. Also known to include foreign drugs. The Merck Index (C) focuses on precise, comprehensive information on chemicals, drugs, and biologicals, whereas the Merck Manual focuses on diseases. Remington (D) is considered the pharmacy encyclopedia for pharmacology, theoretical science, sterilization, and practical pharmacy practice.

181. E

All three options provide solubility data on potassium gluconate. USP-NF (II) has official monographs for drug structure, solubilities, assays, and therapeutic category, but provides limited information on dosage and dosage forms. The other two options are described in the previous question.

182. B

Ferrous sulfate 5 grain (B) is equivalent to 325 mg and is available on the market. The metformin dose in choice (A) does not exist. Synthroid's highest dose (C) is 200 mcg. Boniva 3.5 mg (D) is not available; however, Boniva is available in once-daily dosing at 2.5 mg/day. Lisinopril's highest dosage form (E) is 40 mg.

183. **B**

Simvastatin is half as potent as Lipitor (atorvastatin), so simvastatin 20 mg is the correct answer. Rosuvastatin (A) is twice as potent as Lipitor (atorvastatin). Pravastatin (C) is one-fourth as potent at atorvastatin and would require 40 mg to be equivalent.

184. **D**

St. John's wort is commonly used by patients for mild to moderate depression. However, it is not void of side effects or drug interactions. It is metabolized by CYP P450 3A4 enzyme, which is the most prominent hepatic isoenzyme involved in drug interactions. As a result, warfarin is metabolized by 3A4. Sertraline interacts with St. John's wort because both inhibit the reuptake of serotonin, which could result in serotonin syndrome. Pravachol is the only statin not metabolized by 3A4.

185. **C**

This is a classic NAPLEX question which guides you to assess each complaint of the patient. There is no need to overtreat with an unneeded medication such as pseudoephedrine (III); the patient is not experiencing any congestion. Diphenhydramine (I) is used for the runny nose and sneezing, and the acetaminophen (II) is for the pain of the headache. Thus, options (I) and (II) are appropriate, making choice (C) correct.

Part Six

Appendix

Appendix

As the number of prescription medications continues to grow, it becomes increasingly challenging for pharmacists to remain familiar with brand and generic names of medications. Although it is unrealistic to memorize ALL of the medication names, it is essential that a new graduate know both trade and generic names for the most commonly prescribed medicines, better known as the Top 200. These lists represent the 200 medications (brand name and generic) that have been prescribed the most in the previous year.

When studying for the NAPLEX, focusing on these drugs will best prepare you for passing the exam. You will also find references to the lists throughout the chapters in the drug charts.

TOP 200 GENERIC DRUGS BY UNITS IN 2007

Rank	Product	Total Rxs (add 000)	Rank	Product	Total Rxs (add 000)	Rank	Product	Total Rxs (add 000)
1.	Hydrocodone/APAP	117,200	36.	Paroxetine	15,650	71.	Glipizide	6,672
2.	Lisinopril	61,704	37.	Trazodone HCl	15,473	72.	Benazepril	6,622
3.	Amoxicillin	52,987	38.	Lovastatin	15,309	73.	Metronidazole Tabs	6,459
4.	Levothyroxine	49,677	39.	Fluticasone Nasal	14,985	74.	Amlodipine Besylate/	6,356
5.	Hydrochlorothiazide	45,777	40.	Zolpidem Tartrate	14,613	75.	Metoclopramide	6,325
6.	Azithromycin	45,279	41.	Acetaminophen w/Cod	14,092	76.	Quinapril	6,265
7.	Atenolol	42,180	42.	Potassium Chloride	13,683	77.	Glipizide ER	6,167
8.	Simvastatin	41,496	43.	Amitriptyline	13,462	78.	Propranolol HCl	6,154
9.	Alprazolam	40,914	44.	Diazepam	13,460	79.	Hydroxyzine	6,129
10.	Furosemide Oral	37,094	45.	Naproxen	13,249	80.	Diclofenac Sodium	5,751
11.	Metformin	36,786	46.	Enalapril	12,976	81.	Estradiol Oral	5,719
12.	Sertraline	28,037	47.	Ranitidine HCl	12,654	82.	Gemfibrozil	5,678
13.	Metoprolol Tartrate	27,486	48.	Fluconazole	12,438	83.	Oxycodone ER	5,536
14.	Ibuprofen	24,656	49.	Carisoprodol	11,907	84.	Doxazosin	5,523
15.	Amlodipine Besylate	23,489	50.	Allopurinol	11,495	85.	Meclizine HCl	5,361
16.	Oxycodone w/APAP	23,443	51.	Doxycycline	11,198	86.	Mirtazapine	5,129
17.	Prednisone Oral	23,053	52.	Methylprednis Tabs	11,104	87.	Ntrofrntin Mnohy Mcr	4,952
18.	Cephalexin	22,354	53.	Clonidine	10,958	88.	Glybrid/Metfrmin HCl	4,948
19.	Fluoxetine	22,266	54.	Trimethoprim/Sulfa	9,712	89.	Acyclovir	4,776
20.	Triamterene w/HCTZ	21,335	55.	Promethazine Tabs	9,689	90.	Amphetamine Salt Cmb	4,761
21.	Propoxyphene-N/APAP	21,330	56.	Isosorbide Mononitrt	9,345	91.	Cartia XT	4,626
22.	Warfarin	21,111	57.	Pravastatin	9,225	92.	Fentanyl Transdermal	4,524
23.	Lorazepam	21,022	58.	Meloxicam	9,082	93.	Buspirone HCl	4,520
24.	Omeprazole	20,562	59.	Verapamil SR	8,747	94.	Nabumetone	4,498
25.	Clonazepam	20,078	60.	Folic Acid	8,481	95.	Diltiazem CD	4,489
26.	Amoxicillin/Pot Clav	19,608	61.	Glyburide	8,387	96.	Promethazine/Codeine	4,390
27.	Albuterol Aerosol	18,973	62.	Sulfamethoxazole/Tri	8,335	97.	Methotrexate	4,385
28.	Ciprofloxacin HCl	18,905	63.	Penicillin VK	8,112	98.	Bisoprolol/HCTZ	4,384
29.	Metoprolol Succinate	18,865	64.	Spironolactone	8,068	99.	Oxycodone	4,375
30.	Cyclobenzaprine	18,814	65.	Temazepam	7,878	100.	Butalbital/APAP/Caf	4,330
31.	Tramadol	18,526	66.	Glimepiride	7,725	101.	Phentermine	4,312
32.	Gabapentin	18,074	67.	Albuterol Neb Soln	7,645	102.	Clotrimazl/Betamthsn	4,290
33.	Fexofenadine	17,907	68.	Triamcinln Acet Top	7,327	103.	Minocycline	4,249
34.	Lisinopril/HCTZ	16,806	69.	Clindamycin Systemic	7,100	104.	Nifedipine ER	4,186
35.	Citalopram HBR	16,246	70.	Metformin HCl ER	6,956	105.	Cefdinir	4,181

Rank	Product	Total Rxs (add 000)	Rank	Product	Total Rxs (add 000)	Rank	Product	Total Rxs (add 000)
106.	Terazosin	4,075	141.	Ketoconazole Topical	2,855	176.	Dexamethasone Oral	1,939
107.	Bupropion SR	3,953	142.	Phenobarbital	2,834	177.	Torsemide	1,907
108.	Mupirocin	3,793	143.	Nystatin Systemic	2,821	178.	Erythromycin Ophth	1,895
109.	Felodipine ER	3,743	144.	Cefuroxime Axetil	2,753	179.	Captopril	1,891
110.	Potassium Chloride E	3,708	145.	Nystatin Topical	2,672	180.	Nadolol	1,828
111.	Ramadol HCl/APAP	3,677	146.	Fosinopril Sodium	2,656	181.	Nifedipine	1,793
112.	Tizanidine HCl	3,668	147.	Labetalol	2,630	182.	Methylphenidate	1,785
113.	Ferrous Sulfate	3,664	148.	Carbidopa/Levodopa	2,626	183.	Promethazine DM	1,785
114.	Phenytoin Sodium Ext	3,644	149.	Hydrocortison Top Rx	2,618	184.	Sotalol	1,780
115.	Methadone HCl Non-In	3,626	150.	Fluocinonide	2,591	185.	Cefprozil	1,764
116.	Digoxin	3,569	151.	Hydroxyzine Pamoate	2,539	186.	Diphenoxylate w/Atro	1,745
117.	Lithium Carbonate	3,566	152.	Vitamin D	2,523	187.	Oxybutynin Chl ER	1,743
118.	Methocarbamol	3,551	153.	Indomethacin	2,495	188.	Bumetanide Non-Inj	1,741
119.	Benzonatate	3,502	154.	Prednisone Intensol	2,481	189.	Prednisolne Acet Oph	1,713
120.	Famotidine	3,485	155.	Benztropine	2,479	190.	Nystatin/Triamcinoln	1,701
121.	Atenolol Chlorthal	3,402	156.	Oxybutynin Chloride	2,464	191.	Tamoxifen	1,671
122.	Phenazopyridine HCl	3,377	157.	Amiodarone	2,440	192.	Indapamide	1,654
123.	Chlorhexidine Glucon	3,326	158.	Hydrocodone/Ibprofen	2,394	193.	Metolazone	1,620
124.	Nitroquick	3,220	159.	Medrxyprgsterone Tab	2,388	194.	Cyanocobalamin	1,597
125.	Etodolac	3,155	160.	Nitrofurantoin Mcroc	2,386	195.	Clopidogrel	1,562
126.	Colchicine	3,147	161.	Polyethylene Glycol	2,370	196.	Bupropion ER	1,559
127.	Finasteride	3,146	162.	Hydralazine	2,265	197.	Imipramine HCl	1,524
128.	Aspirin,Enteric-Coat	3,120	163.	Morphine Sulfate ER	2,242	198.	Cilostazol	1,511
129.	Clarithromycin	3,111	164.	Clindamycin Topical	2,238	199.	Hydromorphone HCl	1,503
130.	Nortriptyline	3,105	165.	Tetracycline	2,233	200.	Polymyxin B/Trimeth	1,494
131.	Clobetasol	3,093	166.	Nifedical XL	2,094	All Others		223,693
132.	Hydroxychloroquine	3,093	167.	Doxepin	2,072			
133.	Dicyclomine HCl	3,039	168.	Carbamazepine	2,070			
134.	NovoLog	3,007	169.	Naproxen Sodium	2,066			
135.	Hyoscyamine	2,988	170.	Diltiazem SR	2,066			
136.	Prednisln Sd Phs Orl	2,972	171.	Piroxicam	2,042			
137.	Carvedilol	2,947	172.	Benazepril/HCTZ	2,038			
138.	Nitroglycerin	2,917	173.	Prochlorperaz Mal	1,983			
139.	Baclofen	2,911	174.	Docusate Sodium	1,978			
140.	Cheratussin AC	2,859	175.	Mometasone Topical	1,949			

Source: Verispan VONA, Full year 2007

TOP 200 NAME BRAND DRUGS BY UNITS IN 2007

Rank	Product	Total Rxs (add 000)	Rank	Product	Total Rxs (add 000)	Rank	Product	Total Rxs (add 000)
1.	Lipitor	55,122	36.	Adderall XR	9,19	71.	Evista	4,693
2.	Singulair	27,255	37.	Lotrel	8,914	72.	NuvaRing	4,656
3.	Lexapro	27,023	38.	Actonel	8,784	73.	Omnicef	4,534
4.	Nexium	26,425	39.	Ambien CR	8,765	74.	Niaspan	4,530
5.	Synthroid	25,526	40.	Cozaar	8,587	75.	Tri-Sprintec	4,502
6.	Plavix	22,336	41.	Coreg	8,404	76.	Boniva	4,408
7.	Toprol XL	21,042	42.	Valtrex	8,028	77.	Flovent HFA	4,371
8.	Prevacid	20,397	43.	Lyrica	7,907	78.	Avelox	4,302
9.	Vytorin	19,396	44.	Concerta	7,821	79.	Abilify	4,227
10.	Advair Diskus	18,181	45.	Ambien	7,696	80.	Avalide	4,215
11.	Zyrtec	17,936	46.	Risperdal	7,654	81.	Requip	4,008
12.	Effexor XR	17,200	47.	Digitek	7,487	82.	Zyrtec Syrup	3,916
13.	Protonix	16,066	48.	Topamax	7,416	83.	Coumadin Tabs	3,902
14.	Diovan	15,199	49.	Chantix	7,302	84.	Zyprexa	3,849
15.	Fosamax	15,096	50.	Avandia	7,127	85.	Depakote ER	3,849
16.	Zetia	14,264	51.	Lamictal	6,861	86.	Nasacort AQ	3,748
17.	Crestor	13,758	52.	Ortho Tri-Cyclen Lo	6,820	87.	Skelaxin	3,695
18.	Levaquin	13,553	53.	Xalatan	6,570	88.	Allegra-D 12 Hour	3,664
19.	Diovan HCT	12,868	54.	Aciphex	6,508	89.	Humalog	3,587
20.	Klor-Con	12,788	55.	Hyzaar	6,456	90.	Vigamox	3,577
21.	Cymbalta	12,551	56.	Spiriva	6,396	91.	Endocet	3,537
22.	Actos	12,298	57.	Wellbutrin XL	6,370	92.	Budeprion SR	3,494
23.	Premarin Tabs	11,785	58.	Lunesta	6,318	93.	Depakote	3,484
24.	ProAir HFA	11,253	59.	Benicar	6,229	94.	Namenda	3,466
25.	Celebrex	11,078	60.	Benicar HCT	5,892	95.	Lidoderm	3,444
26.	Flomax	11,041	61.	Aricept	5,817	96.	Strattera	3,421
27.	Seroquel	10,991	62.	Avapro	5,732	97.	Aviane	3,415
28.	Norvasc	10,910	63.	Detrol LA	5,571	98.	Patanol	3,207
29.	Nasonex	10,889	64.	Trinessa	5,225	99.	Proventil HFA	3,162
30.	Tricor	10,471	65.	Cialis	5,182	100.	Clarinex	3,017
31.	Lantus	10,395	66.	Combivent	5,145	101.	Thyroid, Armour	2,956
32.	Viagra	10,384	67.	Budeprion XL	4,808	102.	Astelin	2,893
33.	Altace	10,213	68.	Yaz	4,757	103.	Zyrtec-D	2,879
34.	Yasmin 28	9,664	69.	Glycolax	4,723	104.	Tussionex	2,861
35.	Levoxyl	9,195	70.	Imitrex Oral	4,707	105.	Caduet	2,787

Rank	Product	Total Rxs (add 000)	Rank	Product	Total Rxs (add 000)	Rank	Product	Total Rxs (add 000)
106.	Avodart	2,767	141.	OxyContin	2,005	176.	Uroxatral	1,405
107.	Keppra	2,754	142.	Mirapex	1,959	177.	Estrostep Fe	1,404
108.	Januvia	2,730	143.	Prometrium	1,930	178.	Sular	1,399
109.	Kariva	2,719	144.	Humulin 70/30	1,908	179.	Lescol XL	1,399
110.	Prempro	2,669	145.	Ciprodex Otic	1,907	180.	Novolin 70/30	1,373
111.	Rhinocort Aqua	2,660	146.	Restasis	1,899	181.	Epipen	1,341
112.	Levitra	2,658	147.	Suboxone	1,888	182.	Actoplus Met	1,332
113.	Ortho Evra	2,653	148.	Zymar	1,846	183.	M-Oxy	1,328
114.	Low-Ogestrel	2,640	149.	Arimidex	1,825	184.	Rozerem	1,306
115.	Vivelle-DOT	2,604	150.	Sprintec	1,795	185.	Enablex	1,299
116.	Apri	2,579	151.	Dilantin Kapseals	1,794	186.	Jantoven	1,294
117.	Loestrin 24 Fe	2,578	152.	Fluzone	1,768	187.	Catapres-TTS	1,276
118.	Levothroid	2,577	153.	BenzaClin	1,768	188.	Junel FE	1,266
119.	Necon 1/35	2,568	154.	Vesicare	1,752	189.	Coreg CR	1,231
120.	Fosamax Plus D	2,533	155.	Asacol	1,742	190.	Ortho Tri-Cyclen	1,224
121.	Byetta	2,530	156.	Avandamet	1,718	191.	Primacare One	1,222
122.	Pulmicort Respules	2,493	157.	Lanoxin	1,650	192.	Zovirax Topical	1,205
123.	Paxil CR	2,491	158.	Travatan	1,634	193.	Trilyte	1,204
124.	Glipizide XL	2,465	159.	Zoloft	1,615	194.	Aldara	1,194
125.	Provigil	2,458	160.	Bactroban	1,605	195.	Necon 0.5/35E	1,183
126.	Trileptal	2,450	161.	Tamiflu	1,582	196.	Arthrotec	1,149
127.	Humulin N	2,440	162.	Guaifenex PSE	1,570	197.	Ultram ER	1,135
128.	Lumigan	2,402	163.	Differin	1,535	198.	Ceron-DM	1,130
129.	Alphagan P	2,396	164.	Premarin Vaginal	1,528	199.	Ethedent	1,123
130.	Xopenex HFA	2,371	165.	Pseudovent 400	1,526	200.	Elidel	1,115
131.	Tobradex	2,358	166.	Vagifem	1,509	All Others		236,944
132.	Trivora-28	2,346	167.	Levora	1,506			
133.	Atacand	2,318	168.	Relpax	1,474			
134.	Xopenex	2,313	169.	Allegra-D 24 Hour	1,472			
135.	Cosopt	2,233	170.	Methylin	1,463			
136.	Geodon Oral	2,226	171.	AndroGel	1,446			
137.	Micardis	2,210	172.	Aggrenox	1,428			
138.	Lovaza	2,082	173.	Propecia	1,425			
139.	Micardis HCT	2,057	174.	Asmanex	1,416			
140.	Focalin XR	2,017	175.	NovoLog Mix 70/30	1,415			

Source: Verispan VONA, Full year 2007

INDEX

A

a_1-receptor antagonist, 11
a_2 agonists
    medication chart, 270
    POAG treatment, 268
a_2 agonists
    medication chart, 270
    POAG treatment, 268
Abortive treatment, 147
Absorption, 401-05, 416
Absorption rate constant, 425
ABVD (adriamycin, bleomycin, vinblastine, dacarbazine), 177
Accumulation factor, 427-30
ACE inhibitors
    medication chart, 31
    MI prevention, 36
    STEMI management, 35
    UA/NSTEMI management, 34
ACE-Is. *See* ACE inhibitors, 21
Acetaminophen
    osteoarthritis guidelines, 230
    osteoarthritis treatment, 250
    pain management guidelines, 254
    patient education, 236
    storage/administration, 263
Acetylcysteine, 304
Acid suppressants, 158
Acne
    definitions, 291
    diagnosis, 291
    guidelines, 291
    medication charts, 293-94
    medication storage/administration, 295
    patient education, 295
    signs/symptoms, 291
ACS. *See* Acute coronary syndrome
Activated charcoal, 305, 311
Active transport, 403-04
Acute coronary syndrome, 32
Acute lymphocytic leukemia, 178
Acute myeloid leukemia, 178, 179
Acute pain management, 253
Acute poisoning, 304

Adalimumab, 241
Adverse drug reaction resources, 467
AED. *See* Anti-epileptic drugs
AIDS (acquired immune deficiency syndrome), 53
Aldosterone receptor antagonist
    heart failure guidelines, 19
    medication chart, 23
    MI prevention, 36
Alefacept, 299
Alemtuzumab, 179
ALL. *See* Acute lymphocytic leukemia
Allergic rhinitis
    guidelines, 358
    signs/symptoms, 357
Alligation, 443-44
Allopurinol, 247, 248, 250
Alpha agonists, 334
Alpha antagonist, 334
Alpha blocker, 337
Alpha reductase inhibitors, 337
Alprostadil, 392
Alprostadil intracavernosal, 333
Alprostadil intraurethral, 333
Amantadine, 141
Amenorrhea, 120
American College of Cardiology staging system, 19
American Heart Association staging system, 19
Aminoglycosides, 67
Aminosalicylates
    inflammatory bowel disease, 166, 172
    medication chart, 167
Amitriptyline
    storage/administration, 263
    migraine headache guidelines, 148
AML. *See* Acute myeloid leukemia
Amorphous solids, 380-381
Amoxicillin
    H. pylori treatment, 171
    PUD guidelines, 159
Amphostericin B, 79
Anaerobes, 85
Anakinra, 241
Analgesics
    adjuncts medication chart, 262
    migraine headache guidelines, 147

narcotic medication chart, 260-61

STEMI management, 35

UA/STEMI management, 33-34

Anemia, 193

Anemia of chronic kidney disease

definitions, 281

diagnosis, 281

guidelines, 282

medication chart, 283

medication storage/administration, 284

patient education, 284

signs/symptoms, 281

Angiotension-converting enzyme, 371

Angiotension-converting enzyme inhibitor, 8

Angiotension II receptor blocker

heart failure treatment, 23

medication chart, 9

Anhydrous absorption, 391

Animal Pharmacology and Toxicology Studies, 478

ANOVA, 459

Anovulation, 120

Antacids

administration, 171

GERD guidelines, 158

medication chart, 160

Antagonist, 303

Anthracycline

AML guidelines, 179

breast cancer guidelines, 183

Anthralin, 296

Antiandrogens

in PCOS, 120

prostate cancer guidelines, 185

Antiarrhythmic drugs, 27-31, 40-41

Antibacterial agents, 62-75

Antibiotics

acne guidelines, 292

H. pylori treatment, 171

oncology support, 193

PUD guidelines, 159

therapy principles, 45-46, 85

Anticholinergics

administration, 152

patient education, 337

Parkinson's disease recommendations, 141

urinary incontinence, 334, 337

Anticoagulants

medication chart, 38

STEMI management, 36

UA/STEMI management, 35

Anticonvulant medication, 148

Antidepressants

medication charts, 203-9

migraine headache guidelines, 148

Antidiarrheals

inflammatory bowel disease, 166

medication chart, 365

Antidotes

action, 303-4

activated charcoal, 305

acute poisoning, 304

definitions, 303-4

gastric lavage, 306

ipecac, 305

medication charts, 307-10

medication storage/administration, 311

patient education, 311

whole bowel irrigation, 306

Antiemesis drugs, 194

Anti-epileptic drugs

drug-drug interactions, 138-39, 152

medication chart, 135-38

options, 152

patient education, 140

seizure guidelines, 133-34

Antiestrogensm, 183

Antifungal agents

medication chart, 76-81

oncology support, 193

Antihistamines

definitions, 357

guidelines, 357-58

medication chart, 359-60

Antihypertensive medication, 148

Anti-ischemic therapy

guidelines, 33-34

STEMI management, 35

Antimetabolite therapy, 296, 299

Antimicrobials, 295

Antiplatelet therapy

STEMI management, 35-36

UA/NSTEMI management, 34-35

Antipsychotics, 221-25

Antiretroviral agents, 55-61

Antispasmodics, 166

Antithyroid medication, 117

Antiviral agents, 82-84
Anxiety
    definition, 210
    diagnosis, 210
    medication charts, 212-15
    medication storage/administration, 2316
    patient education, 216
    signs/symptoms, 211
    treatment recommendations, 211
Anxiolytics, 212-15
Apothecary system, 437, 438
Aprepitant, 192, 199
Area under the curve, 424-25
Aripiprazole, 217
Aromataxe inhibitors, 183
Aspirin
    MI prevention, 36
    STEMI management, 35
    storage/administration, 263
    UA/NSTEMI management, 34
Asthma
    definitions, 89
    diagnosis, 89-90
    guidelines, 90-91
    medication charts, 92-94
    medication storage/administration, 95
    patient education, 95
    peak flow meter, 101
    signs/symptoms, 90
Atenolol, 148
Athlete's foot
    definitions, 369
    diagnosis, 369
    guidelines, 369
    medication chart, 370
    signs/symptoms, 369
    treatment, 371
Atomic weight, 444
Atropine, 303
Atypical antipsychotics
    medication charts, 224-25
    schizophrenia treatment, 226
AUC. *See* Area under the curve
Avoirdupois system, 437, 438
Azathioprine
    inflammatory bowel disease, 166
    patient education, 171
Azole antifungals, 76-77

B
Balsalazide, 172
Benzodiazepine
    antidote for, 311
    anxiety treatment, 211, 226
    oncology support, 192, 199
Benzoyl peroxide
    acne guidelines, 292
    acne treatment, 299
β-blocker
    medication chart, 7, 22, 269
    MI prevention, 36
    opthalmic cautions, 274
    POAG treatment, 268
    STEMI management, 35
    UA/NSTEMI management, 33
β-lactams
    carbapenem, 66
    cephalosporin, 64-65
    monobactam, 66
    penicillin, 62-63
Bevacizumab
    breast cancer guidelines, 183
    colorectal cancer guidelines, 182
    lung cancer guidelines, 181
Bexxar, 192
Biaxin, 450
Bile acid resins
    medication chart, 15
    storage/administration, 17
Biliary excretion, 415
Bioavailability, 402
Bioavailable fractions, 421
Biologic agents
    rheumatoid arthritis guidelines, 237
    rheumatoid arthritis treatment, 250
    medication chart, 170
Biopharmaceutics
    absorption, 401-5
    drug liberation, 401-5
Biostatistics
    general definitions, 455-57
    statistical test selection, 458
Biotransformation, 407-13
Bipolar disorder
    definition, 216
    diagnosis, 216

guidelines, 217

medication chart, 218

medication storage/administration, 219

patient education, 219

signs/symptoms, 217

Bismuth, 159

Bisphosphonates

osteoporosis guidelines, 243

osteoporosis treatment, 250

patient education, 246

storage/administration, 246

Black cohosh, 350

Bone and joint disorders

gout, 246-50

osteoarthritis, 229-36

osteoporosis, 242-46

rheumatoid arthritis, 236-41

Brand name drugs, top 180, 562-63

Breakthrough pain, 253

Breast cancer

definitions, 182

diagnosis, 183

guidelines, 183

Bronchodilators, 393

Budesonide

administration, 171

inflammatory bowel disease, 166

Bupropion

depression guidelines, 202

depression treatment, 226

Buspirone, 211

Busulfan, 179

Butorphanol, 147

C

Calcipotriene, 296

Calcitonin

osteoporosis guidelines, 243

patient education, 246

storage/administration, 246

Calcium, 243

Calcium channel blocker, 10

Calculations

alligation, 443-44

compounding, 449-51

concentration, 442-43

density, 438-39

dilution, 442-43

dimensional analysis, 436

dosage, 442

electrolyte solutions, 444-48

estimation, 436

formula reduction/enlargement, 439-40

measurement systems, 437-38

percentage, 441-42

ratio-proportion, 435-36

ratio strength, 441-42

specific gravity, 438-39

Cancer pain management, 253

Capacity-limited systems, 431

Capsaicin cream

administration, 236

osteoarthritis guidelines, 230

patient education, 236

Capsules, 385

Captopril, 26

Carbamazepine

bipolar disorder guidelines, 217

epilepsy options, 152

seizure guidelines, 134

Carbapenem, 66

Carbidopa/levodopa

administration, 152

extended release tablets, 146

PD recommendations, 141

Carbonic anhydrase inhibitors

cautions, 274

medication chart, 271

POAG treatment, 268

Cardiovascular disorders

dyslipidemia, 12-17

heart failure, 18-25

hypertension, 3-12

ischemic heart disease, 32-39

lab tests, 345

Carrier-mediated transport, 403-4

Carvedilol, 26

Catopril, 26

CBC. *See* Complete blood count

CCR5 antagonist, 60

Cefadroxil reconstitution, 450

Central a_2-receptor antagonist, 11

Cephalosporin, 64-65

Cetuximab, 183

CHD. *See* Coronary heart disease

Chemical instability, 379-380

Chi-square test, 458

Chlamydia

    diagnosis, 51

    signs/symptoms, 52

    treatment, 52

Cholesterol absorption inhibitor, 16

Cholinergic agonists

    medication chart, 271

    POAG treatment, 268

Chondroitin, 350

CHOP (cyclophosphamide, doxorubicin, vincristine, prednisolone), 177

Chronic lymphocytic leukemia, 178

Chronic myeloid leukemia, 178, 179

Chronic obstructive pulmonary disease

    definitions, 95

    diagnosis, 95

    guidelines, 96

    medication charts, 97

    medication storage/administration, 98

    patient education, 98

    signs/symptoms, 96

    smoking cessation, 101

Chronic pain management, 253, 263

Cimetidine, 172

Ciprofloxacin, 166

Cisplatin-based combination therapy, 181

Civil monetary penalties, 476

Claritan, 362

Clarithromycin

    H. pylori treatment, 171

    PUD guidelines, 159

Class Ia antiarrhythmics, 27

Class Ib antiarrhythmics, 28

Class Ic antiarrhythmics, 29

Class II antiarrhythmics, 29

Class III antiarrhythmics, 30-31

Class IV antiarrhythmics, 31

Clearance calculation, 423

Clinical lab tests

    cardiology, 345

    electrolyte concentrations, 341

    endocrine system, 344

    hematology, 346

    hepatic function, 343

    renal function, 342

Clinical Protocols and Investigator Information, 478-79

Clinical trials, 479-82

CLL. *See* Chronic lymphocytic leukemia

Clomiphene citrate, 120

Clopidogrel

    MI prevention, 36

    STEMI management, 35

    UA/NSTEMI management, 34

Clozapine, 141

Clycoprotein IIb/IIIa receptor blocker, 37

CML. *See* Chronic myeloid leukemia

CMP. *See* Civil monetary penalties

Coal tar, 296

Cocoa butter, 381

Codeine

    cough suppressant guidelines, 362

    oncology support, 193

    storage/administration, 263

CoEnzyme Q10, 350

Colchicine, 247, 248

Collodions, 391

Colony-stimulating factors, 193, 197

Colorectal cancer

    definitions, 181

    diagnosis, 181

    guidelines, 182

    signs/symptoms, 181-2

Common cold, 354, 357, 358

Common liquid measurement, 437

Compartmental modeling, 420-21

Complete blood count, 346

Compounding calculations, 449-51

Compounding recipes, 439-40

Compounding resources, 468

COMT inhibitors, 141

Concentration, 442-43

Confidence interval, 457

Constant IV infusion, 429

Constipation

    causes of, 371

    definitions, 366

    diagnosis, 366

    guidelines, 367

    medication chart, 368

    signs/symptoms, 366

Contact dermatitis
    guidelines, 357
    signs/symptoms, 357
Contraception
    definition, 315
    hormonal imbalance effects, 316
    medication charts, 317-23
    medication storage/administration, 324
    patient education, 324, 337
    therapy advantages/disadvantages, 316
    therapy selection, 315-16
Conversion factors, 452
COPD. *See* Chronic obstructive pulmonary disease
Coronary heart disease, 13
Correlation, 457
Corticosteroids
    gout treatment, 247
    inflammatory bowel disease, 166
    medication chart, 168
    MS guidelines, 128
    oncology support, 192, 199
    patient education, 198
    psoriasis treatment, 296
    rheumatoid arthritis guidelines, 237
Cough suppressants
    cough classification, 361
    cough signs/symptoms, 361
    definitions, 361
    guidelines, 361, 362
    medication chart, 363
Creams, 391
Crohn's disease. *See* Inflammatory bowel disease
Crystallization, 380-81
CSF. *See* Colony-stimulating factors
CVP (cyclophosphamide, vincristine, prednisolone), 177
Cyanocobalamin, 287
Cyclic lipopeptides, 73
Cyclooxygenase-2 inhibitor, 159
Cyclosporine
    inflammatory bowel disease, 166
    psoriasis treatment, 296
CYP enzymes, 411-12
Cytarabine, 179
Cytomegalovirus, 83

D

Darbepoetin, 193
Decongestants
    allergic rhinitis, 371
    colds and, 371
    common cold signs/symptoms, 354
    definitions, 354
    guidelines, 354-55
    medication chart, 356
    postnasal drip signs/symptoms, 354
Degradation, 379-380
Delavirdine, 61
Density, 448
Depression
    definition, 201
    diagnosis, 201-2
    guidelines, 202
    medication charts, 203-9
    medication storage/administration, 210
    patient education, 210
    signs/symptoms, 202
Dermatological disorders
    acne, 291-95
    psoriasis, 295-99
Desipramine, 202
Dextromethorphan, 362
Diabetes mellitus, Type 1
    definitions, 105
    diagnosis, 105-6, 123
    guidelines, 106-7
    medication charts, 109-12
    medication storage/administration, 113
    patient education, 113
    signs/symptoms, 106
Diabetes mellitus, Type 2
    definitions, 107
    diagnosis, 107, 123
    guidelines, 108
    medication charts, 109-12
    medication storage/administration, 113
    patient education, 113
    signs/symptoms, 108
Dialysis, 281-82
Diarrhea
    definitions, 364
    diagnosis, 364
    guidelines, 364

medication chart, 365

signs/symptoms, 364

Dietary Supplement Health and Education Act,
349-50, 371

Digoxin

heart failure guidelines, 20

medication chart, 22

storage/administration, 311

Dihydroergotamine, 147

Dilatant materials, 382

Dilution, 442-43

Dimensional analysis, 436

Diphenhydramine, 362

Dipivefrin, 268

Dipyridamole, 403

Direct vasodilator, 11

Discrete-dose device, 393

Disease-modifying drugs

medication chart, 130-31

MS guidelines, 128, 129

rheumatoid arthritis guidelines, 237

Disintegration testing, 382

Dissolution rate, 378

Dissolution testing, 382

Distribution volume, 406

Diuretics, 6

Divalproex sodium, 140

DMARD. *See* Disease-modifying antirheumatic drug

Docetaxel, 181

Dolasetrone, 198

Dopamine agonist, 141

Dosage calculations, 442

Dosage forms

considerations, 383

injectable delivery, 394-96

ocular delivery, 396-97

oral delivery liquids, 388-90

oral delivery solids, 384-88

otic delivery, 396-97

parenteral delivery, 394-96

pulmonary delivery, 393-94

topical delivery, 390-92

transdermal delivery, 397

vaginal, 392

Doxazosin, 334

Doxycycline, 295

DPI. *See* Dry-powder inhalers

Drip rate calculation, 451

Drug absorption, 416

Drug distribution, 405-7

Drug excretion, 413-15

Drug identification resources, 468

Drug information

adverse drug reaction, 467

compounding, 468

drug identification, 468

drug interactions, 467

foreign drug information, 468

general resources, 465-66

internal medicine, 467

lactation, 469

OTC drug, 469

parenteral compatibility/stability, 467

pediatric, 469

pharmacology, 468

pharmacotherapy, 466

pregnancy, 469

primary literature, 471

resource comparisons, 470-71

resources, 465-66

secondary literature, 471

tertiary literature, 471

Drug interacton resources, 467

Drug metabolism, 407-13

Drug transport, 403-4

Dry-powder inhalers, 393

Dutasteride, 334

Dyslipidemia

definitions, 12

diagnosis, 13

guidelines, 14

medication charts, 15-16

medication storage/administration, 17

patient education, 17

signs/symptoms, 14

therapy objectives, 40

E

Echinacea

common usage, 350

patient education, 198

Echinocandins, 78

ED. *See* Erectile dysfunction

Efalizumab, 299

Eflornithine, 120

Electrolytes, 341

Electrolyte solutions, 444-48

Elimination half-life calculation, 423

Elimination rate constant, 422

Emergency use IND, 478

Emulsions, 390, 391

Endocrine disorders

    diabetes mellitus, type 1, 105-7, 109-13

    diabetes mellitus, type 2, 107-13

    hyperthyroidism, 116-19

    hypothyroidism, 113-16

    polycystic ovarian syndrome, 119-23

    lab tests, 344

Endocytosis, 404

Enfuvirtide, 61

Enterohepatic recycling, 415

Enzyme induction, 409-11, 416

Epilepsy

    definitions, 132

    diagnosis, 133

    guidelines, 133-34

    medication charts, 135-38

    medication storage/administration, 140

    patient education, 140

    signs/symptoms, 133

Erectile dysfunction

    definition, 329

    diagnosis, 329

    guidelines, 330

    medication charts, 331-32

    medication storage/administration, 333

    patient education, 333

    signs/symptoms, 330

Ergotamine, 147

Erthropoietin, 193

Erythropoiesis-stimulating agents, 193

Esomeprazole, 164, 172

Estimation, 436

Etanercept, 241, 299

Ethosuximide, 134

Evinsa, 198

Excretion, 413-15

Extended release tablets, 386-87

F

Facilitated diffusion, 404

FDA regulatory process, 477-482

Federal Food, Drug, and Cosmetic Act, 478

Felbamate, 134

Fentanyl

    oncology support, 193

    storage/administration, 263

Fibric acid derivatives

    for dyslipidemia, 15

    storage/administration, 17

Fibrinolytic agents, 39

Fibrinolytic therapy, 36

Fick's first law of diffusion, 403

Finasteride

    storage/administration, 123

    urinary incontinence, 334

First-order degradation, 380

Fish oil, 16, 350

5a reductase inhibitor, 334

5-FU, 192

5HT3 antagonist, 192, 199

Fluidity, 382

Flumazenil, 311

Fluoroquinolones, 72

Fluoxetine

    migraine headache guidelines, 148

    PCOS guidelines, 120

Folic acid, 172

Fomepizole

    antidote action, 304

    storage/administration, 311

Foreign drug information resources, 468

Formula reduction/enlargement, 439-40

Friability testing, 383

Fusion inhibitor

    HIV guidelines, 54

    medication chart, 60

G

Gabapentin

    migraine headache guidelines, 148

    seizure guidelines, 134

GAD. *See* Generalized anxiety disorder

Gastric lavage, 306

Gastroesophageal reflux disease

    definitions, 155

    diagnosis, 156

    guidelines, 157-58

    medication charts, 160-62

medication storage/administration, 164

patient education, 164

signs/symptoms, 157

Gastrointestinal disorders

gastroesophageal reflux disease, 155-64

inflammatory bowel disease, 164-71

peptic ulcer disease, 155-64

Gaussian distribution, 458, 459

Gels, 392

Gemtuzumab ozogamicin, 179

Generalized anxiety disorder. *See* Anxiety

Generic drugs, top 200, 560-61

Genetic variability, 411-13

Genetic variations, 416

GERD. *See* Gastroesophageal reflux disease

Ginger, 350

Glatiramer acetate

MS guidelines, 129

patient education, 132

storage/administration, 132

Glaucoma, 267-74

Glitazone, 123

Glomerular filtration, 413

Glomerular filtration rate, 414

Glucosamine, 350

Glucosamine sulfate, 230

Glucose 6-phosphate dehydrogenase, 412-13

Glutathione, 304

Glycoprotein IIb/IIIa receptor blocker

medication chart, 37

STEMI management, 35

UA/NSTEMI management, 34-35

Glycylcyclines, 70

Gonorrhea

diagnosis, 51

signs/symptoms, 52

treatment, 52

Gout

definition, 246

diagnosis, 247

medication chart, 249

medication storage/administration, 250

patient education, 250

signs/symptoms, 247

treatment recommendations, 247-48

GPB. *See* Glycoprotein IIb/IIIa receptor blocker

Granules, 384-5

Grave's disease. *See* Hyperthyroidism

Guaifenesin, 362

Gynecologic/obstetric

contraception, 315-24

hormone replacement therapy, 324-29

H

H_2 antagonists

administration, 171

drug-drug interactions, 172

H_2 receptor antagonists

GERD guidelines, 158

medication chart, 160

PUD guidelines, 159

Half-life

calculation, 423

equation, 380

Hardness testing, 383

HD. *See* Hodgkin's disease

Health Insurance Portability and Accountability Act, 475-77, 483

Health policy

FDA regulatory process, 477-482

HIPAA, 475-77

JCAHO accreditation process, 483

Heartburn

guidelines, 358

signs/symptoms, 357

Heart failure

antiarrhythmic drugs, 27-31

classification of, 19

definition, 18

diagnosis, 18

guidelines, 19-20

medication charts, 21-25

medication storage/administration, 26

patient education, 26

signs/symptoms, 18

treatment guidelines, 40

Helicobucter pylori

medication chart, 163

patient education, 164

PUD treatment regimens, 163

treatment regimen, 159, 171

Hematologic disorders

anemia of kidney disease and dialysis, 281-84

iron deficiency anemia, 277-281

pernicious anemia, 284-87

Henderson-Hasselbalch equation, 379

Heparin antidote, 311

Hepatic extraction ratio, 421-22

Herbals

    common usage, 350-51

    definitions, 349-50

    medication chart, 352-53

Herpes simplex virus, 82

HF. *See* Heart failure

HIPAA. *See* Health Insurance Portability and
    Accountability Act

Hirsutism, 120

HIV (human immunodeficiency virus)

    definition, 53

    diagnosis, 53

    guidelines, 53-54

    medication charts, 55-61

    medication storage/administration, 61

    patient education, 61

    signs/symptoms, 53

HMG-CoA reductase inhibitors, 16

Hodgkin's disease

    definition, 175

    diagnosis, 176

    guidelines, 177

    signs/symptoms, 176

    staging, 176

Hormone replacement therapy

    definitions, 324

    diagnosis, 325

    drug interactions, 329

    guidelines, 325

    indications, 337

    medication charts, 326-28

    medication storage/administration, 329

    patient education, 329

    signs/symptoms, 325

Household liquid measurement, 437

HRT. *See* Hormone replacement therapy

HTN. *See* Hypertension

Hyaluronate injections, 230

Hydralazine/isosorbide dinitrate

    heart failure guidelines, 20

    medication chart, 24

Hydrocarbon/oleaginous base, 391

Hydrolysis, 379

Hydromorphone

    oncology support, 193

storage/administration, 263

Hydrophilic-lipophilic balance, 390

Hypertension

    definitions, 3

    diagnosis, 3-4

    guidelines, 4-5

    medication charts, 6-11

    medication storage/administration, 12

    patient education, 12

    signs/symptoms, 4

    treatment regimen, 40

Hyperthyroidism

    definitions, 116

    diagnosis, 116

    guidelines, 116-17

    medication chart, 118

    medication storage/administration, 119

    patient education, 119

    side effects, 123

    signs/symptoms, 116

Hypothyroidism

    definitions, 113

    diagnosis, 113

    guidelines, 114

    medication chart, 115

    medication storage/administration, 116

    patient education, 116

    side effects, 123

    signs/symptoms, 113

I

IBD. *See* Inflammatory bowel disease

Ibuprofen, 263

IDA. *See* Iron deficiency anemia

IHD. *See* Ischemic heart disease

Immediate release tablets, 386

Immunosuppressants

    medication chart, 169

    psoriasis treatment, 296, 299

IND. *See* Investigation New Drug

Indinavir, 61

Indomethacin, 263

Infectious disease

    human immunodeficiency virus, 53-54

    medication charts, 55-84

    meningitis, 50-51

    pneumonia, 48-49

sexually transmitted disease, 51-52
urinary tract infection, 46-48
Inflammatory bowel disease
definitions, 164
diagnosis, 165
guidelines, 165-66
medication charts, 167-70
medication storage/administration, 171
patient education, 171
signs/symptoms, 165
Infliximab
inflammatory bowel disease, 166
patient edcuation, 171
storage/administration, 171, 172, 241
Influenza, 84
Infusion rate, 451
Injectable delivery, 394-96
Insomnia
guidelines, 358
signs/symptoms, 357
Insulin, 109
Insulin-sensitizing agents, 120
Integrase inhibitors, 61
Interferon agents
CML guidelines, 179
MS guidelines, 129
patient education, 132
storage/administration, 132
Intermittent IV infusion, 429
Intermittent oral dosing, 430
Internal medicine resources, 467
Interval scale, 458
Intravenous drugs, 25
Investigation New Drug, 477-78
Investigator IND, 478
Ionization behavior, 378-79
Iontophoresis, 397
Ipecac, 305
Iron deficiency anemia
definitions, 277
diagnosis, 277-78
guidelines, 278-79
medication chart, 280
medication storage/administration, 281
patient education, 281
signs/symptoms, 278
Ischemic heart disease
acute pharmacologic management, 35-36

antiplatelet therapy, 34-35
definitions, 32
diagnosis, 32
guidelines, 33-34
medication charts, 37-39
signs/symptoms, 32
treatment, 41
Isoniazid, 101
Isotonicity, 445-48
Isotretinoin, 292, 299

J

JCAHO. *See* Joint Commission on Accreditation of Healthcare Organizations
Joint Commission on Accreditation of Healthcare Organizations, 482

K

Kadian, 198
Kaplan-Meier statistical test, 458
Keratolytics, 296
Ketoconazole, 403
Ketolides, 68-69
Ketoprofen, 263
Ketoralac, 263

L

Lactation resources, 469
LADME (liberation, absorption, distribution, metabolism, excretion), 401
Lamotrigine
bipolar disorder guidelines, 217
epilepsy options, 152
seizure guidelines, 134
Lansoprazole, 164
Lapatinib, 183
Latanoprost, 273
Leucovorin, 199
Leukemia
definitions, 178
diagnosis, 178
guidelines, 178-79
signs/symptoms, 178
Levetiracetam, 134
Levodopa therapy, 141
LH-RH agonists, 185

Liberation, 401-5

Liniments, 391

Lipophilicity, 378

Liquid dosage forms, 388-90

Lithium

    bipolar disorder guidelines, 217

    bipolar treatment, 226

Liver function, 343

Loading doses, 428, 432

Loop diuretics, 21

Loo-Riegelman method, 426

Lopinavir/ritonavir solution, 61

Lung cancer

    definitions, 180

    diagnosis, 180

    guidelines, 180-1

    signs/symptoms, 180

Luteinizing hormone-releasing-hormone agonists, 183

Lymphoma, 175-76

M

Macrogol, 306

Macrolides, 68-69

Manufacturing Information, 478

MAOI. *See* Monoamine oxidase inhibitor

Mast cell stabilizers, 393

MDF. *See* Multiple dosing factor

MDI. *See* Metered-dose inhalers

Mean, 459

Measurement scales, 458

Measurement systems, 437-38

Medroxyprogesterone acetate, 120

Medroxyprogesterone conception injection, 123

Megoblastic anemia, 284

Melatonin, 350

Meningitis

    common organisms, 50

    diagnosis, 50

    empiric treatment, 51

    signs/symptoms, 50

Meperidine, 263

Mesalamine

    administration, 171

    inflammatory bowel disease, 166, 172

Metabolism, 407-13

Metastable polymorphs, 381

Metered-dose inhalers, 393

Metformin, 120

Methadone, 263

Methimazole, 117, 119

Methionine, 304

Methotrexate

    inflammatory bowel disease, 166, 172

    patient education, 171

    psoriasis treatment, 296

    rheumatoid arthritis guidelines, 237

    storage/administration, 241

Methylprednisolone, 128

Metoclopramide

    GERD guidelines, 158

    oncology support, 192

Metoprolol, 148

Metric system, 438

Metronidazole

    inflammatory bowel disease, 166

    PUD guidelines, 159

Michaelis-Menten equation, 431

Migraine headache

    definitions, 146

    diagnosis, 146-47

    guidelines, 147-48

    medication charts, 149-51

    medication storage/administration, 152

    patient education, 152

    signs/symptoms, 147

Milliequivalents, 444-45

Millimoles, 444-45

Minocycline, 295

Misoprostol

    administration, 164

    PUD guidelines, 159

Mitoxantrone

    MS guidelines, 129

    storage/administration, 132

Molar solution, 444-45

Molecular weight, 444

Moles, 444

Monoamine oxidase inhibitor, 202, 210

Monobactam, 66

Mood stabilizers

    bipolar treatment, 226

    medication chart, 218

Morphine

    oncology support, 193

patient education, 198
STEMI management, 35
UA/NSTEMI management, 33
MRSA treatment, 85
Mucosal protectant, 162
Multicompartmental models, 420-21
Multiphase liquid dosage forms, 389
Multiple dosing factor, 427-30
Multiple drug dosing, 426
Multiple sclerosis
definitions, 127
diagnosis, 127
disease modifying drugs, 152
guidelines, 128-29
medication charts, 130-31
medication storage/administration, 132
patient education, 132
signs/symptoms, 128

N

Naloxone
antidote action, 303
storage/administration, 311
NAPLEX
blueprint, *xviii*
CAT format, *xv-xvi*
content/structure, *xiii-xiv*
practice test, 489-56
registration, *xvii*
scoring, *xiv-xv*
strategies, *xix-xx*
taking exam, *xvii-xviii*
what is, *xiii*
Narcotic analgesics
medication chart, 260-61
osteoarthritis guidelines, 230
overdose symptoms, 263
patient education, 236
Nasal delivery, 394
Nasolacrimal occlusion, 273
Natalizumab
MS guidelines, 129
patient education, 132
storage/administration, 132
NDA. *See* New Drug Application
Nebulizers, 394
Neurological disorders

epilepsy, 132-40
migraine headache, 146-52
multiple sclerosis, 127-32
Parkinson's disease, 140-46
Neuropathic pain, 253
Neutropenia, 193
New Drug Application, 477
New York Heart Association functional
classification, 19
Newtonian materials, 382
NHL. *See* Non-Hodgkin's lymphoma
Niacin
medication chart, 15
storage/administration, 17
Nitroprusside infusion, 26
NNRTI. *See* Non-nucleoside reverse transcriptase
inhibitors
Nominal scale, 458
Non-Hodgkin's lymphoma
definition, 176
diagnosis, 176
guidelines, 177-78
signs/symptoms, 177
staging, 176
Non-Newtonian materials, 382
Non-nucleoside reverse transcriptase inhibitors,
54, 55
Nonlinear pharmacokinetics, 430-32
Nonnarcotic oral drugs, 256-59
Nonrenal excretion, 415
Nonspecific adrenergic agonists, 272
Nonsteroidal anti-inflammatory drugs
administration, 236
gout treatment, 247
medication chart, 256-59
migraine headache guidelines, 147
osteoarthritis guidelines, 230
pain management guidelines, 254-55
patient education, 236, 250
rheumatoid arthritis guidelines, 237
storage, 241
Nortriptyline, 202
Norvir, 381
Notice, 477
NRTI. *See* Nucleoside reverse transcriptase inhibitors
NSAID. *See* Nonsteroidal anti-inflammatory drugs
NSTEMI, 32-39
NTG. *See* Sublingual nitroglycerin

Nucleoside reverse transcriptase inhibitors
    HIV guidelines, 54
    medication chart, 58-59
Nucleotide inhibitor, 60
Null hypothesis, 456, 458
Numerical scale, 458
Nutritional calculation, 451

O

OA. *See* Osteoarthritis
OCR. *See* Office for Civil Rights
Ocular delivery, 396-97
ODA. *See* Orphan Drug Act
Office for Civil Rights, 475-76
Office of Orphan Products Development, 482, 483
Ointment bases, 391
Olanzapine, 217
Olsalazine, 172
Omega-3 fatty acids, 16, 350
Omeprazole, 158
Omeprazole suspension, 164
Oncology
    hematologic malignancies, 175-79
    medication charts, 187-91
    medication charts, 194-97
    solid tumors, 180-86
    supportive care, 192-93
One-compartment model, 420, 421
OOPD. *See* Office of Orphan Products Development
Ophthalmic preparations, 273
Ophthalmic suspensions, 273
Ophthalmologic disorders, 267-74
Opiods
    oncology support, 192-93, 199
    pain management guidelines, 255
Oral contraceptives, 120
Oral dosing, 425-26
Ordinal scale, 458
Orphan Drug Act, 482, 483
Osmolarity, 445-48
Osteoarthritis
    definition, 229
    diagnosis, 229
    guidelines, 230
    medication charts, 231-35
    medication storage/administration, 236
    patient education, 236

signs/symptoms, 230
Osteoporosis
    definition, 242
    diagnosis, 242
    guidelines, 242-43
    medication charts, 244-45
    medication storage/administration, 246
    patient education, 246
    signs/symptoms, 242
Otic delivery, 396-97
Ovarian cancer
    definitions, 185
    diagnosis, 185
    guidelines, 186
    signs/symptoms, 185
Over-the-counter medications
    antidiarrheals, 364-65
    antihistamines, 357-60
    athlete's foot medications, 369-70
    constipation medications, 366-68
    cough suppressants, 361-63
    decongestants, 354-56
    drug resources, 469
    proton pump inhibitors, 357-60
    top 10 herbals/supplements, 349-53
Ovulation induction, 120
Oxazolidinones, 71
Oxcarbazepine
    epilepsy options, 152
    oral suspension storage/administration, 140
    seizure guidelines, 134
Oxidation, 379
Oxycodone, 193, 263
Oxymorphone, 193

P

Pain management
    cancer support, 192-93, 195-96
    definitions, 253
    diagnosis, 254
    guidelines, 254-55
    medication onset of action, 263
    medication storage/administration, 263
    patient education, 263
    signs/symptoms, 254
Panic disorder. *See* anxiety
Pantoprazole, 164, 172

Parenteral delivery, 394-96
Parenteral drug compatibility/stability resources, 467
Parkinson's disease
    definitions, 140
    diagnosis, 140
    medication charts, 141-45
    medication storage/administration, 146
    patient education, 146
    signs/symptoms, 140
    treatment recommendations, 141
Paroxetine, 148
Passive diffusion, 403
Pastes, 392
Patches, 397
Patient controlled administration, 255, 263
PCA. See Patient-controlled administration
PCOS. See Polycystic ovarian syndrome
PD. See Parkinson's disease
PDE5. See Phosphodiesterase-5 inhibitor
Peak-to-trough ratio, 24-28
Pediatric drug information resources, 469
Penicillin, 62-63
Peptic ulcer disease
    causes, 171
    definitions, 155-56
    diagnosis, 156
    guidelines, 157, 159
    medication charts, 160-63
    medication storage/administration, 164
    patient education, 164
    signs/symptoms, 157
Percentage, 441-42
Permetrexed, 181
Pernicious anemia
    definitions, 284
    diagnosis, 284
    medication chart, 286
    medication storage/administration, 287
    patient education, 287
    signs/symptoms, 284
    treatment summary, 285
Pharmaceutics resources, 468
Pharmacokinetics
    basic parameters, 421-25
    compartmental modeling, 420-21
    nonlinear, 430-32
    plasma drug concentration profiles, 419-20
Pharmacology resources, 468

Pharmacotherapy resources, 466
Phase I reactions, 408
Phase I trials, 479-480
Phase II reactions, 408-09
Phase II trials, 480
Phase III trials, 481
Phase IV trials, 481-82
Phenobarbital, 134
Phenytoin
    epilepsy options, 152
    seizure guidelines, 134
    storage/administration, 140
Phodiesterase inhibitors, 337
Phosphodiesterase-5 inhibitor, 330
Photochemical decomposition, 380
Physical pharmacy, 377-383
PI. See Protease inhibitors
Pioglitazone, 120
PK modeling, 420-21
Plasma drug concentration profiles, 419-20
Plasma level calculation, 422
Plasma protein binding, 406-7
Plastic materials, 382
Platinum therapy, 186
Pneumonia
    common organisms, 48
    diagnosis, 48
    guidelines, 48-49
    signs/symptoms, 48
POAG. See Primary open-angle glaucoma
Polycystic ovarian syndrome
    definitions, 119
    diagnosis, 119
    guidelines, 120
    medication charts, 121-22
    medication storage/administration, 123
    patient education, 123
    signs/symptoms, 120
Polymorphism, 381
Postnasal drip, 354
Powders, 384
Power, 457, 459
PPI. See Proton pump inhibitors
Prazosin, 334
Prednisone
    administration, 171
    inflammatory bowel disease, 166
    MS guidelines, 128

Prefabricated dosage forms, 449, 452
Preformulation, 377-80
Pregnancy resources, 479
Primary literature, 471
Primary open-angle glaucoma
    definitions, 267
    diagnosis, 267
    guidelines, 268
    medication charts, 269-72
    medication storage/administration, 273
    patient education, 273
    signs/symptoms, 268
    treatment overview, 268
Primidone, 134
Privacy Rule, 475-76
Probenecid, 250
Problem-solving techniques, 435-36
Prochlorperazine, 192
Progestin, 120
Promotility
    GERD guidelines, 158
    medication chart, 161
Prophylactic agents, 148
Propranolol, 148
Propylthiouracil
    hyperthyroidism guidelines, 117
    patient education, 119
Prostaglandin analogs
    cautions, 274
    medication chart, 162, 270
    POAG treatment, 268
Prostate cancer
    definitions, 184
    diagnosis, 184
    guidelines, 184-85
    signs/symptoms, 184
Protamine
    antidote action, 311
    storage/administration, 311
Protease inhibitors
    HIV guidelines, 54
    medication chart, 56-57
Protected health information, 476
Proton pump inhibitors
    administration, 164, 172
    GERD guidelines, 158
    H. pylori treatment, 171
    medication chart, 161

PUD guidelines, 159
Pseudomonas, 85
Pseudoplastic materials, 382
Psoraisis
    definitions, 295
    diagnosis, 295
    guidelines, 295
    medication charts, 297-98
    medication storage/administration, 299
    patient education, 299
    signs/symptoms, 295
    treatment recommendations, 296
Psoralens, 296
Psoriatic arthritis, 295
Psychiatric disorders
    anxiety, 210-16
    bipolar disorder, 216-19
    depression, 201-10
    schizophrenia, 219-20
PUD. See Peptic ulcer disease
Pulmonary delivery, 393-94
Pulmonary disorders
    asthma, 89-95
    COPD, 95-98
    tuberculosis, 98-101
P-value, 456-57, 459

Q

Quality assurance tests, 382-83
Quetiapine
    bipolar disorder guidelines, 217
    Parkinson's disease recommendations, 141

R

RA. See Rheumatoid arthritis
Rabeprazole, 164
Radioactive iodine, 117
Raloxifene, 243
Randomization, 481
Rate equation, 380
Ratio scale, 458
Ratio-proportion, 435-36
Ratio strength, 441-42
Reconstitution calculations, 450
Rectal suppositories, 392
Renal clearance, 415
Renal function, 342

Renin inhibitor, 9

Reservoir device, 393

Residuals, 426

Retinoids

acne guidelines, 292

acne treatment, 299

psoriasis treatment, 296

Rheology, 381-82

Rheumatoid arthritis

definition, 236

diagnosis, 236

guidelines, 237

medication charts, 238-40

medication storage/administration, 241

patient education, 241

signs/symptoms, 236

Risperidone, 217

Ritonavir, 381

Ritonavir capsule, 61

Rituximab

ALL/CLL guidelines, 179

non-Hodgkin's lymphoma guidelines, 177

Rosglitazone, 120

Rotigotine patch

administration, 146

patient education, 146

S

Saw palmetto, 350

Schizophrenia

definition, 219

diagnosis, 219

guidelines, 219-20

medication chart, 221-25

medication storage/administration, 226

patient education, 226

signs/symptoms, 219

SCLC. *See* Small cell lung cancer

Secondary literature, 471

Seizures. *See* Epilepsy

Selective alpha 1A antagonist, 334

Selective serotonin reuptake inhibitors

anxiety treatment, 211

depression guidelines, 202

Selegiline, 146

Serotonin agonists, 147, 152

Sertraline, 148

Sexually transmitted disease

causative organism, 51

diagnosis, 51

guidelines, 52

signs/symptoms, 52

Sildenafil, 333

Single-agent chemotherapy, 178

Single-phase liquid dosage forms, 388-89

6-mercaptopurine

inflammatory bowel disease, 166

patient education, 171

Small cell lung cancer, 180

Social Security Act, 475

Solid dosage forms

capsules, 385

extended release, 386-87

granules, 384-85

immediate release, 386

powders, 384

rapid release, 387-88

tablets, 385-86

traditional release, 384-86

Solid-state properties, 380-81

Solubility, 378

Solvates, 381

Solvents, 388

Specific gravity, 438-39

Spironolactone

PCOS guidelines, 120

storage/administration, 123

SSRI. *See* Selective serotonin reuptake inhibitors

Stability, 379-380

Stanford V, 177

Statins

medication chart, 16

medication storage/administration, 17

MI prevention, 36

Statistical significance, 456-57

Statistical test, 458

Stavudine solution, 61

Steady-state equation, 427-28

Steady-state plasma level, 426

STEMI, 32-39

Sterilization methods, 395

Steroids metered-dose inhalers, 393

St. John's wort, 350

Streptogramins, 71

Sublingual nitroglycerin
    STEMI management, 35
    UA/NSTEMI management, 32, 33
Sucralfate, 164
Sulfasalazine
    administration, 172
    patient education, 171
Sulfinpyrazone, 250
Sulfonamides, 73
Sumatriptan injection, 152
Sumatriptan nasal spray, 152
Superposition, 426
Supplements, 352-53
Suppositories, 392
Suppository calculations, 449
Surfactant, 390
Suspensions, 389-90
Syphilis
    diagnosis, 51
    signs/symptoms, 52
    treatment, 52

T

Tablets, 385-86
Tacrolimus, 296
Tadalafil, 333
Tamoxifen, 183
Tamsulosin, 334
Taxanes
    breast cancer guidelines, 183
    ovarian cancer guidelines, 186
Terazosin, 334
Teriparatide
    osteoporosis guidelines, 243
    patient education, 246
    storage/administration, 246
Tertiary literature, 471
Testoderm, 333
Testosterone gel, 333
Tetracycline
    medication chart, 70
    PUD guidelines, 159
    storage/administration, 295
Thiazolidinediones, 120
Thixotropic products, 382
Thyroid disease. *See* Hyperthyroidism;
    Hypothyroidism

Thyroidectomy, 117
Tiagabine
    migraine headache guidelines, 148
    seizure guidelines, 134
Tinea pedis. *See* Athlete's foot
Tonicity, 447-48
Topical agents
    patient education, 295
    psoriasis treatment, 296
Topical delivery, 390-92
Topiramate
    migraine headache guidelines, 148
    seizure guidelines, 134
Total parenteral nutrition, 451
TPN. *See* Total parenteral nutrition
Transdermal delivery, 397
Trapezoidal rule, 424
Trastuzimala, 183
Treatment IND, 478
Tricyclic antidepressants
    anxiety treatment, 211
    urinary incontinence treatment, 334
T-tests, 458, 459
Tuberculosis
    definitions, 98
    diagnosis, 98
    guidelines, 99
    medication charts, 100
    medication storage/administration, 101
    patient education, 101
    signs/symptoms, 99
Tubular reabsorption, 414, 416
Tubular secretion, 414
Two-compartment model, 420
Typical antipsychotics, 221-23
Tyrosine kinase inhibitors, 179

U

UA. *See* Unstable angina
Ulcerative colitis. *See* Inflammatory bowel disease
Ultrasound, 397
Unstable angina, 32
Urethral suppositories, 392
Uricosuric drugs, 248
Urinary incontinence
    definitions, 333
    diagnosis, 333

guidelines, 334

    medication charts, 335-36

    medication storage/administration, 337

    patient education, 337

    signs/symptoms, 333-34

    treatment recommendations, 334

Urinary tract infection

    common organisms, 46

    diagnosis, 46

    guidelines, 47

    signs/symptoms, 46-47

Urologic disorders

    erectile dysfunction, 329-33

    urinary incontinence, 333-37

UTI. *See* Urinary tract infection

V

Vaginal dosage forms, 392

Valproate, 217

Valproic acid

    epilepsy options, 152

    migraine headache guidelines, 148

    seizure guidelines, 134

    storage/administration, 140

Vardenafil, 333

Varicella-Zoster virus, 82

Venlafaxine

    anxiety treatment, 211

    depression guidelines, 202

Viscosity, 382

Vitamin B_{12}, 284-85, 287

Vitamin D, 243

Vitamin K, 311

Volume of distribution, 424

W

Wagner-Nelson method, 426

Warfarin, 311

Water-soluble base, 391

Whole bowel irrigation, 306

Z

Zero-order kinetics, 380

Zevalin, 192

Ziprasidone, 217

Zofran ODT, 198

Zoledronic acid solution, 246

Zonisamide, 134

Zyrtec, 18